D1426399

Magnetic Resonance Imaging of Congenital Heart Disease

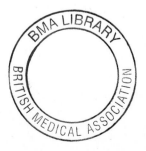

Mushabbar A. Syed • Raad H. Mohiaddin

Editors

Magnetic Resonance Imaging of Congenital Heart Disease

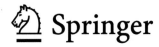 Springer

Editors

Mushabbar A. Syed, M.D., FACC
Department of Medicine and Radiology
Stritch School of Medicine
Loyola University Chicago
IL
USA

Raad H. Mohiaddin M.D., Ph.D., FRCR,
FRCP, FESC
Magnetic Resonance Unit
Royal Brompton Hospital
London
UK

Cardiovascular Imaging
Heart and Vascular Institute
Loyola University Medical Center
Maywood
IL
USA

ISBN 978-1-4471-4266-9   ISBN 978-1-4471-4267-6   (eBook)
DOI 10.1007/978-1-4471-4267-6
Springer London Heidelberg New York Dordrecht

Library of Congress Control Number: 2012951637

Printed on acid-free paper

Springer is part of Springer Science+Business Media (www.springer.com)

To my parents with utmost gratitude and love, may they rest in peace. To my wife, Humaira, for her unwavering love and support and our wonderful children, Daneyal, Ameena and Aleena, who taught me what's truly important in life.

Mushabbar A. Syed

To my parents for their tremendous sacrifices, and to my wife, Khalida, and my children, Hasan, Zain, and Reema, for their support and understanding.

Raad H. Mohiaddin

Foreword

As a cardiologist with a career interest in congenital heart disease in adults, I was delighted to have the opportunity to read *Magnetic Resonance Imaging of Congenital Heart Disease* and write a foreword for it. Over past two decades, CMR has come to occupy an ever more important place in the assessment and management of patients with congenital heart defects (CHD) and other cardiovascular disorders. Thus, this new text will be of broad interest to both imagers and clinicians who deal with cardiovascular disease. Cardiovascular MRI offers an ever-expanding amount of information about the heart and circulation. It can provide outstanding images of cardiovascular morphology and function. It is increasingly being used to detect pathologic fibrosis and has an expanding role in the assessment of myocardial viability. Amazing though CMR is, its limitations and weaknesses also need to be clearly understood. As CMR has evolved, it has challenged other imaging modalities to improve and evolve, all of which improves the understanding that we clinicians have of our patients and consequently the care we can offer them. In many ways, cardiovascular CMR has offered important new insights that clinicians and imagers a generation ago would have considered impossible.

The editors and their expert contributors have taken a large step towards making detailed information about CMR accessible to those working in the field and to those who use the information derived from CMR in their clinical practices. The field is ever changing and ever improving. This text offers an excellent foundation for the reader who is not familiar with the field, and up to date descriptions of where we stand with imaging a broad range of cardiovascular diseases. The text is well referenced without being overwhelming, and the illustrations are generally outstanding, including many movie images.

The opening chapter reviews the general principles of CMR, including information about the physics of the technique, and the hardware used. It reviews such useful subjects as remaining motionless in the scanner, and the use of sedation and anesthesia. It provides important information relating to how to structure a study of various congenital cardiovascular conditions. The second chapter deals with the important issue of MRI safety, culminating (as in many chapters) with a series of "practical pearls". Chapter 3 provides an introduction to the anatomy of CHD. The next seven chapters cover the subject of CMR in CHD in all its various forms. A particular emphasis is given to the role of CMR of septal defects, tetralogy of Fallot, Ebstein anomaly, transposition of the great arteries, and single ventricle/Fontan circulations. Chapter 12 focuses on aortic abnormalities including aortic coarctation, PDA, aortic aneurysms, and vascular rings. Chapter 13 deals with inherited cardiomyopathies. Including hypertrophic cardiomyopathy, dilated cardiomyopathy, left ventricular non-compaction, and arrhythmogenic right ventricular dysplasia. Chapter 14 addresses coronary artery anomalies and discusses the appropriate roles of CMR and CT angiography in assessing such patients. The next two chapters deal with pericardial diseases and cardiac tumors. Chapter 17 discusses CMR in children, and Chap. 18 describes the current status of interventional CMR, an area with exciting potential. The final chapter explores the emerging roles for CMR in ACHD electrophysiology. These last two chapters represent an exciting marriage of differing imaging and therapeutic modalities that move the field forward.

Overall, the text offers the reader an exciting and comprehensive voyage through the place of CMR in a broad range of cardiovascular diseases with a special focus on congenital heart disease. It succeeds in describing the technical details of MRI techniques in sufficient detail to also help the clinician understand the most important elements of CMR in assessing and managing their patients. We readers are indebted to the editors and their contributors for having put together such an excellent and much needed text on this topic.

Gary Webb, M.D.

Contents

Contributors

Sonya V. Babu-Narayan, MBBS, B.Sc., MRCP, Ph.D. National Heart and Lung Institute, Imperial College, London, UK

NIHR Cardiovascular Biomedical Research Unit, Royal Brompton and Harefield NHS Foundation Trust, London, UK

Frédérique Bailliard, M.D., M.S. Centre for Cardiovascular Imaging, Great Ormond Street Hospital for Children NHS Trust, London, UK

Bailliard Henry Pediatric Cardiology, Raleigh, NC, USA

Puja Banka, M.D. Department of Cardiology, Harvard Medical School, Boston, MA, USA

Department of Cardiology, Boston Children's Hospital, Boston, MA, USA

Emanuela R. Valsangiacomo Buechel, M.D., FESC Division of Paediatric Cardiology, University Children's Hospital Zurich, Zurich, Switzerland

Sylvia S.M. Chen, MBBS, M.D., FRACP Cardiovascular Magnetic Resonance Unit, The Royal Brompton Hospital, London, UK

Andrew M. Crean, M.D., B.Sc., BM, MRCP, M.Sc., FRCR, M.Phil. Departments of Medicine (Cardiology) & Medical Imaging, Peter Munk Cardiac Center, Toronto General Hospital, Toronto, Canada

Sabine I.S. Ernst, M.D., Ph.D., FESC National Heart and Lung Institute, Imperial College, London, UK

J. Paul Finn, M.D. Department of Radiology Sciences, David Geffen School of Medicine, Ronald Reagan UCLA Medical Center, Los Angeles, CA, USA

University of California Los Angeles (UCLA), Los Angeles, CA, USA

Department of Radiology, Diagnostic Cardiovascular Imaging Section, UCLA, Los Angeles, CA, USA

Mark A. Fogel, M.D., FACC, FAHA, FAAP Department of Cardiology and Radiology, University of Pennsylvania School of Medicine, Philadelphia, PA, USA

Division of Cardiology, The Children's Hospital of Philadelphia, Philadelphia, PA, USA

Tal Geva, M.D. Harvard Medical School, Boston, MA, USA

Department of Cardiology, Children's Hospital Boston, Boston, MA, USA

Marina L. Hughes, DPhil, MRCP, FRACP Centre for Cardiovascular Imaging, Great Ormond Street Hospital for Children NHS Trust, London, UK

Cardiorespiratory Unit, Great Ormond Street Hospital for Children Foundation Trust, London, UK

Henryk Kafka, M.D., FRCPC, FACC Departments of Cardiology and Radiology, Queen's University, Kingston General Hospital, Kingston, ON, Canada

Jennifer Keegan, B.Sc., M.Sc., Ph.D. National Heart and Lung Institute, Imperial College, London, UK

Philip J. Kilner, M.D., Ph.D. Cardiovascular Magnetic Resonance Unit, Royal Brompton Hospital and Imperial College, London, UK

Steve W. Leung, M.D. Department of Medicine and Radiology, Division of Cardiovascular Disease, University of Kentucky, Lexington, KY, USA

Roger Luechinger, Ph.D. Institute for Biomedical Engineering, University and ETH Zurich, Zurich, Switzerland

Edward T. Martin, M.S., M.D., FACC, FACP, FAHA Department of Cardiovascular MRI, Oklahoma Heart Institute, Tulsa, USA

Raad H. Mohiaddin, M.D., Ph.D., FRCR, FRCP, FESC, FACC Cardiovascular Magnetic Resonance Unit, Royal Brompton Hospital and National Heart and Lung Institute, Imperial College London, London, UK

Vivek Muthurangu, M.D., MRCPCH UCL Centre for Cardiovascular MR, University College London, London, UK

Rory O'Hanlon, M.D., MRCPI Department of Cardiology, St. Vincent's University Hospital, Dublin, Ireland

Centre for Cardiovascular Magnetic Resonance, Blackrock Clinic, Dublin, Ireland

Michael A. Quail, B.Sc. (hons), MB ChB (hons), MRCPCH Academic Clinical Fellow, Pediatric Cardiology, Centre for Cardiovascular Imaging, UCL Institute of Cardiovascular Sciences and Great Ormond Street Hospital for Children, London, UK

Subha V. Raman, M.D., MSEE CMR/CT, The Ohio State University, Columbus, OH, USA

Pierangelo Renella, M.D. Department of Radiology Sciences, David Geffen School of Medicine, Ronald Reagan UCLA Medical Center, Los Angeles, CA, USA

Department of Pediatric Cardiology, UC-Irvine College of Medicine, Children's Hospital Orange County, Orange, CA, USA

University of California Los Angeles (UCLA), Los Angeles, CA, USA

Sharon L. Roble, M.D. Department of Cardiology, The Ohio State University, Columbus, OH, USA

Anna N. Seale, MB BChir, MRCP Department of Paediatric Cardiology, Royal Brompton Hospital, London, UK

Cardiovascular Magnetic Resonance Unit, Royal Brompton Hospital and Imperial College, London, UK

Mushabbar A. Syed, M.D., FACC Department of Medicine and Radiology, Stritch School of Medicine, Loyola University Chicago, IL, USA

Cardiovascular Imaging, Heart and Vascular Institute, Loyola University Medical Center, Maywood, IL, USA

Oliver Richard Tann, MBBS, B.Sc., MRCP, FRCR Cardio-Respiratory Unit, Great Ormond Street Hospital, London, UK

Andrew M. Taylor, M.D., FRCR, FRCP Cardio-Respiratory Unit, UCL Institute of Child Health and Great Ormond Street Hospital for Children, London, UK

Joel R. Wilson, M.D. Department of Cardiac Energetics, National Heart, Lung and Blood Institute, National Institutes of Health, Bethesda, MD, USA

Mark A. Fogel

1.1 Introduction

A basic understanding of the underlying principles of cardiovascular magnetic resonance (CMR) and methods used to form images is important if one is to successfully apply this technique in clinical practice or research and interpret it correctly. This section will provide a brief overview of the fundamentals and some techniques in CMR imaging. For more information, the reader is referred to the references in this chapter or the larger textbooks on fundamentals of magnetic resonance imaging as well as other chapters in this book [1].

1.2 Physics and CMR Harware

The crux of CMR is nuclear magnetic resonance where a signal is emitted by a sample of tissue after radiofrequency energy is applied to it. This signal is emitted by tissue molecules; contrast this to X-ray imaging where the tissue or contrast agents attenuate externally applied radiation. At the atomic level, it has been well known that spins and charge distributions of protons and neutrons generate magnetic fields. Only certain nuclei can selectively absorb and subsequently release energy since it requires an odd number of protons or neutrons to exhibit a magnetic moment associated with its net spin. The hydrogen atom is the one used in CMR imaging since it consists of a single proton with no neutrons which gives it a net spin of ½ as well as its large magnetic moment and its abundance in the body (water and fat). Although each magnetic moment of individual hydrogen

M.A. Fogel, M.D., FACC, FAHA, FAAP
Department of Cardiology and Radiology, University of Pennsylvania School of Medicine,
Philadelphia, PA 19004, USA

Division of Cardiology, The Childrens Hospital of Philadelphia, 8th Floor, NW Tower, Room 8NW46, 34th Street and Civic Center Boulevard, Philadelphia, PA 19004, USA
e-mail: fogel@email.chop.edu

protons themselves is small, the additive effect of the many magnetic moment vectors because of its abundance makes it detectable in CMR.

Generally, the net magnetization of a tissue in the body is zero as there is a random orientation of the individual protons or "spins"; stochastically, the odds greatly favor a zero magnetization. However, when the body is placed in a strong magnetic field (Fig. 1.1) such as 1.5 or 3 T MRI systems (for comparison, the Earth's magnetic field is approximately 0.05 mT at the surface), the spins align themselves with the applied field either parallel or anti-parallel to the field. In addition, the atoms undergo a phenomenon known as precession (such as the motion of a spinning top as it loses its speed) whose axis is based around the direction of the magnetic field (Fig. 1.1a); this precession, described as cycles per second, is described by the most famous equation in CMR and MRI – the Larmor equation, $\omega = \gamma B_0$, where ω is the frequency of precession of protons in an external magnetic field, γ is a constant called gyromagnetic ratio and B_0 the external magnetic field (the magnetic field generated by the MRI system). There is a different gyromagnetic ratio for each atom; for hydrogen, it is 42.58 MHz/T which generates a frequency of approximately 64 MHz at 1.5 T (Larmor frequency for a 1.5 T magnet is $1.5(T)*42.56(MHz\ T^{-1}) = 63.8\ MHz$). When a radiofrequency pulse is applied which just happens to match the Larmor precessional frequency, some of the protons will flip to a high energy state. For protons at field strengths used for CMR, radiofrequencies in range of "very high frequency" or VHF can be used which is non-ionizing, contributing to the inherent safety of MRI when compared to X-rays.

To get from here to how a signal is generated from tissue, two more concepts must be introduced. As mentioned, the hydrogen spins are either in the low or high energy spin states with only slightly more spins in the low energy state. The number of excess spins is directly proportional to the total number of spins in the sample and the energy difference between states (Boltzman equilibrium probability). The formula used to determine this difference is $N^-/N^+ = e^{-E/kT}$ where

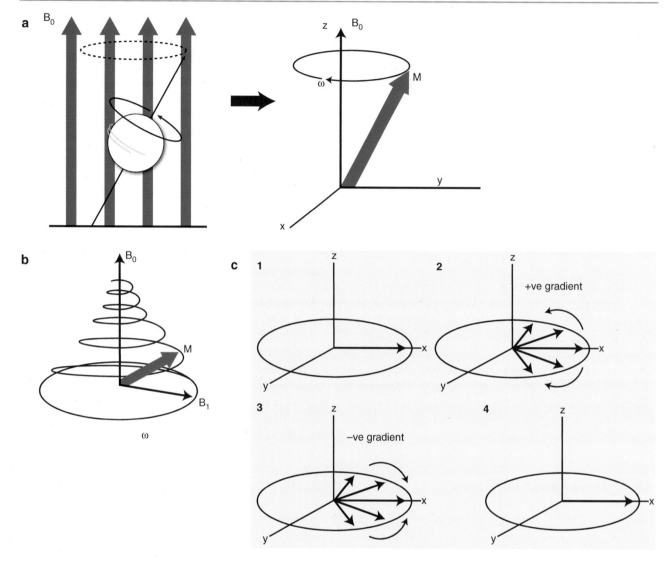

Fig. 1.1 (**a**) Protons spin and precess like a top wobbling (*left*). If the proton is at the (0,0,0) coordinate of an x,y,z coordinate system (*right*), its axis is represented by the *blue* vector M and wobbles around the z axis which is in line with B$_0$ at a frequency ω. (**b**) After energy is inputted into the system, the axis flips (in this particular instance, 90°) and then slowly returns to its original position. (**c**) In *1* the protons are flipped 90 with subsequent "dephasing" of the spins in *2* which can be increased by a gradient (i.e. faster protons and slower protons will separate). In *3*, energy can be inputted into the system to flip the protons to an exact mirror image so that the faster spins are not behind the slower spins. Finally, the faster spinning protons catch up to the slower spins to create a large detectable signal (in *4*)

N$^-$ is the number of spins in high energy state, N$^+$ is number of spins in the lower energy state, k is Boltzmann's constant (1.3805 × 10^{-23} J/K), T is the temperature (in Kelvin) and E is the energy difference between the spin states. The second concept is that the energy of a proton (E) is directly proportional to its Larmor frequency υ (in Hz), such that E = hυ, where h is Plank's constant (h = 6.626 × 10^{-34} J s). By substituting into the Larmor equation, this yields the relationship between E and the magnetic field B$_0$, E = hγB$_0$. When energy is inputted into the system and it matches the energy difference between the lower and higher energy spin states, atoms from the lower energy states get flipped up to the higher energy states. As these atoms then return to the lower energy state, they release energy and this signal, the resonance

phenomenon, can be detected (Fig. 1.1b). This is how the MRI signal is generated.

It follows that only those excess spins in the low energy state can be excited to the high energy state and generate the MRI signal. It is amazing that there are only approximately nine more spins in the low energy state compared to the high energy state for each two million spins at 1.5 T! However, one must also realize that since each ml of water contains nearly 10^{23} hydrogen atoms, the Boltzman distribution discussed above predicts over 10^{17} spins contributing to the MRI signal in each ml of water! It is interesting to note that the higher the magnetic field strength, the greater the number of excess spins in low versus high energy state; it follows that as the field strength increases, so does the magnitude of the

MRI signal. Hence, there is a push by manufacturers to create larger and larger magnetic fields from the 1.5 T fields most commonly used today. Indeed, many 3 T systems have been deployed and 7 T systems have been discussed for clinical use.

When the radio frequency energy is applied that matches the Larmor frequency, some of the protons in the low energy state jump up to the high energy level as noted above. This radiofrequency pulse has a magnetic field itself, B_1, which is perpendicular to the direction of B_0 and of mT order of magnitude. It tilts the longitudinal magnetization (M_z) a certain amount depending upon the duration of the RF pulse and the strength of B_1 field. If an RF pulse is applied to tilt the net magnetization from the longitudinal plane (Z plane) totally to the transverse (XY) plane (called a 90° RF), the transverse component of the net magnetization is the one that will generate an induced voltage in a receiver antenna (the MR signal). The way this occurs is through what is termed "relaxation" where the protons return from their excited state to a low energy state (Fig. 1.1b). The duration of the induced voltage is a function of the time it takes to undergo relaxation and is described by relaxation time constants termed T1 and T2 which describe the changes in longitudinal magnetization (M_z) and transverse magnetization (M_{xy}) respectively.

1.2.1 T1 Relaxation

When the protons are flipped to transverse plane, the Mz component of magnetization decreases to near zero (Fig. 1.1b, c); the time for return of this magnetization Mz after the RF pulse is turned off is measured by the time constant T1 which is defined as the time necessary to recover 63 % of the equilibrium magnetization M_0 after the 90° RF pulse (Fig. 1.2): $M_z(t) = M_0(1 - \exp(-t/T1))$. Physically, the return of longitudinal magnetization is a function of how fast the spins release their energy to the tissue which is termed the "lattice" hence T1 being called spin-lattice relaxation. As one might guess, this process depends in part on the physical properties of the tissue where the frequency of precession of the spins need to overlap the frequencies of the molecules in the lattice. In addition, the process is also dependent on the main magnetic field strength; at higher fields, the frequencies of spins precession increases with less overlap of frequencies in the lattice, resulting in a longer T1. Water, however, has a frequency range that is large.

1.2.2 T2 Relaxation

When the protons are flipped to transverse plane, the M_{xy} component of magnetization becomes maximized as all the protons precess with the same phase, called phase coherence

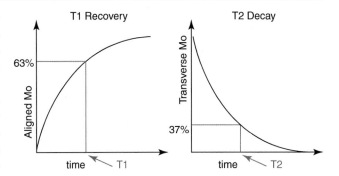

Fig. 1.2 T1 relaxation or recovery (*left*) is the return of magnetization Mz, to the equilibrium magnetization Mo; the time constant is defined as recovering to 63 %. T2 relaxation or decay (*right*), is the decay in the transverse plane

(Fig. 1.1b, c). The spins of each proton in the general vicinity of each other interact with each other, however, and in time, this coherence is lost resulting in a decrease in the net magnetization (Fig. 1.1c) and induced voltage in the receiver antenna. This is appropriately called spin-spin relaxation or transverse relaxation and is measured by the T2 time constant. The transverse magnetization (M_{xy}) will decay exponentially from M_z by the following formula (Fig. 1.2): $M_{xy}(t) = M_z(0)\exp(-t/T2)$. The time constant is defined as decaying to 37 % of its initial value. This relaxation is highly dependent on the make-up of the tissue; small molecules in a generally unstructured tissue have long T2 values because fast and rapidly moving spins average out the intrinsic magnetic field inhomogeneities while large molecules in densely packed tissue have shorter T2 values. Unfortunately, there are other factors responsible for decay of magnetization in the transverse plane; imperfections of the main magnetic field, susceptibility differences between nearby tissues can and do contribute to the loss of phase coherence (Fig. 1.1c). This is measured by the time constant T2*. In general, T1 is always greater than T2 which is always greater than T2*.

1.2.3 Image Formation

Now that the basic physical properties are defined, the discussion can turn to creating images. To create images, a magnetic field gradient must be formed. Within the main magnetic field, B_0, all protons precess at the same frequency (Fig. 1.1a). The Larmor equation tells us that this precession is a function of this field strength; by changing the magnetic field ever so slightly by position and time, the precession of the protons can be changed ever so slightly by position and time. Using this information, localization of the MR signal from the precise part of the body can be accomplished and images can be generated. This precision controlled alteration of the magnetic field is created by gradient coils, which generate linear variations in the main magnetic field strength in three orthogonal planes (Figs. 1.1c and 1.3a). By using these coils simultane- ously, a linear magnetic field gradient can be generated in any direction. This gradient changes the precession frequency of the protons at precise locations in a linear fashion.

To select a certain plane (slice) in the body (Fig. 1.3b), an RF pulse is applied and it follows that if the RF pulse center frequency is shifted to match a specific location along the gradient, it will selectively excite the protons at that region. A slice of arbitrary thickness, orientation and location along the direction of the "slice select gradient" can therefore be selectively excited to generate the signal used to form the MR image and the signal detected by the MRI receiver coil will come from the excited slice only (Fig. 1.3b). The ampli- tude of the signal is directly proportional to its thickness, practically limiting the thickness at approximately 2 mm.

After selecting the slice, the image itself needs to be cre- ated in two-dimensions in the xy plane (practically speaking in two orthogonal planes of the bore of the magnet – right/left and up/down when looking into the bore). This creates the pixels (two-dimensional picture elements); in three-dimen- sional imaging, this is called voxels (three-dimensional vol- ume elements). As with choosing the slice, linear field gradients and the Larmor relationship between field strength and precessional frequency are used to encode spatial loca- tion information into the MRI signal. After a slice-selective RF pulse, a linear magnetic field gradient is switched on in one of the in-plane directions of the image, perpendicular to the "slice select gradient;" this gradient changes the preces- sional frequency in a linear distribution along the gradient direction allowing the identification of every location along the gradient by the frequency of the signal (Fig. 1.3). This is called *frequency encoding*. The MR signal is detected and put through an analog-to-digital converter; remembering that we have encoded the slice and one direction in the plane of the image at this point, the signal is thus the amalgamation of all of these frequencies. Therefore, the signal varies with posi- tion, also called its "spatial frequency;" this is called "k-space." If one looks at the distribution of the signal, it creates a sinu- soidal distribution of phase across the direction of the gradi- ent; this describes a single spatial frequency kx (important in phase encoding in the next step). A special mathematical technique called the "Fourier transformation" is used to sepa- rate out the individual frequency components in the detected signal, decoding the signal into individual signals coming from locations along the frequency encoding gradient. The Fourier transformation can be used to translate the signal from "k-space" to the image and vice versa (Fig. 1.3).

Finally, the third spatial dimension (second in-plane dimension) must also be encoded (if frequency encoding is the "x," the "y" in the "xy" plane must also be created); the technique used is called "phase encoding" (Fig. 1.4) and is also based on the Larmor equation. Phase encoding is accom- plished with the application of a number of gradient pulses of differing amplitudes which encode a specific spatial

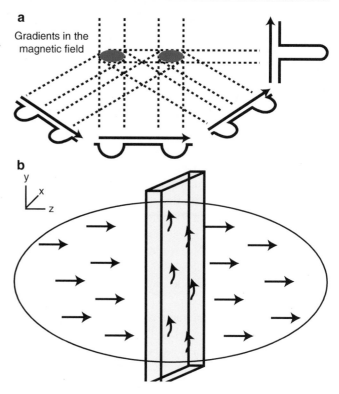

Fig. 1.3 By altering the magnetic field in three orthogonal planes, gra- dients can isolate a plane in space (**a**). This is accomplished by flipping the protons only in the plane desired (**b**)

frequency, k_y (Fig. 1.4). This phase encode gradient pulse is changed to encode a different spatial frequency component prior to each frequency encoding gradient. In this manner, by successive phase encoding pulses, and "y" part of the image is built up and a matrix is formed; this matrix is referred to as *k-space*, and the numerous gradient pulses "fill" the k-space until the image is complete. The two-dimensional Fourier transform is utilized to convert the spatial frequencies cre- ated by the phase encoding steps into an image (Figs. 1.4 and 1.5). Phase-encoding can also be used in the slice direction to encode thinner slices than possible with the slice selection gradient technique; so called 3D data acquisition.

1.2.4 MRI Hardware

Once all the components of generating an MR signal are known, it is important to review the equipment needed. There is of course the main magnet (B_0 or B_z field), the RF transmit- ter coil (B_1 field), the gradient coils (G_x, G_y, G_z fields) and receiver coils which "listen" for the signal. In addition, there are second-order shim coils which are often used to achieve a more homogeneous B_0 field. There are a number of computer systems including those which are used to control the MRI magnetic field-generating units and those used to reconstruct the acquired data. There is also a system which provides an interface for the user and the other systems.

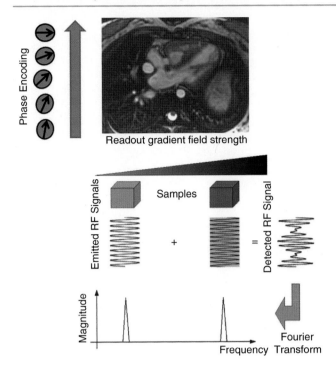

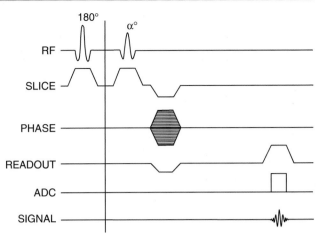

Fig. 1.5 A typical pulse sequence diagram includes (**a**) when the radiofrequency (*RF*) pulse is applied (*top line*) and at times, how much of a flip angle (in this case, 180°), (**b**) when the slice selection gradient (*Gz or slice*) is turned on (*second line*), (**c**) when the phase encoding gradient (Gy) is turned on (*third line*), when the frequency encoding gradient (*readout or Gx*) is turned on (*fourth line*), and when the analog to digital converter is turned on (*fifth line*) and the signal is created (*sixth line*). This is an example of a magnetization prepared gradient echo pulse sequence

Fig. 1.4 The image is created by a combination of frequency encoding in one direction (in this case, in the x plane or the horizontal portion of the image) and phase encoding in the other dimension (in this case, in the y plane or the vertical portion of the image). For frequency encoding, a gradient is applied to change the magnetic field in that direction (*right triangle*). Different frequencies correspond to different positions (different colors and waves on the diagram) which produce a detected radiofrequency (RF) signal which is a combination of all the frequencies of the various positions (*rightmost signal*). When put through the Fourier transform, signals can be separated into their different positions (*lower graph*). The vertical portion of the image is created by changing phases of the radiofrequency pulses (phase encoding, see text). The cardiac magnetic resonance image is of a "4-chamber" view of a patient with single ventricle after Fontan

1.2.5 Pulse Sequences

This is the sequence of events which control all the various factors involved in creation of an image. It is important to note that these times are on a microsecond scale and need to be controlled by computer for precise timing. Timing of all the gradients switching on and off, the phase encoding, the RF pulses, the analog to digital converting data sampling and control of transmitter and receiver operation are all defined by the pulse sequence. As there are a limitless amount of pulse sequences, it is impossible to describe all of them, however, to understand them, a pulse sequence diagram is used which details the timing of each component; a representative pulse sequence diagram is shown in Fig. 1.5. To simplify the concepts, it should be noted that there are five broad concepts with regard to pulse sequences which may be understood to aid in examining many of the pulse sequences in use. They are as follows:

1. *Magnetization preparation* is a technique employed, usually at the beginning of the sequence, which changes the

tissue characteristics prior to actually creating the image (Fig. 1.5). T2 preparation, for example, can be employed to suppress myocardial muscle and is used in visualizing coronary arteries (Fig. 1.6). The inversion recovery technique uses a 180° RF pulse to magnify differences in different tissue characteristics of T1; the saturation recovery technique uses a 90° RF pulse prior to image. The inversion recovery technique is used in delayed-enhancement (Fig. 1.7) as well as dark blood imaging [2] (Fig. 1.8) while saturation recovery is used in first-pass perfusion imaging (Fig. 1.9).

2. *Echo Formation*: This is the "echo" referred to above and various types of echo formation is used in cardiac MR. An older technique of echo formation which still has applicability today is called spin-echo, which is used most often in dark blood imaging for morphology and tissue characterization (e.g. myocardial edema) (Fig. 1.8). Another technique of echo formation, gradient-echo imaging (Fig. 1.10) is used in a whole host of applications such as
   - cine imaging for cardiac function including myocardial tagging (Figs. 1.11 and 1.12)
   - assessing valve morphology (Fig. 1.13), valve regurgitation as well as valve or vessel stenosis
   - in delayed-enhancement (Figs. 1.7 and 1.10) and first-pass perfusion (Fig. 1.9) for myocardial scarring and myocardial perfusion respectively
   - phase contrast velocity mapping to determine blood flow (Figs. 1.14 and 1.15).
   - Steady-state free precession imaging (or SSFP) (Figs. 1.15, 1.16, and 1.17), is also utilized for a whole

RCA   aneurysm

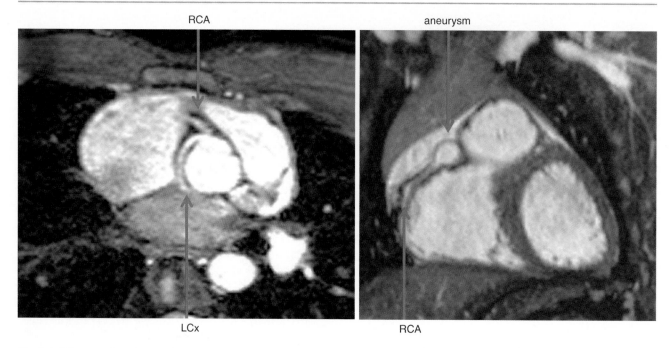

LCx   RCA

Fig. 1.6 T2 prepared steady state free precession to visualize coronary arteries. The image on the *left* demonstrates a right coronary artery (*RCA*) giving rise to a left circumflex coronary artery (*LCx*). The image on the *right* demonstrates right a coronary artery aneurysm from Kawasaki's disease

RV

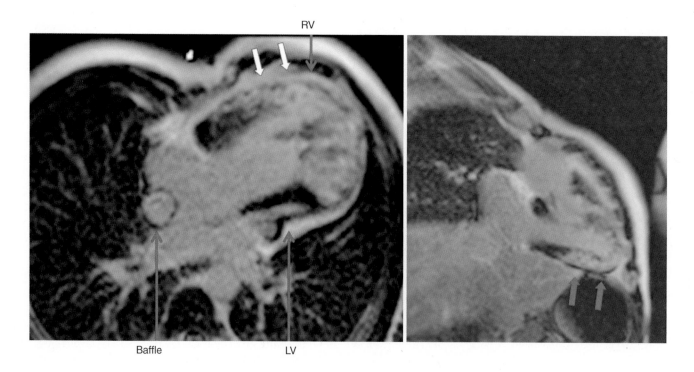

Baffle   LV

Fig. 1.7 Delayed enhancement imaging from a "4-chamber" (*left*) and long axis view (*right*) of a patient with hypoplastic left heart syndrome after Fontan. *White arrows* in red outline demonstrate some of the areas of myocardial scarring. On the right, areas of scarring are identified by *red arrows*

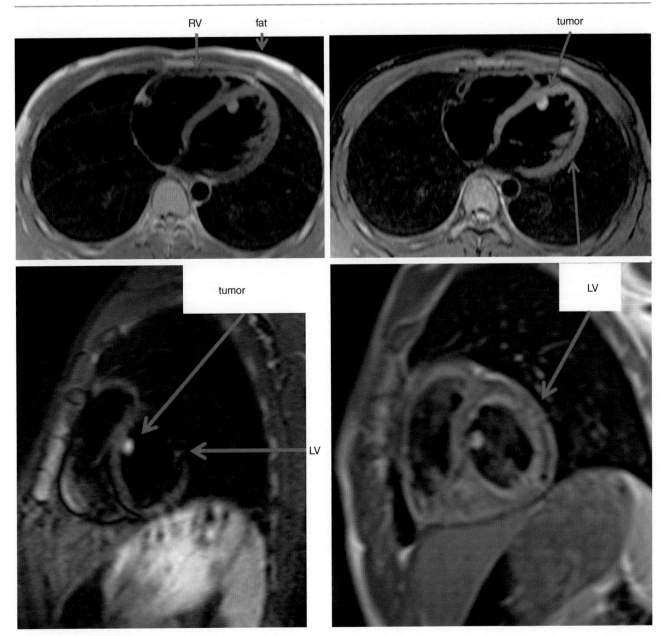

Fig. 1.8 Dark blood imaging in a patient with a left ventricular hemangioma (*tumor*). *Upper left panel* is a dark blood T1 weighted image of the tumor demonstrating slight hyperenhancement; note the fat in the chest wall. *Upper right panel* is the same dark blood T1 weighted image with a "fat saturation" pulse applied prior to imaging (prepulse). Note how the fat in the chest wall is not present on this image because the prepulse destroyed all the spins of the fat, however, the tumor is still present, indicating there are no fatty elements in the tumor (it is not a lipoma). *Lower left panel* demonstrates hyperenhancement on T1 weighted imaging after gadolinium administration. The *lower right image* is a T2 weighted image with fat saturation demonstrating hyperenhancement indicating increased water content

host of applications similar to the ones gradient echo imaging is used above (except for phase contrast velocity mapping). It is more commonly used than gradient echo due to its high signal to noise, blood to myocardium contrast and imaging efficiency [3].

- Echo-planar imaging is used as a method for perfusion imaging due its high efficiency.

3. *Filling k-space*: As noted above, k-space is filled with each phase encoding step. Most sequences employ what is known as Cartesian k-space sampling, where there is a linear filling of k-space which each phase encoding step. There are, however, other methodologies which have come into existence and are used. A "radial" filling of k-space has some advantages over Cartesian sampling when it comes to efficiently filling the matrix and has been used in cine imaging [4]. A "spiral" filling of k-space trajectory has been utilized for coronary artery imaging, because it has some advantages in speed and most

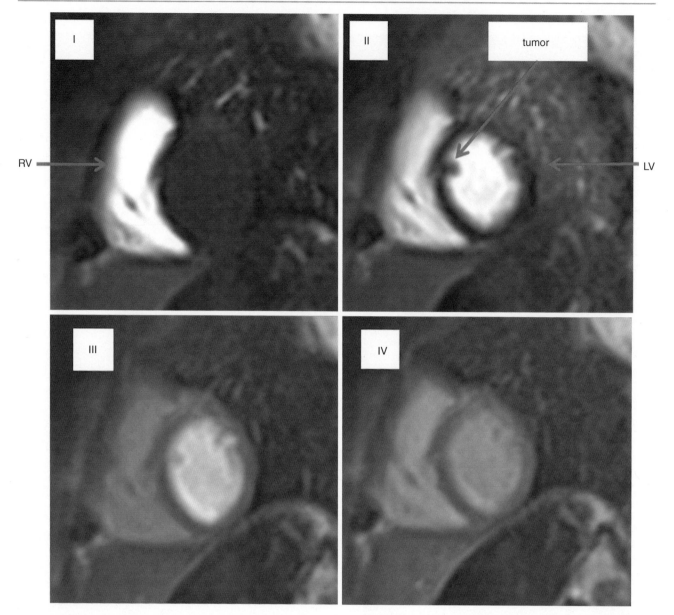

Fig. 1.9 Perfusion imaging in the patient in Fig. 1.8 with a left ventricular hemangioma (*tumor*). Four frames during first pass myocardial perfusion imaging demonstrate contrast in the right ventricular (*RV*) cavity (**I**), the left ventricular (*LV*) cavity (**II**) where the tumor can be seen, and phases (**III** and **IV**) where the contrast enters the LV myocardium. Note how the tumor becomes signal intense in (**III** and **IV**); so much so that it is indistinguishable from the cavity (somewhat in **III** and indistinguishable in **IV**). The tumor can be visualized in **II** as the contrast is in the cavity but not in the myocardium where presumably the tumor receives its blood supply from

importantly, insensitivity to motion; unfortunately, it is highly sensitive to field inhomogeneities and therefore, has not gained in popularity.

4. *Segmentation*: This refers to the number of lines of k-space filled per cardiac cycle [5]. If one line of k-space is filled per cardiac cycle, that pulse sequence is said to be "non-segmented;" if all the lines are filled in one cardiac cycle, that pulse sequence is said to be "single-shot." There are of course gradations of segmentation between the two and the degree of segmentation is referred to by the number of lines of k-space filled per heartbeat (e.g. 3, 5, 7 segments

or views, etc). Any level of segmentation can be used with any of the methods of magnetization preparation, echo formation or the ways of filling k-space. It generally follows that if the more lines of k-space filled in a heartbeat, the less time it will take to form the image while the reverse is true with the less lines of k-space per heartbeat (i.e. the number of segments inversely proportional to the time it takes to create the image). It is also true, however, that the more lines of k-space acquired per heartbeat, the worse the temporal resolution will be (i.e. the number of segments inversely proportional to the number of time

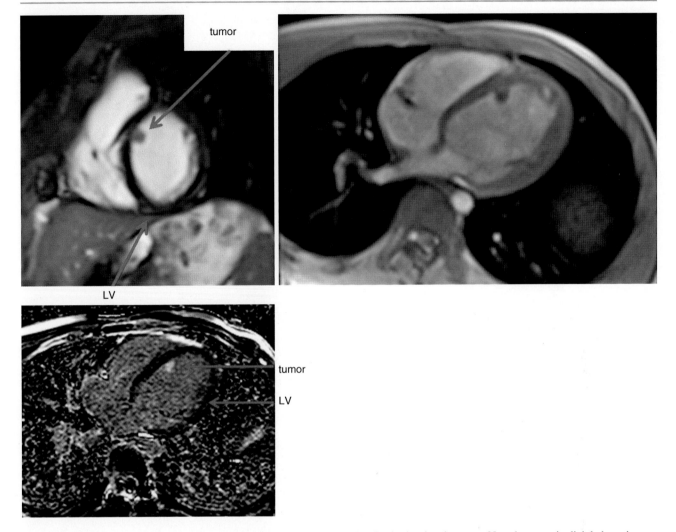

Fig. 1.10 Tissue characterization in the patient in Figs. 1.8 and 1.9 with a left ventricular hemangioma. The *upper left panel* is a steady state free precession image in short axis clearly showing the spherical tumor while the *upper right panel* is an axial gradient echo sequence also clearly showing the tumor. Note the tumor is slightly hyperintense with cardiac muscle on steady state free precession and the hypoenhancement on gradient echo imaging. The *lower image* is a delayed enhancement image of the tumor demonstrating hyperenhancement

points that can be created in the cardiac cycle) in retrospective gating (see below). Tradeoffs are part of CMR and for most applications such as phase contrast velocity mapping and flow, image creation can be obtained in a breath-hold. It is important to realize that a regular cardiac rhythm is needed to ensure that lines of k-space from each cardiac cycle is acquired during the same point in time of the cardiac and respiratory cycles; in patients with arrhythmias or an inability to breath-hold, single-shot methods are commonly used.

5. *Image Reconstruction*: As mentioned above, the Fourier transformation is used to create an image from the lines of k-space which is acquired from the MR signal. A technique called "partial Fourier" or "partial k-space" has been used for many years which reduces scan time with a lower signal-to-noise than using a "full" Fourier transformation. Parallel imaging with names such as SENSE, [6] SMASH,

GRAPPA, and TSENSE [7] use multiple coils and multiple channels and have become an ubiquitous in many sequences; they sample only a fraction of the full k-space but yet allow for a full field-of-view and resolution images with significant time savings at the cost of signal-to-noise.

1.3   Prospective Triggering/ Retrospective Gating

Because the heart needs to be at the same phase of the cardiac cycle with any segmented technique, as noted above, a way is needed to determine this phase. This is nearly universally the R-wave of the ECG. A static or non-moving image uses the R wave to signal the beginning of systole as is the touchstone of the cycle; the CMR sequence then begins. This technique is called prospective triggering since the sequence

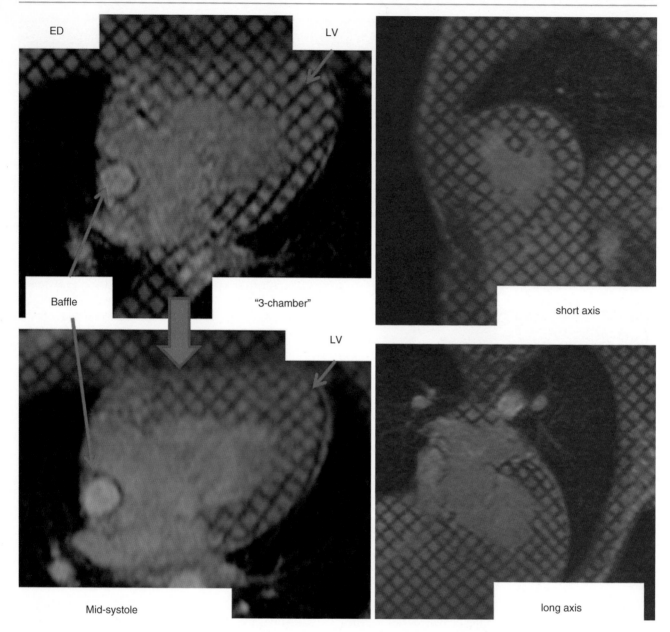

Fig. 1.11 Myocardial tagging in the "3-chamber" (*upper* and *lower left*), short axis (*upper right*) and long axis views (*lower right*) of a patient with a single left ventricle after Fontan. This is an example of spatial modulation of magnetization (SPAMM) where a grid is laid down on the myocardium and deformation can be visualized. Note the deformation from end-diastole (*ED, upper left*) to mid-systole (*lower left*) in the "3-chamber" view. It is the equivalent of speckle tracking in echocardiography except by CMR, the "speckles" are purposefully created in a certain geometry for strain and wall motion assessment

is initiated by the R wave; lines of k-space are then acquired. Phases of the cardiac cycle are defined by a fixed time after the R-wave, so small perturbations of rhythm will put the heart at a slightly different point in the cardiac cycle; this generally does not affect the image too much. In addition, there is generally some "dead space" prior to the next R wave so very late diastole is usually not imaged or utilized. Cine or moving images, are acquired by either this method or the method of retrospective gating. With retrospective gating, lines of k-space are acquired continuously regardless of the phase of the cardiac cycle while the ECG is simultaneously recorded; after image acquisition, the software "bins" the lines of k-space relative to the ECG and cardiac cycle. In this way, each cardiac phase is defined as a certain percentage of the cardiac cycle, allowing the actual duration of each phase to vary flexibly with variation in cardiac cycle. In addition, no "dead space" is left prior to the next phase which can be important in assessing flows or ventricular function.

The above paragraph makes a distinction between static and dynamic techniques. Static ones are generally used for

4-chamber

RV long axis

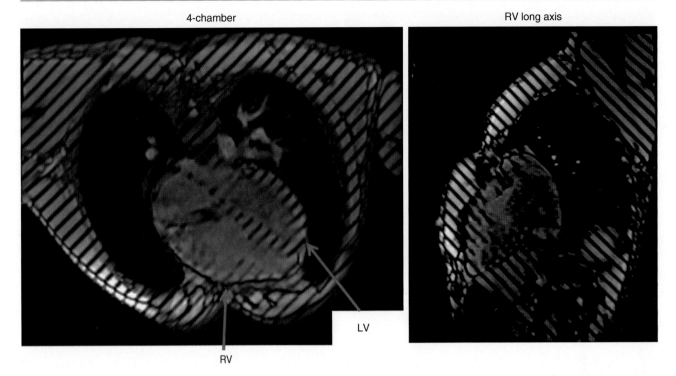

LV

RV

Fig. 1.12 Myocardial tagging in the "4-chamber" (*left*) and long axis of the right ventricle (*right*) in a patient with pulmonic stenosis after balloon dilation. Note how this differs from Fig. 1.11 with one set of parallel lines laid down on the myocardium – the so called "1-dimensional" tagging

cardiovascular anatomy or characterizing tissue. Dynamic techniques are used to assess function or flow in addition to anatomy. A run of single shot images, acquired quickly, can be strung together as motion and this is termed "real-time" and is asynchronous with the cardiac cycle; this can be used in cine imaging, phase contrast velocity mapping or dynamic 3D angiography. First-pass perfusion imaging can be thought of as a hybrid between static and dynamic imaging, where each image depicts a different phase of the cardiac cycle over time.

1.4   ECG Signal

For many years, the upstroke of the R wave on the ECG signal was used to trigger the scanner and used as a marker for end-diastole; unfortunately, artifacts occurred because of the high magnetic field strength and radiofrequency pulses which precluded reliable detection of the true R wave. Bizarre T waves and spikes during the ST segment of the ECG would cause the triggering to falsely detect these waves as the R wave. This is especially true in congenital heart disease where abnormal QRS axes and bundle branch blocks from surgery can make the distinction of the R wave even more problematic in the scanner. On most systems in use today, detection of the R wave as a trigger has been replaced by the use of vectorcardiography (VCG), which is less susceptible to distortion from the magnetic field and of

flowing blood in the thoracic aorta which can act as a conductor. Although wired connection between the VCG and the imaging systems is still used, there is an increasing use of wireless transmission which allows for more flexibility in the scanner.

There are alternatives to the direct connection between the "MRI ECG" and the patient. The ECG signal from external monitoring systems such as the anesthesia equipment can be used which can generate a signal contemporaneous with the R-wave to the MR scanner. Alternatively, the ECG signal can be discarded for "peripheral pulse triggering" where a finger or ear pulse may also be used; obviously, this requires good peripheral circulation. If the patient is cold or has a coarctation, this will often be unsuccessful. It also should be noted that because there is a delay in transmission of the pulse to the distal part of the body that is being monitored, the waveform will be delayed by 200–300 ms when compared with the ECG; this needs to be taken into account during the analysis and interpretation phase of the examination. Peripheral pulse gating is especially useful in patients where a good detection of the R wave cannot be obtained otherwise. Another alternative is the use of non-triggered steady state free precession (e.g. true FISP) sequences where lines of k-space are continually being obtained by the imaging system without regard to the ECG or respiration (see below). With the use of parallel imaging in the spatial or time domains, a temporal resolution as high as 30–40 ms can be acquired. This type of

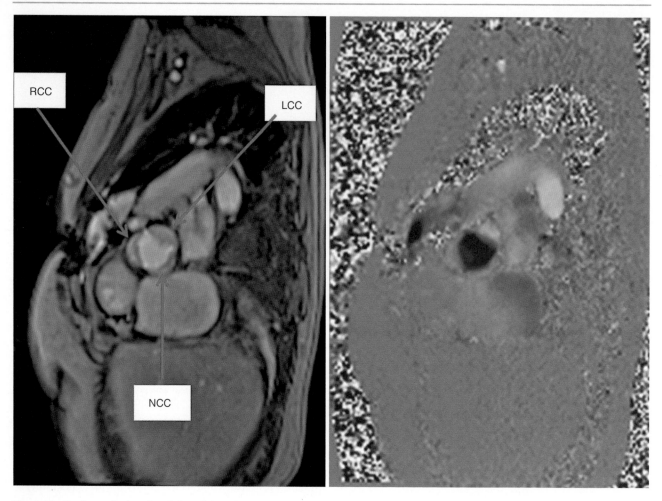

Fig. 1.13 Gradient echo imaging (*left*) and through plane phase encoded velocity mapping (*right*) of the aortic valve. Note how the right (*RCC*), left (*LCC*) and non-coronary commissures are easily visualized on both images, demonstrating the trileaflet valve

imaging can be used in patients with arrhythmias to obtain functional information when triggering to the ECG is problematic (see below). Finally, recent advances in hardware and software has enabled the use of "self gating" sequences, where a coil is used to monitor the motion of the ventricle which acts as a signal for ventricular contraction and relaxation. This approach allows the heart itself to be monitored and act as its own signal for the imager; retrospective analysis of the lines of k-space can then be "binned" to construct moving images.

A special note is required on patients with arrhythmias. With frequent premature ventricular contractions, runs of supraventricular tachycardia or trigeminy for example, it is unclear what an ejection fraction, cardiac index or end-diastolic volume would mean given that these ventricular performance parameters can change from beat-to-beat. A qualitative assessment using real time steady state free precession is one way to get a handle on ventricular function. Nevertheless, there may be instances when some quantitative information may be needed; in these particular cases, "arrhythmia rejection" can be used. With this approach, a range of heart rates or R-R intervals can be set and the imaging system will only allow those lines of k-space which meet these requirements into the final image; the rest of the lines of k-space which fall outside these heart rates are ignored. This approach is inefficient, however, in this manner, quantitative ventricular performance information can be obtained for a range of heart rates. For example, if the range is set between an RR of 700 and 800 ms, the resulting cardiac index can be said to be present for heart rates between 75 and 86 beats/min.

1.5 Respiration

Besides cardiac phases, respiration must be dealt with as it causes positional variation of the heart from movement of the lungs and diaphragm; if not taken into account, this will lead to motion artifacts. There are a number of ways in which this is dealt with in CMR:

(a) Breath-holding, where the patient's breath is held during image acquisition. For many common applications

RVOT

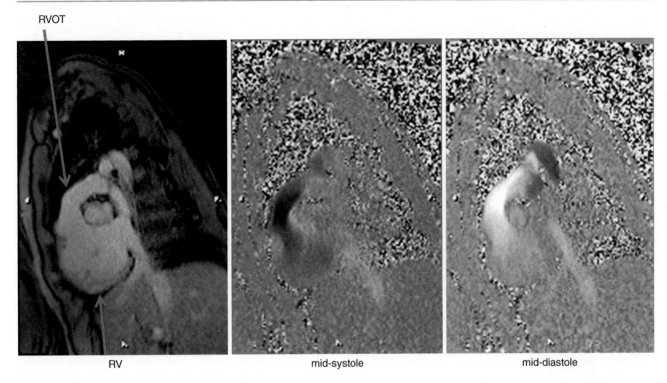

RV   mid-systole   mid-diastole

Fig. 1.14 In-plane phase encoded velocity mapping in a patient with double outlet right ventricle after a right ventricle to pulmonary artery conduit. On the *left* is a magnitude image of the right ventricular (*RV*) outflow tract (*RVOT*). In the *middle* is a mid-systole frame of the in-plane phase encoded velocity map in the exact orientation and position as the image on the left where flow cephalad is signal poor (*dark* on the image); on the *right* is a mid-diastolic frame where flow caudad is signal intense indicating severe conduit insufficiency

such as cine and phase contrast velocity mapping, image acquisitions are fast enough to be performed in a reasonably short breath-hold. This can be done in adults or in children under anesthesia who are paralyzed, intubated and mechanically ventilated. These pulse sequences are widely available and commonly used routinely.

(b) Signal averaging, also termed multiple excitations, where the signal from the complete image is "averaged" over many respiratory and cardiac cycles, "averaging out" the respiratory motion and making the image sharper than without this technique but less sharp than breathholding. This can be used in small children unable to voluntarily breath-hold or adults who cannot cooperate.

(c) Respiratory gating, where the motion of the diaphragm or the chest wall is tracked by either a navigator pulse (which tracks diaphragmatic motion, the equivalent of an "M-mode" of the diaphragm on echocardiography) or respiratory bellows which is placed around the chest wall. Lines of k-space are continuously acquired during the cardiac cycle and only those lines of k-space which fall within certain positional parameters of the diaphragm or chest wall are incorporated into the image; the others are discarded. Although this is a very inefficient method of imaging, it is very effective and used in

imaging coronary arteries for example where high resolution is needed and the navigator echo method is employed. Coronary imaging is unsuitable for single shot (see below) imaging. Whole heart angiography is also unsuitable for anything but respiratory gating.

(d) Single shot imaging, where all the lines of k-space are acquired within a single heartbeat. Advances in hardware and parallel imaging have dramatically improved the speed and quality of these single-shot and real-time techniques and are now often used for scanning patients unable to breath-hold.

1.6   Contrast Agents

These agents offer another important source of distinguishing tissues from each other besides the intrinsic properties of T1, T2 and T2* for example. The most commonly used imaging agents, the paramagnetic chelates of gadolinium (Gd^{3+}), generally work by predominantly shortening T1 and to a certain extent T2; they generally enhance the signal on T1 weighted images. Gadolinium, which has a very large magnetic moment, has unpaired orbital electron spins and shortens T1 by allowing free protons to become bound creating a hydration layer, which helps energy release from

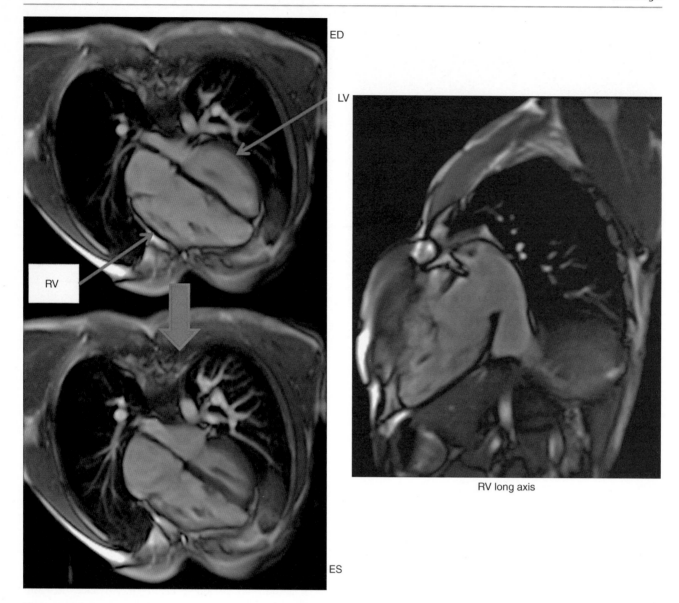

Fig. 1.15 Steady-state free precession imaging in the four chamber view (*left*) at end-diastole (*ED, upper*) and end-systole (*ES, lower*) in a patient with tetralogy of Fallot. The long axis of the right ventricle (*RV*) is on the *right*. *LV* left ventricle

excited spins and accelerates the return to equilibrium magnetization. For other contrast agents which predominantly shorten T2, the reverse is true; shortened T2 leads to decreased signal on T2 weighted images. The effects of these agents can be described by the following formulae:

$$\frac{1}{T1} = \frac{1}{T1_o} + r_1 C$$

$$\frac{1}{T2} = \frac{1}{T2_o} + r_2 C$$

where $T1_o$ and $T2_o$ are the relaxation times prior to and T1 and T2 are the relaxation times after contrast agent adminis-

tration, C is the concentration of the agent and r_1 and r_2 are the longitudinal and transverse "relaxivities" of the individual agent (which are field strength dependent). CMR applications which utilize these agents include delayed enhancement, first pass perfusion, coronary angiography in certain sequences and characterization of tumors and masses.

1.7 Remaining Motionless in the CMR Scanner – Anesthesia and Sedation

The degree of cooperation necessary for successful performance of CMR is generally greater than that of any other type of MRI examination; scans require no significant movement,

End-diastole   End-systole

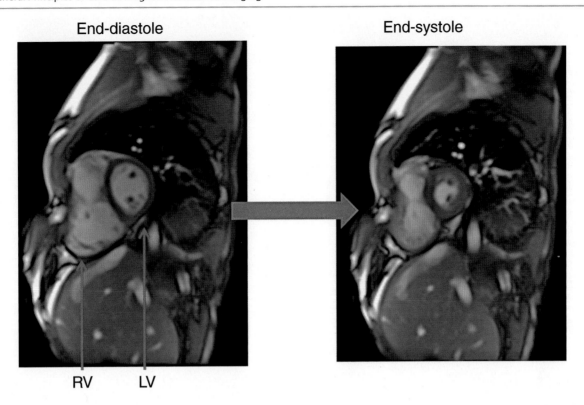

RV   LV

Fig. 1.16 Steady-state free precession imaging in the short axis view at end-diastole (*ED*, *left*) and end-systole (*ES*, *right*) in the patient with tetralogy of Fallot in Fig. 1.15

repeated breath-holds at the same point of the respiratory cycle over a period 45 min to an hour and can be lengthy. Couple this with the strange environment of the scanning room, it is no wonder that both adults and children alike find this very intimidating. Therefore, the use of medication may be required; either conscious sedation or general anesthesia is generally administered so that children who are too young to cooperate or adults with congenital heart disease who may not want to cooperate for one reason or another (e.g. claustrophobia) can still undergo successful CMR. With conscious sedation, patients continue to breathe throughout the scan and imaging has to be substantially altered because of this whereas in a paralyzed, intubated and mechanically ventilated patient under general anesthesia, the effect of "breath-holding" can be created by having the anesthesiologist temporarily suspend ventilation. This is not to say that anytime a patient undergoes general anesthesia in the CMR environment that suspending respiration should be performed but rather that this technique is available to the CMR imager. It should be noted that imaging using sedation or general anesthesia with free breathing is much more physiologic than imaging with positive pressure mechanical ventilation and breathholding and therefore, may be more advantageous than the minor increase in image fidelity with breathholding. For example, a single ventricle patient after Fontan depends upon both cardiac and respiratory effects to allow for pulmonary blood flow; suspending respiration may

alter the physiology artificially and therefore, although accurate for suspended respiration, the physiology is not reflective of the patient's true state, In addition, because systemic venous return changes during the respiratory cycle, imaging during suspended respiration will obtain data only in that state while if the patient is imaged during free breathing, the loading conditions across the respiratory cycle is "averaged" into the image and is more reflective of the patient's true physiologic state.

There is no definitive cut-off age for the age range where medication is needed to remain motionless for a successful CMR study, however, in general, most children greater than or equal to 10–12 years old can cooperate. Of course, this is just a rule of thumb as there can be 7 year olds who are very mature and can follow directions while there are some 15 year olds who will just not cooperate and will require pharmacology. Limited scans with reduced times may be possible with younger patients who would normally require conscious sedation or general anesthesia and this may be considered; it is all in the judgment and purview of the family, physicians and other health care providers caring for the patient. Preparation of the child prior to the scan is important; the involvement of child life experts or the presence in the scanner room of a supportive parent or other regular caregiver can reduce anxiety and be the difference between a scan under medication, without medication or a successful versus an unsuccessful scan.

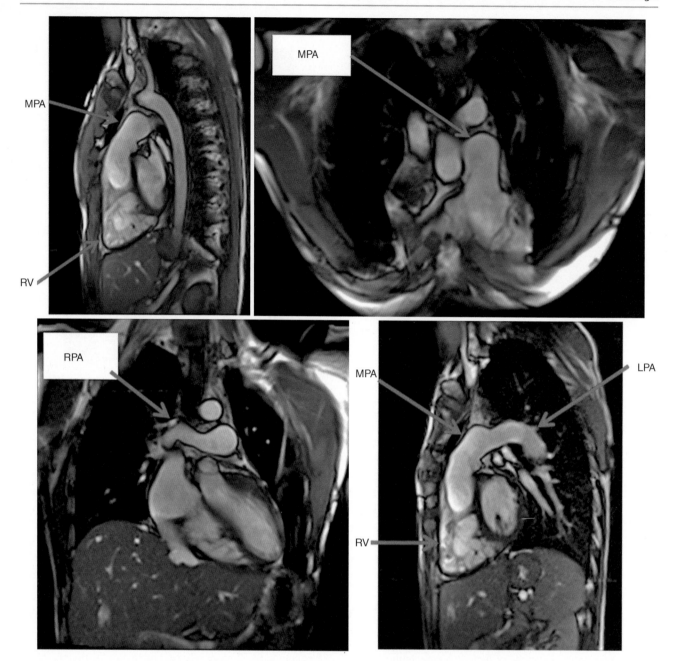

Fig. 1.17 Various steady-state free precession cines of the patient in Figs. 1.15 and 1.16 with tetralogy of Fallot. The right ventricular outflow tract views are seen in the *upper panels* in off-axis sagittal (*left*) and coronal (*right*) views which are orthogonal to each other. The right (*RPA*) and left pulmonary arteries (*LPA*) are seen in long axis in the *left lower* and *right lower panels* respectively. *MPA* main pulmonary artery, *RV* right ventricle

As the CMR environment can be a challenging one for the anesthesiologist or the pediatrician/nurse sedation specialist, monitoring is extremely important since the patient's body will be mostly within the scanner itself, direct visualization during the study is not possible without removing the patient from the bore of the magnet and removing the coil. Many centers utilize a direct video feed with cameras designed to work within the CMR environment and placed in critical positions. For example, a camera pointed down the bore of the magnet is essential along with cameras in other areas to get a good view of what is occurring in the scan room. In addition, extensive physiological monitoring of subjects using equipment specifically designed to be operated in the MR scan room is essential for the safe conduct of the study. Pulse oximetry, limb-lead ECG, blood pressure monitoring, inspiratory and expiratory gas analysis such as end-tidal carbon dioxide and temperature monitoring (especially in young children) should all be available and used.

The monitoring systems should be available wherever the anesthesiology/sedation teams are positioned; this is generally either in the control room or scan rooms. Many facilities position the anesthetic equipment and gas tanks directly outside the scan room, with the gas lines passing through "wave guides" in the wall of the scanner room installed for just this purpose. This arrangement has two advantages: (A) there is reduced risk of inadvertently introducing non-CMR compatible equipment into the scan room and (B) communication between the anesthesiology/sedation team and imaging teams is much easier in this setup. It should be noted, however, that this comes at the cost of increased compliance in the anesthetic circuit. If the decision is made to keep monitoring and anesthetic equipment in the scan room, there is usually a minimum distance that this equipment must be kept from the magnet within which it may not operate correctly, may interfere with the images and might even be attracted into the scanner bore. Careful establishment of this distance from the manufacturer is mandatory before the equipment is first introduced into the scan room. Even consideration to the use of physical restraints to prevent incursion of the equipment within such a distance, and thus avoid accidents should be considered. Direct verbal communication between the anesthesiology/sedation teams and the imaging teams should be on-going at all times with visual contact preferably as well.

Neonates and very small infants less than 6 months of age may undergo CMR successfully while sleeping using a "feed and swaddle" technique. The patient usually is kept awake for a while prior to scanning (3–4 h); when the child enters the preparation area, the intravenous is inserted and the ECG leads are placed. At this point, the baby is very fussy, however, feeding the infant and subsequently swaddling with a warm blanket in a quiet and dimly–lit environment prior to the study will allow the patient to fall asleep; the patient is subsequently transported to the scanner room. Vacuum-shaped support bags can also be utilized to reduce patient motion; placing ear plugs, a hat over the head and ears as well as blankets around the head all aid in keeping the child comfortable and asleep. Imaging sequences that allow for free breathing must be used.

Whether to use deep sedation or anesthesia to perform CMR has been debated for many years. Consideration should be given to how long the CMR scan is likely to take, the patient's age, the flexibility of CMR scanner time and the availability of anesthesiology staffing and/or the availability of specialized sedation teams which include nurses and pediatricians. The practice is obviously a matter for individual institutional and patient preferences. Anesthesia is much more predictable when it comes to onset of action and duration/depth of impaired consciousness; this is advantageous in scheduling CMR examinations and running the schedule smoothly. Deep sedation use has been associated with reduced image quality in some studies [8] but not in others [9], and in some institutions, is far more likely to fail than anesthesia [10], though failure rates can be reduced to close to zero [9] by careful use of expert personnel and strict sedation regimes [9, 11–14]. Imaging performed under anesthesia can be shorter "in theory" because of the ability to breath-hold; in practice, however, the scanning time difference is marginal at best and breathholding, as mentioned above, is less physiologic. Anesthesia has been reported to be marginally safer than deep sedation in some studies [8, 15] and equal in others [9], but there is no doubt that it is more costly and invasive. There are numerous pediatric centers with many years of experience at performing CMR under deep sedation with excellent safety records [9, 11, 12, 14]. The end result is that both techniques are likely to remain in practice for a while.

1.8 The Standard Pediatric/Congenital Heart Disease Examination

There are numerous protocols for a standard CMR examination of the heart, many equally as valid as the other. The one presented in this chapter is meant to be as complete and as efficient as possible, however, it should be recognized that this is not the only one. As each phase of the protocol is delineated, the technique utilized will be expanded upon in detail to give the basics of the different types of CMR.

1. **Axial imaging** (Fig. 1.18): The initial part of the examination begins with a set of static steady state free precession (bright blood) images in the axial (transverse plane) extending from the thoracic inlet to the diaphragm. Generally, 45–50 contiguous end-diastolic slices are obtained of 3 (for babies) to 5 mm in thickness; end-diastole is acquired by placing a "delay" after the R wave of the ECG. At this point in the cardiac cycle, the heart is relatively motionless, allowing for high fidelity imaging. This set of data, which usually takes two and a half to four and a half minutes to acquire (depending upon the patient's heart rate and size), is utilized as a general survey of the anatomy and may be used as a localizer for subsequent, higher fidelity cine imaging, flow measurements, etc. These images are usually acquired with multiple averages (generally 3) during free breathing. In babies, to maintain signal to noise but nevertheless obtain thinner slices, overlapping slices can be used; the cost is prolonged acquisition time.

   (a) From this survey, a number of features may be gleaned with regard to cardiovascular structure in congenital heart disease [16]. (1) The position of the heart in the chest and in which direction the apex is pointing, (2) normal cardiac segments (atria/ventricles/great arteries), (3) the intersegmental connections (atrio-ventricular

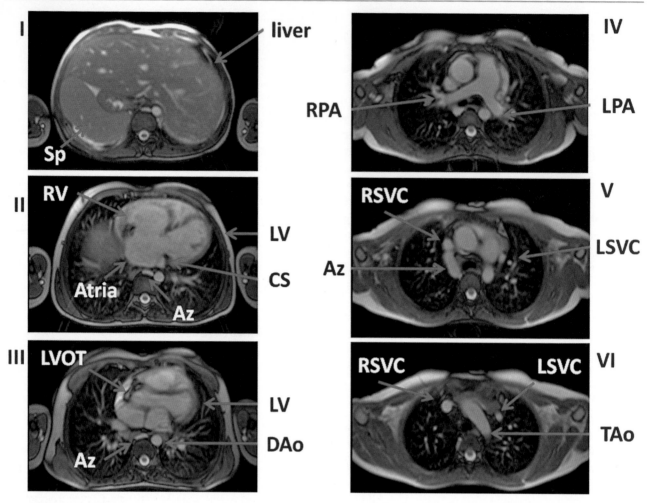

Fig. 1.18 Selected initial axial images of a patient with heterotaxy and complete common atrioventricular canal. Note how much can be gleaned from the first set of static steady state free precession images. Images progress from inferior to superior as the roman numerals increase from top to bottom and from left to right. In (**I**), a transverse abdominal view shows a midline liver and spleen (*sp*) on the right. In (**II**), note the complete common atrioventricular canal, the dilated coronary sinus (*CS*) and dilated mildline azygous (*Az*). In (**III**), note the widely patent left ventricular outflow tract. (**IV**) (*top right*) demonstrates the main pulmonary artery as well as the right (*RPA*) and left pulmonary artery (*LPA*) being confluent. In (**V**), note how the dilated AZ enters the right superior vena cava (*RSVC*) as well as the presence of a left superior vena cava (*LSVC*). Finally, in (**VI**), note the left aortic arch along with the RSVC and LSVC without a bridging vein. *TAo* transverse aortic arch

and ventriculo-arterial) (4) veno-atrial connections, (5) aortic arch anatomy such as coarctation of the aorta and sidedness of the aortic arch, (6) pulmonary arterial tree (such as pulmonary stenosis, pulmonary sling), (7) extra cardiac anatomy and its relationship with the cardiovascular system such as the trachea and tracheobronchial tree, abdominal situs such as the position of the liver, spleen and stomach, qualitative assessment of lung size (e.g. important in Scimitar syndrome). For lesions such as main and branch pulmonary artery stenosis and coarctation of the aorta off-axis imaging planes are necessary to confirm and better display these findings, however, these lesions can often be inferred from the stack of axial images. Qualitative assessment of lung hypoplasia and unbal-

anced pulmonary blood flow can be roughly estimated by the pulmonary vascular markings. If the study is ordered to determine if the patient has a vascular ring, the diagnosis is nearly always readily obtained using this stack of images using the feed and swaddle technique if an infant [17]. Image acquisition time for the three dimensional dataset can be accomplished in 20–30 s depending on the patient's heart rate.

(b) There are drawbacks to using the axial stack when using it for diagnostic purposes. Smaller anatomic structures such as the pulmonary veins may not be visualized well or seem to appear to be connected anomalously but really be connected normally because of partial volume effects; followup with off-axis imaging is mandatory.

HASTE Images

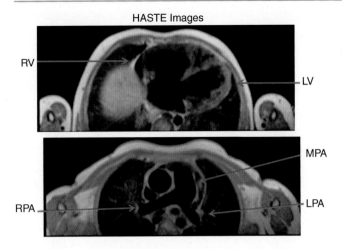

Fig. 1.19 Two initial axial HASTE images of the patient in Fig. 1.18 with heterotaxy and complete common atrioventricular canal. The *upper* and *lower panels* are equivalent to panel II and IV in Fig. 1.18; compare these images with those of Fig. 1.18

(c) In addition to the axial stack of SSFP images, a set of HASTE (Half-Fourier-Acquired Single-Shot Turbo Spin Echo) axial images (Fig. 1.19) can be very useful and are usually obtained while multiplanar reconstruction is being performed on the SSFP images (see below). HASTE is a dark blood, single shot (image obtained in one heart beat) technique which is low resolution and acquired during free breathing, generally obtained in 1–2 min. If the RR interval of the patient is under 600 ms, the images are generally acquired every other heartbeat (doubling the acquisition time) to allow the protons to relax further. HASTE images are less susceptible to flow artifacts and metal artifacts. For example, turbulence in the systemic to pulmonary artery shunt (Blalock-Taussing shunt) or Sano shunt in a single ventricle patient after Stage I Norwood reconstruction will demonstrate signal loss in the shunt itself and the pulmonary arteries on SSFP imaging. Turbulent flow occurs in diastole as well as systole in this scenario and recalling that the static SSFP images are acquired in diastole, these structures are difficult if not impossible to see on the SSFP images. These structures, are however, readily visualized on the HASTE images. Multiple patients can present with braces on their teeth which is common in adolescents as well as stents in their great arteries or other blood vessels; these metallic objects can and generally do produce artifacts which appear on the SSFP imaging, but not on the HASTE images. Note, however, that because of the "cage effect," (see below in the dark blood section) direct measurement of the cavity of the stent is not possible. HASTE imaging can also be useful with visualizing regions of the coronaries and in characterizing masses, however, dedicated subsequent imaging of these structures are mandatory; the HASTE images gives the imager a "first pass" at the problem.

2. **Multiplanar Reconstruction**: During the acquisition of the HASTE images, multiplanar reconstruction is performed on the axial SSFP images. When the SSFP images contain artifacts or are not of high quality, the HASTE images are used. Multiplanar reconstruction is the act of taking the contiguous stack of images and reconstructing these images into other planes (e.g. axial images being resliced as coronal images or in a double oblique angle to obtain the "candy cane" view of the aorta). Most scanners today come with software which allows this to be readily performed. The purpose of this is obviously to obtain orientation and slice positions for dedicated images of the anatomy in question, functional imaging and blood flow. Further anatomy can be obtained with cine, the various types of dark blood imaging or three-dimensional gadolinium images (see below). For the three-dimensional gadolinium slab, these axial images act to ensure that the anatomy in question is covered by the slab. Ventricular function and blood flow are obtained using cine and phase-contrast magnetic resonance (PCMR) (see below). Off-axis imaging planes can be used, for example, to profile the ventricular outflow tracts, the atrio-ventricular valves, major systemic and pulmonary arteries and veins and all their connections to the heart.

3. **Dark Blood Imaging** (**Figs**. 1.8 **and** 1.20): High resolution dark blood imaging (as compared to the low resolution HASTE images) is static in nature and is used sparingly because it is time consuming; 1–2 images can be obtained in a breathhold. There are numerous types of dark blood imaging such as T1 weighting, T2 weighting, spin echo imaging, turbo spin echo imaging, double or triple inversion recovery, etc; this technique is generally utilized for tissue characterization and to define anatomy when turbulence or artifacts get in the way of bright blood techniques. The blood from the heart cavities and blood vessels are black while soft tissue is signal intense. Most dark blood imaging in children utilize either T1 or T2 weighted imaging with the double inversion approach. The details of how each type of dark blood imaging is created is beyond the scope of this chapter, however, a simple example is instructive. The double inversion T1 weighted dark blood technique is utilized to maximally suppress signal from blood and begins with a non-selective inversion pulse which can be thought of as flipping all the protons 180° throughout the body, destroying all the signal from these spins. This is subsequently followed by a selective inversion pulse which flips the protons once again 180° but in a selected region of the body (such as the imaging plane needed); a standard T1 weighted spin echo sequence is then run. In this way, all the blood entering the imaging plane is signal poor with the spins

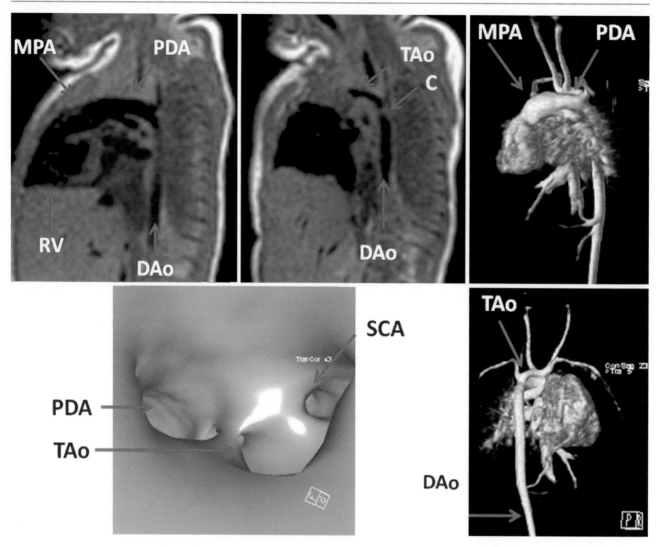

Fig. 1.20 Dark blood, three-dimensional gadolinium and "fly-through" imaging of a neonate with hypoplastic left heart syndrome who has not undergone surgery. The *left upper image* is an off axis sagittal view demonstrating the right ventricular outflow tract giving rise to the main pulmonary artery (*MPA*), patent ductus arteriosus (*PDA*) connecting to the descending aorta (*DAo*). The *upper middle* is similar to the upper left except a few millimeters over to the right demonstrating the hypoplastic transverse aortic arch (*TAo*), the coarctation (*C*) and the DAo.

The *right upper* and *right lower images* are three-dimensional reconstructions from a time-resolved gadolinium sequence which demonstrates the MPA, PDA, hypoplastic TAo and DAo from a sagittal (*top*) and posterior (*bottom*) view. The *lower left* is a "fly-through" image of the three-dimensional reconstruction looking up from the DAo towards the os of the PDA, hypoplastic TAo and subclavian artery (*SCA*)

destroyed in the non-selective inversion pulse and detailed endocardial or endovascular surfaces can be visualized. Dark blood imaging can be used, as mentioned above, to characterize different types of tissue as these will generate different signal. As an example, fat will be intensely bright on T1 weighted imaging while myocardium will be much less so. In addition, special pulses can be used to change the signal intensity and determine if indeed this tissue is what is suggested; taking for example fat as was just mentioned, a "fat saturation" pulse may be coupled with dark blood imaging and will turn the very bright signal of fat without this fat saturation pulse into a very dark signal with the fat saturation pulse, confirming that the

bright signal is indeed fat. This may be useful for lipomas – visualizing this mass on T1 weighted images with and without a fat saturation can confirm the diagnosis. Triple inversion recovery may be used to delineate edema in the tissue from, for example, a myocardial infarction or myocarditis.

Typically, in our imaging protocols, this is performed after the SSFP and HASTE imaging but should not be used after gadolinium administration except for specific applications such as myocarditis or tumor characterization; if used after gadolinium administration, the blood pool will demonstrate signal which is counterproductive to the intent of dark blood imaging in the first place. Uses for dark blood imaging besides myocarditis is to visualize the pericardium, assess for arrhythmogenic right ventricular dysplasia (ARVD) to look for fatty infiltration or RV wall abnormalities (not very reliable for fatty infiltration of the wall, however, since epicardial and pericardial fat can be confused in the thin walled right ventricle and the delineation of fat in the myocardium by MRI is not in the diagnostic criteria), to image the tracheobronchial tree (useful in a vascular ring study) and tumor characterization (with and without gadolinium). As mentioned above, it is useful to image patients when coils, stents, braces, spinal rods and other foreign material cause artifacts on bright blood imaging. Precise measurements cannot be performed within a stent, however, because of the "cage effect." The image artifact caused by the stent prevents the physician from seeing the critical area in and around the stent. This is caused by the fact that a metallic stent behaves as a "Faraday Cage" due to its geometry and material, and the stent additionally creates a magnetic susceptibility artifact due to the material of manufacture of the stent.

4. **Cine** (**Figs.** 1.10, 1.13, 1.15, 1.16, and 1.17): Myocardial motion and blood flow can be visualized with cine imaging to determine congenital function and physiology; it is one of the two workhorses of CMR in this regard (the other being phase contrast velocity mapping which will be discussed next). The two major types of cine imaging are spoiled gradient echo imaging and SSFP; the spoiled gradient echo technique is older but still has a number of uses in state-of-the-art CMR. For example, spoiled gradient echo imaging is useful to determine valve morphology using a high flip angle (Fig. 1.13); in this way, flowing blood into the imaging plane is bright and outlines the leaflets of the valve very well. It is also useful when artifacts plague SSFP as a low TE and high bandwidth gradient echo image is less susceptible to these artifacts. High TE gradient echo imaging will enhance turbulence (where SSFP is less susceptible to turbulence) and may be useful in identifying these areas of flow disturbances.

High resolution SSFP cine imaging (Figs. 1.15, 1.16, and 1.17) can demonstrate exquisite images of the myocardium, valves, blood pool, and vessels and in assessing myocardial function, it is the technique of choice. These cine images provide excellent spatial and temporal resolution for the assessment of global and regional myocardial wall motion. This cine sequences should be retrospectively gated so that wall motion data is available for the entire cardiac cycle; with prospective triggering, the phases prior to the R wave is generally truncated as noted above in the physics section. With retrospective gating, the number of calculated phases should be figured so that there is only one or less interpolated phase between each measured phase; an interpolated phase is one that

shares data between the two measured phases. This is easily performed by doubling the patient's RR interval and then dividing by the "TR" (line TR × number of segments) to get the maximum number of phases or dividing by the number of phases desired to obtain the maximum TR needed.

Temporal resolution should be set to provide, in general, 20–30 phases across the cardiac cycle, depending upon the heart rate. Obviously, in a patient with a heart rate of 150 beats per minute (R-R of 400 ms), 20 frames per heartbeat is more than adequate (20 ms temporal resolution) while if the heart rate is 50 beats per minute (R-R of 1,200 ms), 20 frames per heartbeat is not sufficient (60 ms temporal resolution). This is because systole does not vary too much as a function of heart rate; it is diastole that lengthens or shortens. A 60 ms temporal resolution for a heart rate of 50 beats per minute will not capture enough frames in systole to adequately assess the ventricle.

When an entire ventricular volume dataset is acquired, ventricular volume and mass at end-diastole and end-systole is measured yielding end-diastolic and end-systolic volumes, stroke volume, ejection fraction, cardiac output and mass [18–22]. To perform an entire ventricular volume set, generally a four-chamber view is first obtained by cine (orientation and slice position determined by multiplanar reconstruction as noted above); the four-chamber view is defined as the view that intersects the middle of both atrioventricular valves and the apex of the heart. Subsequently, a series of short axis views are obtained which are perpendicular to the four-chamber view and span from atrioventricular valve to apex. It should be noted that this requires obtaining short axis slices one slice past the atrioventricular valve level and one slice past the apex to ensure the entire volume is obtained; this can be clearly positioned off the four-chamber view at end-diastole. Measurement of ventricular volumes involves contouring the endocardial border of each slice of a given phase (e.g. end-diastole or end-systole) from base to apex and planimeterizing this area. The product of the sum of the areas on each slice encompassing the ventricle and the slice thickness yields the ventricular volume at that phase. This procedure, if performed at end-diastole and end-systole, will yield two values and the difference between these values is the stroke volume; and the ratio of the stroke volume to the end-diastolic volume multiplied by 100 yields the ejection fraction. The cardiac output is obtained by multiplying the ventricular stroke volume and the average heart rate during the cine acquisition. Ventricular mass is similarly measured, generally at end-diastole, by contouring the epicardial border on each slice which contains ventricle and planimeterizing the area which contains both the ventricular volume and mass. This value is subtracted from the ventricular volume measurement at each slice and yields the ventricular mass. Most scanners come with and numerous independent companies sell software which semiautomates this process; ventricular volumes and mass can generally be obtained in a few minutes of post-processing. More tedious is contouring ventricular volumes through every phase of the cardiac cycle, however, this will yield a ventricular volume – time curve which may be useful in some situations. Because CMR can acquire multiple contiguous, parallel tomographic slices, there is no need for geometric assumptions, making the technique an excellent tool for precise measurement of ventricular volumes and mass in congenital heart disease. Ventricular size and shape can vary considerably in various forms of congenital heart disease (e.g. single ventricles, corrected transposition of the great arteries, etc).

Besides ventricular size, mass, and wall motion, cine imaging is excellent for identifying vessel sizes as well as stenosis or hypoplasia including great arteries, along an ventricular outflow tract or in a baffle or conduit. On the flip side, cine can also be used to assess regurgitation of valves of which there should be minimal in the normal heart. All this is determined not only by the shape of the vessel but by loss of signal due to acceleration of flow through a stenotic vessel/valve or a regurgitant valve; a classic example is the flow void through coarctation of the aorta. In addition, shunts can be identified by cine as turbulence visualized across atrial or ventricular septae will indicate interatrial and interventricular communication. A way in which shunting can be accentuated visually is with the use of a pre-saturation tag. When the protons in a plane of tissue are flipped 180° to destroy their spins prior to imaging (similar to an selective inversion pulse in a plane of tissue intersecting the imaging plane), a pre-saturation tag is said to be laid down. This pre-saturation tag labels the tissue it intersects with decreased signal intensity (black on the image). If the presaturation tag is laid down on the left atrium prior to a gradient echo sequence in a patient with an atrial septal defect, blood flowing from left to right will be dark on the bright blood cine and visualized to cross from left to right atria. Similarly, if there is right to left flow, bright signal from the right atrium would be seen to cross to the darkness of the left atrium.

By stringing a series of continuous single shot images together in one plane ("single plane, multiphase" imaging), motion can be captured and this is termed "real time cine CMR." Essentially, the SSFP technique is used to acquire all the lines of k-space needed to create an image continuously in the same plane. "Interactive real time cine CMR" adds the ability to be able to manipulate the real time imaging plane interactively, similar to echocardiographic "sweeps"; this provides a fast way to assess cardiovascular anatomy, function and flow. These images can be used for localization for higher resolution regular cine CMR and has been utilized in the past to actually acquire fetal cardiac motion. It is also used in the event there is too much arrhythmia so that at least a qualitative assessment of the heart can be made. Temporal resolution can be as low as 35 ms using parallel imaging.

CMR techniques in general and cine in particular build the image of multiple heartbeats; if multiple averages (excitations) are used, this can be in the hundreds. The disadvantage to this is the time it takes to acquire the data unlike "real time" CMR cine imaging just mentioned or echocardiography where the cardiac motion is instantaneously obtained. The distinct advantage to this approach, however, is because the image is built over many heartbeats, it represents the "average" of all those heartbeats over the acquisition time. This truly is an advantage as it would be assumed that this "average," embedded in the image, is more reflective of the patient's true physiologic state than the instantaneous images of echocardiography. To perform the equivalent, the echocardiographer would have to view hundreds of heartbeats and "average" it in the imager's mind with all the subjectivity that entails. Picture measuring hundreds of M-mode dimensions of the ventricle (end-diastolic and end-systolic diameters) and then averaging them all together to get a shortening fraction; that is what is obtained with cine CMR in one image when measuring ventricular function parameters!

5. **Phase Contrast (encoded) Magnetic Resonance (Figs. 1.13, 1.14, 1.21, 1.22, and 1.23) [23–31]:** This CMR technique is used to measure flow and velocity in any blood vessel with few limitations (generally 4–6 pixels must fit across the blood vessel in cross-section for it to be accurate); for example, cardiac output may be obtained across the aorta and the pulmonary valve. In the absence of intracardiac shunts, the flows across the aortic and pulmonary valves should be equal – an internal check to the measurement. In another example, relative flows to each lung may be measured by utilizing through-plane velocity maps across the cross-section of the right and left pulmonary arteries, obviating the need for nuclear medicine scans. By placing a through-plane velocity map across the main pulmonary artery, an internal check on the branch pulmonary artery flows is obtain as the sum of the blood flow to the branch pulmonary arteries must equal the blood flow in the main pulmonary artery. In addition, it is also common to utilize phase encoded velocity mapping as a check on cine measurements (e.g. cardiac index of the aorta should be equal to the cardiac index of the left ventricle in the absence of mitral insufficiency). It is clear that this is a strength of CMR – the ability to perform

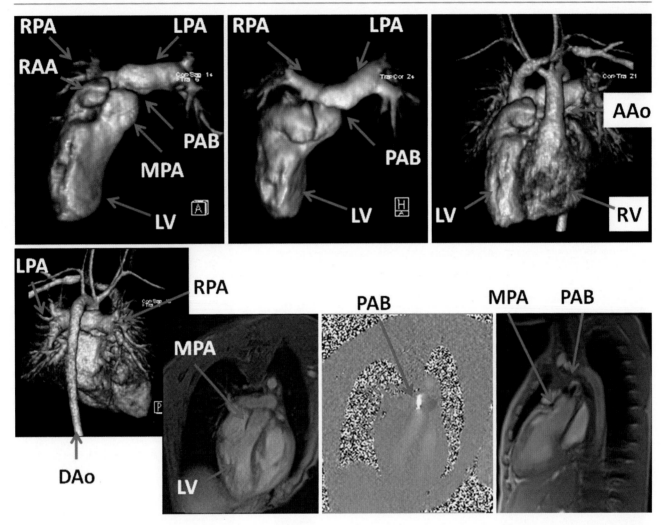

Fig. 1.21 Various types of imaging in an infant with corrected transposition of the great arteries after a pulmonary artery band (*PAB*). The *upper left* and *middle panels* are two views of a three-dimensional gadolinium image of the right sided circulation showing the left ventricle, main pulmonary artery (*MPA*), PAB and the right (*RPA*) and left pulmonary arteries (*LPA*) from anterior (*left*) and anterior tipped up to transverse view (*middle*). Note how the right atrial appendage (*RAA*) is easily seen. The *right upper* and *left lower images* are three-dimensional gadolinium reconstructions of both circulations demonstrating the anterior aorta and branch pulmonary arteries form the anterior (*upper right*) and posterior (*lower left*) views. The *lower panel* second from the left and second from the right are magnitude and in-plane phase images from phase encoded velocity mapping demonstrating the left ventricular outflow tract and showing the jet through the PAB (signal intense is caudad) with a VENC of 400 cm/s. The *right lower image* is an orthogonal view through the left ventricular outflow tract demonstrating the turbulence distal to the PAB

these checks for internal validation of the quantitative data, unlike other imaging modalities.

It is key to understand what the "phase" means in the term "phase encoded velocity mapping" for one to understand how this is used to measure flow. Phase was discussed in the physics section and will be explained in a slightly different way in this section, although it represents the same physical principle. When tissue is excited by radiofrequency energy, the subsequent signal that gets generated when the protons relax (for example, a sine wave) can be described by its frequency (how many cycles per second), its amplitude (the strength of the signal) and its phase (where, in a given time, is the sine wave in its

cycle). Two waves can have the same frequency and amplitude but be in different points in their cycle (i.e. they are identical waves but shifted in time); they are out of phase. Think of two identical sine waves placed one atop the other in a signal amplitude-time graph (signal amplitude on the Y axis and time on the X axis) and then shift one slightly to the right in time; these sine waves are identical but out of phase with each other. Another way to understand this is that the same part of each of the two identical sine wave occurs at a different point of time (e.g. the peak of sine wave "A" occurs prior to the peak of sine wave "B").

The principle underlying phase contrast CMR very simply is that moving tissue within a magnetic field that

Aortic Regurgitation

Cardiac output = 3.8 l/min/m²

Forward flow = 108 cc

Reverse flow = 38 cc

Regurgitant fraction = 35%

Heart rate = 87 BPM

Peak velocity = 3.7 m/s

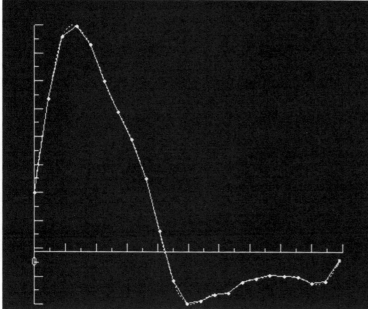

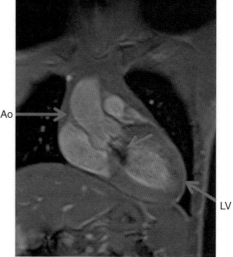

Fig. 1.22 Data and images from a patient with a bicuspid aortic valve, aortic stenosis and insufficiency. The graph of flow versus time is on the *lower left* and on the *upper left* is the relevant data. Gradient echo images of the left ventricular outflow tract in two orthogonal views demonstrating the aortic insufficiency jet during diastole (*short arrows*). *AAo* ascending aorta, *LV* left ventricle

has a gradient applied to it changes phase. Put another way, whenever anything moves along the axis of an applied gradient, the phase of the spinning vectors in that object becomes altered relative to the stationary object. Remember the Larmor equation states the precessional frequency of the protons is directly proportional to the magnetic field; if that magnetic field is altered by position creating a gradient, the precessional frequency will change depending upon position. Any tissue moving across the gradient will change precessional frequency and accumulate phase shift selectively "labeling" itself. Phase contrast velocity mapping utilizes a "bipolar" radiofrequency pulse which is equal in magnitude but opposite in direction (e.g. turns from positive to negative and then from negative to positive); this is done with two back to back

pulses. The sequence has the following effect: Before any radiofrequency pulse is applied, protons are tilted as a function of where they are positioned in the magnetic gradient. When the first radiofrequency pulse is applied, both stationary and moving tissue protons are further tilted; when the second equal and opposite radiofrequency pulse is applied immediately afterwards, protons of the stationary tissue return the tilt of their protons back to their original position and accumulate a net phase of zero (their tilt goes back to their original position since they experienced and equal and opposite radiofrequency pulse and haven't moved position). Protons of the moving tissue, however, do not revert to their original tilt since they have moved and are experiencing a different magnetic field because of the magnetic gradient. These protons are said to have

Aortic flow

Cardiac output = 4.6 l/min/m²

Pulmonary flow

Cardiac output = 10.7 l/min/m²

Qp/Qs = 2.3

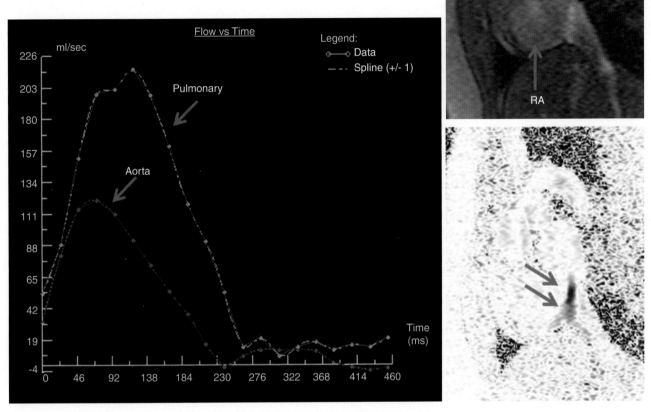

Fig. 1.23 Data and images from a 2 year old with an atrial septal defect (*ASD*) of the inferior vena cava type and anomalous right pulmonary venous connections to the right atrium (*RA*). The off axis sagittal magnitude image (*upper right*) demonstrates the ASD while the in-plane, colorized phase encoded velocity map (*lower right*) in the same orientation as the magnitude image demonstrates left to right flow by the *red color* jet as in echocardiography (*red* is caudad and *blue* is cephalad flow). The aortic and pulmonary flow are both graphed simultaneously (*lower left*); data demonstrates as Qp/Qs = 2.3

accumulated a "phase shift." To summarize, this will yield a zero phase change for stationary objects when both pulses are applied whereas there will be a net accumulation of phase in moving tissue. By subtracting, pixel by pixel, one the phases of one pulse from the other, background phase changes of stationary objects are cancelled out and the phase shift of the moving tissue is amplified. Then, usually, the "phase difference" method is used to map the phase shift angles into signal intensities. Flow is calculated by the formula:

$$\Delta\,phase = g \times v \times T \times A_g Z$$

where g = gyromagnetic ratio, v = velocity, T = duration of the gradient pulse and A_g is the area of each lobe of the gradient pulse.

By tailoring the strength of the radiofrequency pulse to the anticipated velocities, accurate measurement can be obtained; this is called a VENC (velocity encoding) and is the equivalent of the Nyquist limit in echocardiography. Using the VENC and the signal intensity, the velocity of moving tissue in each pixel can then be encoded. This can occur with either blood (hence blood phase encoded velocity mapping) or with myocardial tissue (also called myocardial velocimetry and is the equivalent to Doppler tissue imaging). Spatially, there are two ways to encode velocity in the image: (a) "through plane" where each pixel encodes velocity into and out of the plane of the image and (b) "in-plane", where velocities are encoded in the plane of the image and not into and out of the plane; this is similar to Doppler echocardiography. Unlike Doppler echocardiography, however, velocities are encoded in either the Y- or X-direction of the image. This is advantageous as each pixel can encode velocity in three orthogonal planes. Motion in one direction is mapped onto the anatomic image as increased signal intensity or bright and motion in the other direction appears signal poor and dark; stationary tissue appears gray. Air, such as in the lungs or around the patient, are encoded in a mosaic black and white. Color can be added to make it similar to Doppler echocardiography.

Flow measurements by this methodology utilizes the cross-sectional area of the vessel perpendicular to the transaxial direction of flow. Most MRI companies and some independent software developers have programs which identify of the regions of interest simultaneously on the anatomic or "magnitude" images as well as the "phase" images (which can sometimes be difficult to read at times). The product of the velocity and the area of an individual pixel gives flow through that pixel; summing this across the vessel cross sectional region will yield the flow at a given phase of the cardiac cycle. Integrating this across the entire cardiac cycle (i.e. each phase plotted as a time-flow curve), the flow during one heartbeat is calculated. The product of the heart rate and this flow in one heartbeat will yield the cardiac output.

Through plane phase encoded velocity mapping can also be used to assess the peak velocity for gradient calculations as might be used for coarctation of the aorta or ventricular pressure estimates as with a tricuspid regurgitant jet. If the plane is perpendicular to flow in the region of maximum velocity, the greatest velocity in any pixel in the region of interest in the cardiac cycle is used in the simplified Bernoulli equation. It should be noted that planes not perpendicular to flow or one at a level where the maximum velocity is not present will underestimate this number; generally, this is used in conjunction with in-plane velocity mapping (see below) to measure maximum velocities. This is similar to Doppler echocardiography where, if the plane is angled obliquely to the jet of interest or the sector is not in the area of maximum velocity, an underestimate the maximum velocity will occur.

Encoding velocity parallel to flow ("in-plane" velocity encoding) is predominantly used to measure peak flow velocities which is similar to what Doppler echocardiography measures. The advantage of this type of phase encoding over the through plane technique in measuring maximum velocities is that velocities can be measured along a jet of interest in the direction the jet is pointing (similar to continuous wave Doppler), through plane mapping is placed at a certain level of the jet and the velocity measured which is similar to the range-gating technique of pulse wave Doppler echocardiography. With in-plane velocity mapping, the jet is aligned by rotating the entire field of view to make one side exactly perpendicular to the jet. The peak flow velocities can then be translated into pressure gradients via the simplified Bernoulli equation. The phase maps on present day scanners can give a temporal resolution of about 15–20 ms with non-breathhold techniques.

Phase encoded velocity mapping has limitations. Reliability of both through plane and in plane velocity mapping is a function of a few factors such as slice thickness ("partial volume" effects may induce inaccuracies in velocity calculations) and the angle of the jet (the jet needs to aligned perpendicular to the direction of phase encoding, similar in some sense, to Doppler flow measurements). In addition, if the VENC is not chosen close but not below the maximum velocity anticipated, errors may occur. If the VENC chosen is too low, velocities in the vessel will exceed the ability of the CMR scanner to encode them which is akin to aliasing and exceeding the Nyquist limit in Doppler echocardiography. If the VENC chosen is too high, the lower velocities will not be measured as accurately; this is analogous to the difference when measuring a 4 oz of fluid in an 6 oz measuring cup (appropriate setting of the VENC) versus a gallon measuring cup (in appropriate setting of the VENC). Maxwell terms, eddy currents and whether or not background subtraction is used will also play a role in velocity mapping accuracy.

Phase encoded velocity mapping has many applications in congenital heart disease and in broad categories, they are (A) flow quantification, (B) flow visualization and (C) velocity measurements and (D) myocardial velocimetry:

(A) Flow Quantification:

1. Cardiac output (Figs. 1.22 and 1.23): Measuring cardiac output is an essential factor in assessing cardiovascular performance; this is especially true in patients who have undergone surgical procedures or who have underwent catheter intervention. Lesions such as single ventricles, corrected transposition, tetralogy of Fallot, etc all benefit from measuring an elementary parameter such as cardiac output. This can also be used as an internal check to the ventricular stroke volume measurements.

2. Regurgitant lesions (Fig. 1.22): As flow can be quantified as forward and reverse flow, the regurgitant volumes and fractions can be measured and calculated; lesions such as tetralogy of Fallot after

repair with a transannular patch [32] or in patients with a bicuspid aortic valve and severe aortic insufficiency all require measurement of leaky semilunar valves. These measurements are readily obtained by placing phase encoded velocity map at the sinotubular junction (for the aortic valve) and just above the pulmonary valve and measuring the forward and reverse area under the flow-time curve. The regurgitant fraction is simply the area under the reverse flow (regurgitant volume) divided by the area under the forward flow (forward volume) multiplied by 100. An internal check is the measure flow in the cavae which should be the net cardiac output measured by velocity mapping in across the leaky semilunar valve. To obtain how much leakage there is across an atrioventricular valve, a combination of techniques are used; cine CMR is used to measure the stroke volume of the ventricle and phase encoded velocity mapping to measure the amount of forward flow through the semilunar valve. The difference between the two (assuming no semilunar valve insufficiency) is the regurgitant volume of the atrioventricular valve. Alternatively, the forward flow across the atrioventricular valve during diastole and the forward flow across the semilunar valve in systole can be used (assuming no shunting).

3. Shunts (Fig. 1.23): Many lesions in congenital heart disease have shunting between the circulations present; this shunt flow can be easily calculated by placing velocity maps across the aorta and main pulmonary artery and measuring flow (e.g. Qp/Qs) [33]; if there is a aorto-pulmonary window, branch pulmonary artery flow is generally used instead. Measuring flow in both branch pulmonary arteries can add an internal check on the amount of pulmonary blood flow for intracardiac shunts and the sum of the flow in the cavae can be used as a check on the amount of systemic blood flow assuming no systemic to pulmonary collaterals.

4. Flow Distribution To Each Lung [34]: Altered flow distribution to left and right lungs can be common in many lesions in congenital heart disease such as in single ventricle lesions after Fontan, tetralogy of Fallot or in transposition of the great arteries after arterial switch procedure; all may have branch pulmonary stenosis. Relative flow to each lung is assessed by placing a phase encoded velocity map at each branch pulmonary artery although care must be taken to place the map in the branch pulmonary artery proximal to the takeoff of the first branches to ensure this

blood flow is included. Flow measured in the main pulmonary artery must equal the sum of the flows to each lung in the absence of collaterals and is used as an internal check.

5. Collateral Flow [35]: Patients with single ventricles after bidirectional Glenn or Fontan operation develop aorto-pulmonary collaterals presumably in response to decreased pulmonary blood flow and cyanosis [36]. In addition, patients with relatively long standing coarctation of the aorta can develop aortic collaterals which bypass the obstructed segment. In the former, the amount of collateral flow can be quantified by measuring flow via velocity mapping across the ventricular outflow tract and subtracting measured caval return or measuring flow in the pulmonary veins and subtracting measured flow in the branch pulmonary arteries. In the latter, the amount of collateral flow can be determined by placing phase encoded velocity maps across the aorta just distal to the coarctation site and across the aorta at the level of the diaphragm. Normally, flow at each level will be very similar or the flow at the level of the diaphragm slightly lower (because of flow to the intercostal arteries), however, in the presence of coarctation with collaterals, flow just distal to the coarctation site in the aorta will be lower than flow in the aorta at the level of the diaphragm since collateral flow will present in the latter and not in the former.

(B) Velocity Measurements

1. Pressure gradients: Stenoses of a blood vessel such as a great artery (e.g. coarctation of the aorta, left pulmonary artery stenosis, or a pulmonary artery band (Fig. 1.21)) or of a valve (aortic stenosis in a bicuspid aortic valve) can occur in numerous congenital heart lesions. It is important for many reasons to determine pressure gradients in these lesions; as noted above, the determination of gradients by CMR is similar to Doppler echocardiography, using the simplified Bernoulli equation. A maximum velocity is measured, typically in the vena contracta, and the gradient is simply the product of 4 and the velocity (in meters/second) squared. Measurement of maximum velocities may be performed in two ways: (A) "in-plane" velocity mapping directed parallel to the obstruction to flow and (B) "through plane" velocity mapping perpendicular to flow. Both have their strengths and weaknesses (see above discussion).

(C) Flow Visualization:

1. Septal defects using in-plane velocity mapping: Septal defects at both the atrial and ventricular

level can be visualized with in-plane velocity mapping. The imaging plane needs to be oriented in the direction of the flow across the defect to successfully visualize it; blood flowing one way would be dark and flow the other way would be bright. In addition, color can be superimposed on the image to simulate color Doppler echocardiography.

2. Flow directionality in blood vessels using through plane velocity mapping: A good example of this is isolation or disruption of the subclavian arteries; this may be caused by surgery (e.g. a subclavian flap angioplasty to repair coarctation of the aorta) or may be congenital. When this occurs, the subclavian artery usually is supplied with blood in a retrograde fashion via the vertebral artery; sometimes, with some paraspinal plexuses or other collaterals supply the subclavian artery. Clinically, a "subclavian steal" can occur and CMR velocity mapping techniques can be used to identify retrograde flow in the vertebral arteries. Normally, if an axial through plane velocity map is placed in the neck, both carotid and vertebral arteries will be labeled as either bright or black on the images as they are all flowing in the same direction. With isolation of a subclavian artery, flow in the ipsilateral vertebral artery is retrograde while flow in the other three head vessels (carotid and vertebral arteries) will be antegrade. A velocity map in this scenario will encode the verterbral artery ipsilateral to the isolated subclavian artery in one direction (e.g. dark) and the other three head vessels will be encoded in the opposite direction (e.g. bright), proving the physiology.

3. Valve morphology (Fig. 1.13): Phase contrast velocity mapping is also useful for identifying valve morphology; as through plane phase contrast velocity mapping "tags" flowing blood, this can be used to outline the leaflets tips making a cast of the valve morphology while it opens and closes; the flowing blood is bright or dark and highlights the valve leaflet tips which are gray. Bicuspid, unicuspid and quadracuspid valves are easily seen. Of particular note, bicuspid aortic valve is very common clinically; it can easily be identified by phase contrast mapping and the degree of valvular stenosis and regurgitation assessed [37, 38].

(D) Myocardial velocimetry: This application of phase contrast velocity mapping is the CMR equivalent to Doppler tissue imaging in echocardiography; velocities of the myocardial tissue can be recorded. The phase contrast velocity mapping sequence is configured such that the VENC is set fairly low (15–30 cm/s); modifications in the sequence must be made to keep the TE as low as possible. Doppler tissue imaging can only record myocardial velocities in one direction; that is parallel to the Doppler beam. Myocardial velocimetry, however, is a much more comprehensive measurement of myocardial velocities in that, similar to other phase contrast velocity mapping applications, each pixel can encode velocities in three orthogonal planes; a three-dimensional velocity map of the myocardium can be measured. Both myocardial velocimetry in CMR and Doppler tissue imaging in echocardiography suffer from the same drawback in that both techniques do not truly measure the velocity of a specific piece of myocardium; they identify a point in space and the velocity of myocardium moving into and out of that point is measured. Only CMR myocardial tagging and Doppler spectral tracking truly measures the velocity of a piece of myocardium non-invasively. An excellent review comparing the merits of myocardial velocimetry to myocardial tagging was published in 1996.

6. **Magnetic Resonance Angiography** (MRA) (**Figs**. 1.20, 1.21, 1.24, **and** 1.25): Magnetic resonance angiography, nearly all based on intravenous gadolinium diethylenetriamine pentaacetic acid (Gd-DTPA), is be used to determine detailed anatomy such as major pulmonary and systemic arteries and veins and to glean physiology is a key part of the examination. As discussed above, gadolinium is a paramagnetic element which is administered in a chelated form and is an extracellular agent that changes the magnetic property of the tissue or vessel it is in. It markedly decreases T1 relaxation and which allows its application to distinguish the target structure (e.g. the aorta) from background (e.g. lung, other mediastinal contents). It is considered a highly safe substance with adverse events occurring in one in 200,000–400,000. Usually a "double dose" of contrast is given (for most agents, this is 0.4 cc/kg; please check the labeling of your individual agent).

Recently much attention has been given to the incidence of nephrogenic systemic fibrosis (NSF) in patients with chronic, severe renal failure, first described in 2000 in 15 patients undergoing hemodialysis who presented with "scleromyxoedema-like" skin lesions. A detailed discussion of this entity is beyond the scope of this chapter; suffice it to say that after modifications of gadolinium use, NSF is nearly eradicated. Very few reports of children developing NSF exist and none under 6 years of age.

Generally, with few exceptions such as myocardial perfusion imaging, this portion of the study is performed after cine imaging and before phase contrast velocity

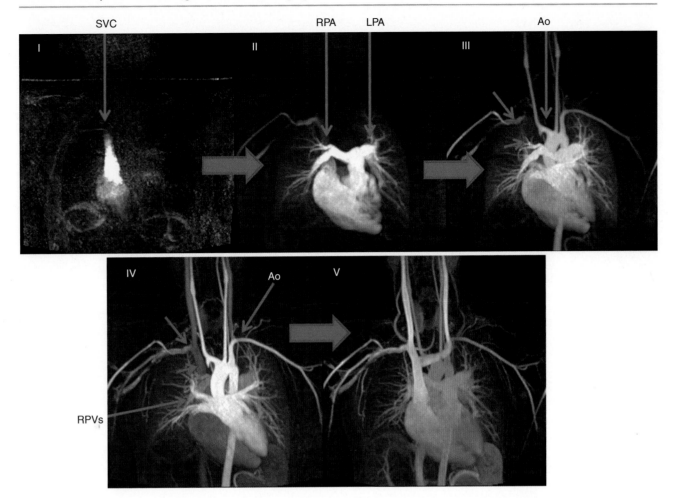

Fig. 1.24 Three dimensional time resolved gadolinium imaging in a coronal view. The images are maximum intensity projections (MIPs) and temporally follow the roman numeral from left to right and from top to bottom. Each phase can be created into a three-dimensional image. Spatial resolution is an isotropic 1 × 1 × 1 mm and temporal resolution is 2.2 s. In (**I**), flow into the superior vena cava (*SVC*) is seen followed by flow into the right side of the heart (**II**). In (**III**), flow is now seen in the pulmonary veins and the beginnings of the aorta (*Ao*). In (**IV**), flow has left the right side of the heart and is now mostly in the pulmonary veins, the left side of the heart and the aorta. In (**V**), flow is seen returning to the heart from the systemic veins. Note the interrupted right subclavian artery in (**III** and **IV**) (*arrows*). *LPA* left pulmonary artery, *RPA* right pulmonary artery, *RPVs* right pulmonary veins

mapping. Since approximately 10 min is needed between gadolinium administration and imaging for delayed enhancement (see below), the time after gadolinium administration is used to perform phase contrast velocity mapping; this is also advantageous as the gadolinium agent boosts the signal from phase contrast velocity mapping, increasing the signal to noise ratio. There are two types of gadolinium techniques commonly used to evaluate three dimensional anatomy:

1. Static three-dimensional imaging can be utilized to create a three-dimension images of the cardiovascular system which can be rotated and cut in any plane desired. The three-dimensional slab (see Physics section) can be acquired in any orientation and can be viewed in its raw data format, as a maximum intensity projection, a shaded surface display or as a volume rendered object. As it is a three-dimensional acquisi-

tion with one frequency encoding and two phase encoding directions, the thickness of the slices can be much thinner than other techniques – on the order of ¾ to 1 mm. As the resolution is higher than other techniques in CMR, this type of imaging is used to visualize smaller vessels (e.g. aortic-pulmonary collaterals in pulmonary atresia/intact ventricular septum, aortic collaterals in coarctation, etc.). Multiple three-dimensional data sets are generally obtained which (a) can separate out the systemic and pulmonary circulations and (b) increases the chances of a successfully imaging what is needed.

With this technique, it is best to know exactly when the contrast agent reaches the target vessel to begin the three-dimensional sequence. This can be performed in either two ways: (a) Bolus tracking, where the target structure (e.g. the pulmonary arteries in the case of

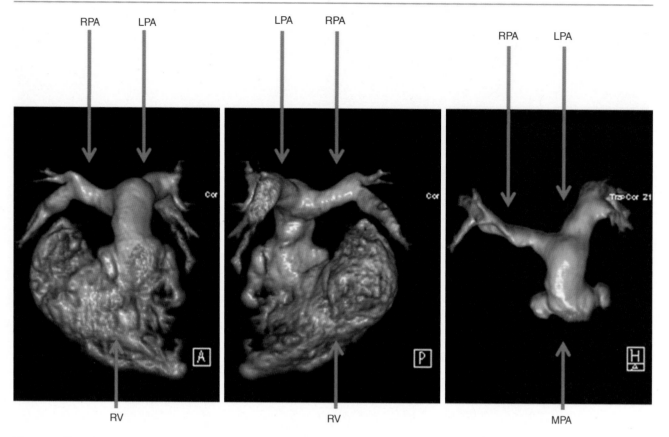

Fig. 1.25 Three dimension right heart reconstructions of the patient in Fig. 1.24. The right ventricle (*RV*), main (*MPA*), right (*RPA*) and left pulmonary artery (*LPA*) are clearly seen from an anterior (*left*), poste- rior (*middle*) and transverse (*right*) view. The RV was removed from the transverse view (*right*) to facilitate visualizing the branch pulmonary arteries

tetralogy of Fallot) is imaged with "real-time" sequence during gadolinium injected – once the contrast agent is seen to arrive at the target structure, the three-dimensional sequence is then obtained. (b) Timing bolus, where a small amount of contrast agent is injected and timed to determine when it will arrive at the target vessel. Injecting the full dose of gadolinium followed by the three-dimensional sequence with a delay placed based on the small amount of contrast agent initially given, is then performed knowing the gadolinium will arrive at the target vessel based on the initial timing bolus. Modifications need to be made, depending upon the three-dimensional sequence, if it is "center weighted k-space" or "front-loaded k-space."

2. Time resolved (dynamic) three-dimensional gadolinium imaging (Fig. 1.24) is similar to the static version mentioned above, however, multiple three-dimensional data sets are obtained in an extremely short period of time (at times, it can be subsecond). These three-dimensional data sets are acquired continuously and the bolus of gadolinium is followed through the cardiovascular system. This can be performed successfully with parallel imaging (multiple coils used), strong gradients and slew rates, and advanced software and

sequences. Each phase of the acquisition can be made into a high resolution (1 mm or less isotropic voxels) three-dimensional image. This approach can be used to image physiology (view shunt flow or small connections) as well as determining lung perfusion (e.g. regions of lung with higher flows will be much brighter than regions of lung with low flow or no flow such as with pulmonary embolism).

In either technique, it is recommended, as best as possible, to acquire isotropic voxels (voxels with the same dimensions in all three directions). When acquiring the data in this manner, the three-dimensional image can be manipulated and resliced in any plane and the resulting image would appear as if it was acquired in that orientation. In neonates and infants where smaller spatial resolution is needed, isotropic voxels are also very important but signal to noise takes on a very important role; as long as the voxel sizes are small, the field of view can remain high (i.e. by keeping the matrix high) and signal to noise will be preserved.

7. **Viability (Delayed Enhancement) (Figs.** 1.7 **and** 1.10) [34, 39, 40]: It is generally believed that infarcted myocardium is less of an issue in congenital heart disease than

it is in adults and there is some truth to this; nevertheless, many lesions in pediatric cardiology, either in the native state or post operatively, are at risk for myocardial necrosis. Diseases as anomalous left coronary artery from the pulmonary artery (native state) or repaired tetralogy of Fallot or single ventricles (post operative) may manifest myocardial infarction and scarring. CMR viability imaging, also known as delayed enhancement, has shown to be effective in the detection of myocardial scarring and can be applied to the infant through adult with congenital heart disease [41–43]. With viability imaging, intravenous gadolinium chelate, which can freely distribute in extracellular water but cannot cross intact cellular membranes, is delivered to the myocardium and accumulates in areas of fibrosis due to increased volume of distribution and slower washout kinetics [44]. This imaging technique distinguishes areas of myocardial scarring with high signal intensity in comparison to viable myocardium.

As examples, many studies have used delayed enhancement to correlate myocardial scarring with heart function and clinical outcome in different diseases. Babu-Narayan et al. correlated delayed enhancement in transposition of the great arteries patients after surgical repair with age, length of time after surgery, higher right ventricle end-systolic volume index and lower RV ejection fraction [45]. Babu-Narayan et al. also showed correlation of scarring with increased QRS duration, QT dispersion, and JT dispersion from ECG exams as well as a significantly higher occurrence of arrhythmia/syncope. Myocardial scarring has also been investigated in tetralogy of Fallot patients after repair [46, 47]. RV delayed enhancement was shown to correlate with decreased exercise tolerance, increased RV indexed end systolic volume, decreased RV ejection fraction, and more documented clinical arrhythmia. Left ventricular delayed enhancement correlated with more arrhythmia, shorter exercise duration, increased LV indexed end-diastolic and end-systolic volume, and decreased LV ejection fraction. Regions of myocardial delayed enhancement have also been known to occur in patients with hypertrophic cardiomyopathy [48, 49] and the extent of delayed enhancement has been associated with clinical markers of sudden death risk and progression to heart failure [50]. Finally, delayed enhancement has found use in many other applications such as a component in characterizing cardiac tumors, in the diagnosis of myocarditis, in arrhythmogenic right ventricular dysplasia, and in infiltrative cardiomyopathy to name a few.

Regions of irreversible myocardial injury will exhibit high signal intensity on T1 weighted images when administered gadolinium which significantly shortens the longitudinal relaxation time. Although the mechanism by which this occurs is open to debate, it is thought that ruptured cell membranes of myocytes allow the gadolinium to be avidly taken up by the scarred myocardium into the intracellular regions; this results in increased tissue concentration of the contrast agent and hence, an increased signal intensity. In addition, with scar tissue, there is increased interstitial space between collagen fibers, allowing for gadolinium to inculcate itself in these regions and become more concentrated. This is opposed to normally perfused myocardium where the gadolinium is subsequently "washed" out by coronary blood flow. The signal intensity-time curves separate, with the infarcted myocardium gadolinium curve becoming signal intense much before perfused myocardium and remaining highly signal intense after 5–20 min whereas normal myocardium becomes much less so. CMR pulse sequences, first described in the literature in the mid-1980s, have taken advantage of this high concentration and slow washout of contrast agent when attempting to image infarcted myocardium. With segmented inversion recovery fast gradient echo sequences and other techniques such as steady state free precession, signal intensity differences between normal and infarcted myocardium can be as high as 500 %. The technique has been shown to accurately delineate the presence, extent and location of acute and chronic myocardial infarction.

After preliminary scout images and cine sequences are obtained, 0.1–0.2 mmol/kg of intravenous gadolinium is administered. The myocardium is then imaged approximately 5–20 min after this injection; as neonates and children wash out the contrast agent quicker, they are usually imaged on the "sooner side" or if imaged later, have a longer inversion time (TI) (see below). The sequence makes use of a non-selective 180° inversion pulse which spoils all the spins in the myocardium (black on the image) and gives it T1 weighting. The magnetization of tissue goes from +1 to −1 by this process. As both the myocardial and scar tissue begin to recover their spins (enabling the myocardial and scar tissue to "give off" signal), because scar tissue shortens the T1, it recovers signal much quicker than normal myocardium. A time delay is placed after the 180° inversion pulse (TI) to image the ventricle at just the point where the normal myocardium is about to regain signal again (and because the scar tissue recovers spins much quicker, can give off signal). That is to say that the TI is chosen between the non-selective 180° pulse and the center of k-space of the sequence so that the magnetization of normal myocardium is near the zero line (i.e. normal myocardium is dark on the image). This allows for maximizing the difference in signal intensity between scared and normal myocardium, the ventricle is imaged in mid-late diastole. TI time can be manually changed as the acquisition time continues. Collections of lines of k-space generally occurs every other heartbeat.

There are a number of recent advances that have further refined the ability of CMR delayed enhancement to detect myocardial fibrosis. Some manufacturers have implemented three-dimensional volumes slabs to allow for thinner slices. Steady state free precession imaging can be used as opposed to gradient echo imaging to decrease the time needed for image acquisition. In addition, "single shot" techniques are available (as opposed to segmented versions) to obtain an entire slice in one heartbeat, further allowing for increased coverage of the myocardium in one breathhold.

Further advances have relied on refining the correct TI time which, as can be surmised, is a critical component to the whole procedure; as mentioned, it is chosen to optimally "null" the myocardium (i.e. the time at which normal myocardium crosses the "zero" point of signal intensity) where the difference between signal intensity between normal and infarcted tissue is maximized. With a TI time that is too short, the normal myocardium will be below the zero point which will cause two issues (a) differences between signal intensities of infracted and normal myocardium will not be maximized and (b) as the image intensity is a function of the magnitude of the magnetization vector, normal myocardium may become hyperenhanced and scar tissue become nulled if the TI is shortened enough. On the other hand, if the TI time is too long, the normal myocardium will be shades of gray with the scar tissue having high signal as well; as one can see, the contrast between the two tissues will be reduced. Finally, as mentioned already, as gadolinium concentration decreases from the myocardium as time progresses, the TI will have to be adjusted upwards the longer the time after injection.

To make better choices of TI times, two advances have improved the process: (1) "TI scouts" have been developed which obtain images at various increments of TI. The imager can choose the TI based on this scout as to image which appears optimal. (2) A phase sensitive inversion recovery approach can be used which provides consistent contrast between normal and scarred tissue over a wide range of TIs. This "auto viability" technique maintains signal polarity; the inversion recovery preparation pulse and phase reference acquisition are interleaved requiring two heart beats.

There are few pitfalls with viability imaging. In patients who cannot hold their breath or with arrhythmias, using certain viability sequences, image quality can be degraded. This may be overcome by utilizing the "single shot" techniques and navigator sequences. In addition, ghosting artifacts can occur from tissue which have long T1 values, such as pericardial effusion.

Other sections of the CMR protocol: There are a number of other techniques in CMR that are not infrequently used but do not fit into the generalized protocol. They should be inserted at appropriate points in the protocol.

- *Coronary artery imaging (Fig. 1.6) [51, 52]*: For CMR to be implemented successfully to image the coronary arteries, two main technical challenges needed to be overcome; that of cardiac motion and respiratory motion. The magnitude of both motions greatly exceed coronary artery diameters and in the absence of motion suppression algorithms, would cause blurring and possibly missing the coronary arteries all together. There are multiple other challenges as well but these two present the most complex ones. Various techniques have been used in the past to overcome these motion related problems and a history of how modern coronary imaging is performed by CMR is beyond the scope of this chapter; suffice it to note that it has been a long road to the present day high quality, high resolution imaging of the coronary arteries.

  To compensate for coronary motion, high quality ECG or vector gating is required; peripheral pulse gating would not be adequate. In addition, if arrhythmias were present and "arrhythmia rejection" algorithms not used, image degradation will be present. In either case, cardiac motion is compensated for by imaging during the "quiescent phase" of the cardiac cycle which is generally mid to late diastole. This is advantageous as well in that this is the phase where the coronaries are most filled with blood. To determine the "quiescent phase" of the cardiac cycle, it has been our practice to perform a four-chamber view and left ventricular outflow tract high temporal resolution cine (30–60 phases depending upon the heart rate), focusing on the atrioventricular groove and aortic annular motion respectively. When both of these regions of the heart remain motionless (usually mid diastole) is considered the beginning of the "quiescent phase." In addition, the length of the "quiescent phase" is measured in both views as well and is timed only as both structures remain motionless; this is helpful in determining how long the "shot time" for each heartbeat is (i.e. the amount of time it takes to acquire the lines of k-space).

  To compensate for respiratory motion, a number of approaches have been used in the past including breathholding, chest wall bellows, etc, however, in the current era, the state of the art is utilizing navigator pulses. A navigator is used to track motion of a structure and in this particular instance, is used to determine respiratory motion. Most navigators in use today for coronary imaging track the right dome of the diaphragm, however, the left hemidiaphragm and the anterior chest wall have also been used. Lines of k-space accepted into image reconstruction is only those that occur when the diaphragm is within certain defined boundaries (i.e. within 2 mm of the end – expiratory position of the diaphragm). Efficiency is the amount of lines of k-space accepted divided by the total lines of k-space. The overwhelming effect of respiration on cardiac motion is in the supero-inferior dimension and at end-expiration, the ratio between cardiac and diaphragmatic displacement ranges from 0.6 to 0.7 and this "tracking factor" is used to shift slice position coordinates.

Finally, two other major pre-pulses are used to suppress the signal from surrounding tissue. As fat has a relatively short T1, a frequency selective fat prepulse can be used to saturate the signal from fat surrounding the coronaries. Because the coronaries also course near the epimyocardium, cardiac muscle needs to be suppressed as well. Unfortunately, blood and myocardium have similar T1 relaxation properties; however, their T2 relaxation differs significantly. T2 preparation pulses are used to enhance the contrast between the blood of the coronaries and the myocardium (it also suppresses deoxygenated venous blood); Magnetization transfer contrast is used to image coronary veins.

Uses in congenital heart disease fall into three basic categories: (a) anomalous coronary artery imaging such as anomalous left coronary artery from the pulmonary artery or anomalous coronary arteries from the opposite sinus, (b) patient who have had coronary manipulation surgically such as transposition of the great arteries after arterial switch or the Ross procedure and (c) acquired coronary artery disease such as Kawasaki's disease or with familial hypercholesterolemia.

Perfusion Imaging (Fig. 1.9): Perfusion imaging of the myocardium with CMR using contrast has the advantage of no radiation, increased spatial resolution (compared to nuclear techniques) and provides functional information. Essentially, the concept of myocardial perfusion imaging is simply the relative changes in myocardial signal intensity are assessed during a bolus administration of gadolinium contrast agent under both pharmacological stress (typically either adenosine or much less commonly in pediatrics, dipyridamole) and at rest. The contrast agent causes increased myocardial signal intensity in proportion to the amount of contrast agent passing through each region of myocardium which is in turn, proportional to the amount of coronary blood flow. Normally perfused myocardium will have a more rapid and intense signal increase under pharmacologic stress as compared with rest, while areas supplied by coronary arteries with flow-limiting stenosis will have slower and less intense rise in signal intensity under stress conditions.

Myocardial perfusion imaging is generally performed as a T1-weighted, segmented gradient-echo or steady-state free-precession implementation. T1-weighting is improved by a preparatory radiofrequency pulse at the beginning of the sequence; inversion recovery preparation has been utilized and provides the greatest contrast

between normal and abnormal myocardium, however, because it is sensitive to arrhythmias a saturation recovery preparatory pulse is now generally utilized that renders the magnetization insensitive to arrhythmias, and allowing quantitative assessment of results. In general, a stack of 3–6 short axis slices and, if possible, four-chamber and long axis views of the ventricle (depending upon the disease and parameters chosen) are acquired under pharmacologic stress and then, approximately 15–20 min later, repeated at rest which is finally followed by delayed enhancement (see above) 10 min afterwards. Images are obtained every beat or every other beat, depending on the sequence.

Analysis of the images depend upon the relative changes in signal intensity (either qualitative or semi-quantitative) to assess for ischemia. Qualitatively, the assessment is performed as a cine and visual analysis is performed of the relative signal intensity in regions of myocardium; a reduced rate of increase in signal intensity or an absolute decrease in signal intensity relative to normal myocardium is abnormal. This can be either because of (a) hypoperfusion, (b) infarction or (c) artifact. To determine the difference between these, stress and rest perfusion images are combined with delayed enhancement imaging. If the region of abnormal signal intensity corresponds to infarcted regions of the ventricle, then the reason for abnormal signal intensity is obvious. If it does not, then hypoperfusion and ischemia is the reason if the stress images show the defect and the rest images do not. It is most likely artifact if the both rest and stress images show the defect (but not always) and there is a typical artifact pattern (susceptibility artifact, Gibbs ringing or excessive motion of the heart). The visual analysis is simple, relatively fast, and has comparable sensitivity and specificity to nuclear techniques. Semi-quantitative and quantitative approaches are more time-consuming which make it less suitable for routine use, however, it is used in some centers and in some studies, improved the accuracy over visual analysis.

Perfusion CMR has been investigated since 1990, however, because of software and hardware advances, has gained the greatest clinical use since ~2000. Since that time, there have been numerous single center studies demonstrating its clinical utility and accuracy. There is limited data in the literature, unfortunately, on patients with congenital heart disease, however, alternatives such as nuclear imaging and cardiac catheterization expose children to radiation; using CMR myocardial perfusion imaging for some of these applications has obvious potential benefits. Potential applications in congenital heart disease include patients who have had coronary artery manipulation (e.g. transposition of the great arteries after arterial switch procedure or patients after the Ross procedure), anomalous coronary arteries, assessment of cardiac tumors and Kawasaski's disease.

- **Myocardial tissue tagging** (*Figs.* 1.11 *and* 1.12) [53–56]: One relatively unique capability of CMR is the ability to purposely magnetically tag tissue, whether it be myocardium or blood. A cine CMR, typically a gradient echo sequence, is modified by numerous prepulses which, by design, destroys all the spins in a given plane resulting in a linear signal void. In Spatial Modulation of Magnetization (or SPAMM for short), there are multiple radiofrequency pulses of 130° separated in time and a series of gradient radiofrequency pulses which produce saturated spins (the hydrogen atoms become incapable of producing a signal) in two sets of parallel lines perpendicular to each other. By applying standard gradient echo cine CMR afterwards, a grid pattern is created which divides the wall into "cubes of magnetization." This is the equivalent of "speckle tracking" in echocardiography where in CMR, the myocardial tissue tagging is creating the speckles. The translation, rotation and deformation of the "cubes of magnetization" can be tracked to assess wall strain, motion and regional wall thickening in both two- and three-dimensions in either systole or diastole. High temporal resolution tagging can be performed, if needed, by interleaving multiple sets of images with trigger delays. This is needed because there is tag degradation and progressive image blurring as the number of acquired images increases, with this degradation apparent in the later images. In practice, however, this high temporal resolution is rarely necessary as 6–7 images in systole or diastole is sufficient to track the motion and deformation with little tag degradation. With 3-T systems, stripe persistence is much greater than with 1.5 T scanners and stripes may persist without degradation throughout the cardiac cycle. Myocardial tissue tagging can be visualized qualitatively to assess subtleties of regional wall motion abnormalities. Strain and wall motion can be assessed using this technique in two ways:

(A) Tracking the grid intersections on the magnitude images: The magnetically tagged grid intersections on all phases are tracked manually or semi-automatically. A triangular grid is created for each image and finite strain analysis on the deforming triangles is applied [57–59]. In addition, the center of each triangle can be used to calculate regional wall motion (linear as well as rotational movements) in relation to any point in space, which is usually the center of mass of the ventricular cavity. Wall twist (using angles), radial wall motion or wall thickening or thinning can be measured. Software to perform this analysis is still not readily available and is generally used only in specialized centers.

(B) Analysis in K-space: By analyzing the tagged images in k-space rather than as a magnitude image, a more rapid evaluation of the images can be performed. Researchers have developed HARP (Harmonic Phase imaging) [60], which, simplistically, takes the raw spectral peaks of k-space in the tagged images. When a single peak is isolated, the inverse Fourier transform can create a HARP image, which has imaginary and real components to it. Through analysis of these HARP images, ventricular strain and wall motion can be measured [61, 62].

By laying down one set of parallel lines rather than two, "one dimensional" tagging can be performed [63]. Some investigators have utilized this type of tagging for strain measurements and have obtained excellent results, similar to the SPAMM technique (Fig. 1.3). This type of tagging, however, has found great utility in labeling relatively thin structures, such as the right ventricular free wall with subsequent analysis of regional myocardial shortening both qualitatively as well as quantitatively. The parallel set of tags need to be laid down perpendicular to the direction of myocardial motion (e.g. in the four-chamber view of the ventricle, the tags are laid down perpendicular to the long axis of the ventricle). For quantification, the distance between the signal poor areas of the tag are measured at end-diastole and end-systole, and a regional shortening fraction is obtained.

T2* for myocardial iron assessment: By the analysis of T2* in patients who may have iron overload (thalessemia, sickle cell disease, etc), the amount of myocardial iron present can be measured. In brief, the sequence obtains multiple images of the same short axis slice at various echo times utilizing a gradient echo sequence. With longer TEs, the myocardium and liver become increasingly dark. Because iron is ferromagnetic, the magnetic properties of the myocardium and liver change with increasing iron concentration, decreasing the measured T2* (which makes the myocardium even darker) relative to normal myocardium. Values <20 ms are considered at risk for decreased ventricular function. Chelation therapy is generally modified in these patients using this information.

A couple of protocols for specific disease states are worth mentioning that use the techniques noted above.

Tumor/Mass characterization (Figs. 1.8, 1.9, and 1.10): Characterization of tumors and masses on CMR are very useful as a high likelihood of what the mass is can be obtained. Many cardiac tumors and masses can be differentiated from each other by their tissue characteristics as well as their location, symptoms and the patient's age. For example, a lipoma will be signal intense on T_1 weighted images and become signal poor after fat saturation. A hemangioma will become signal intense during perfusion imaging and may be indistinguishable from the ventricular cavity on the image which is one of its characteristics. Tumor characterization by CMR include T_1 and T_2 weighted images, images with fat saturation, gradient echo imaging, perfusion (e.g. for hemangiomas), delayed enhancement imaging, T_1 weighted images after gadolinium administration and myocardial tagging. If time permits, functional imaging can be used to assess for effects of the tumor such as obstruction to flow and decreased cardiac output.

Arrhythmogenic right ventricular dysplasia: With fatty or fibrofatty replacement of myocardium, mostly of the right ventricle, arrhythmias can generally result (e.g. left bundle branch block tachycardia). In its severest form, the right ventricle can become dilated and function poorly with dyskinetic wall regions. In addition, there can be right ventricular conduction delay on ECG, inverted T waves and Epsilon waves. As imaging is only one of multiple criteria in the 1994 Task Force manuscript, it cannot be utilized in and of itself to make a diagnosis but must be combined with other criteria. There are criteria for arrhythmogenic right ventricular dysplasia in adults and has been utilized successfully, however, when applied to the pediatric population, there is a question to how useful it truly is. The CMR criteria in adults with arrhythmogenic right ventricular dysplasia vary from study to study but in general, there is (1) fatty substitution of the myocardium, (2) ectasia of the RVOT, (3) dyskinetic bulges or dyskinesia of RV wall motion, (4) a dilated RV, (5) a dilated RA, (6) fixed RV wall thinning with decreased RV wall thickening. The protocol includes T_1 weighted imaging, cine for ventricular function, one-dimensional right ventricular myocardial tagging if needed to assess regional wall motion, phase encoded velocity mapping and DE which has recently shown to be helpful. Interestingly, when looking at the 1994 Task Force Criteria for arrhythmogenic right ventricular dysplasia, evidence of fatty substitution of the myocardium by CMR is not one of the criteria; this must be done by biopsy.

Techniques which will not be discussed in this chapter but the reader should be aware of are:
- XMR – the combination of CMR and cardiac catheterization
- Interventional CMR – performing intervention in the CMR suite
- Exercise CMR – utilizing a "CMR-friendly" exercise bicycle or other technique to obtain ventricular function and flow parameters during exercise.
- Fetal CMR – utilizing CMR for evaluation of the heart in-utero
- Details of CMR at 3T as applied to pediatrics and congenital heart disease.
- Four dimensional phase encoded velocity mapping (Fig. 1.26)

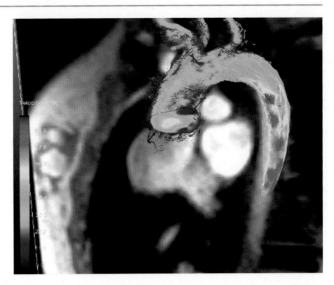

Fig. 1.26 Four-dimensional flow in the candy cane view of the normal aorta by utilizing a stack of three-dimensional phase encoded velocity maps. Color code of the velocity is in the _lower left_ of the image

References

1. Ridgway JP. Cardiovascular magnetic resonance physics for clinicians: part I. J Cardiovasc Magn Reson. 2010;12(1):71.
2. Simonetti OP, Finn JP, White RD, Laub G, Henry DA. "Black blood" T2-weighted inversion-recovery MR imaging of the heart. Radiology. 1996;199:49–57.
3. Carr JC, Simonetti OP, Bundy JM, Li D, Pereles S, Finn JP. Cine MR angiography of the heart with segmented true fast imaging with steady-state precession. Radiology. 2001;219:828–34.
4. Shankaranarayanan A, Simonetti OP, Laub G, Lewin JS, Duerk JL. Segmented k-space and real-time cardiac cine MR imaging with radial trajectories. Radiology. 2001;221:827–36.
5. Atkinson DJ, Edelman RR. Cineangiography of the heart in a single breath hold with a segmented turboFLASH sequence. Radiology. 1991;178:357–60.
6. Pruessmann KP, Weiger M, Scheidegger MB, Boesiger P. SENSE: sensitivity encoding for fast MRI. Magn Reson Med. 1999;42:952–62.
7. Kellman P, Epstein FH, McVeigh ER. Adaptive sensitivity encoding incorporating temporal filtering (TSENSE). Magn Reson Med. 2001;45:846–52.
8. Malviya S, Voepel-Lewis T, Eldevik OP, Rockwell DT, Wong JH, Tait AR. Sedation and general anaesthesia in children undergoing MRI and CT: adverse events and outcomes. Br J Anaesth. 2000;84:743–8.
9. Fogel MA, Weinberg P, Parave E, Harris C, Montenegro L, Concepcion M. Safety and efficacy of deep sedation in infants, children and adolescents undergoing cardiac magnetic resonance. J Pediatr. 2008;152:534–9.
10. Malviya S, Voepel-Lewis T, Tait AR. Adverse events and risk factors associated with the sedation of children by nonanesthesiologists. Anesth Analg. 1997;85:1207–13.
11. Bluemke DA, Breiter SN. Sedation procedures in MR imaging: safety, effectiveness, and nursing effect on examinations. Radiology. 2000;216:645–52.
12. Shepherd JK, Hall-Craggs MA, Finn JP, Bingham RM. Sedation in children scanned with high-field magnetic resonance: experience at the Hospital for Sick Children, Great Ormond Street. Br J Radiol. 1990;63:794–7.

13. Vade A, Sukhani R, Dolenga M, Habisohn-Schuck C. Choral hydrate sedation of children undergoing CT and MR imaging: safety as judged by American Academy of Pediatrics guidelines. Am J Roentgenol. 1995;165:905–9.

14. Volle E, Park W, Kaufmann HJ. MRI examination and monitoring of pediatric patients under sedation. Pediatr Radiol. 1996;26:280–1.

15. Lawson GR. Sedation of children for magnetic resonance imaging. Arch Dis Child. 2000;82:150–4.

16. Didier D, Ratib O, Beghetti M, et al. Morphologic and functional evaluation of congenital heart disease by magnetic resonance imaging. J Magn Reson Imaging. 1999;10:639–55.

17. Fogel MA, Harris M, Harris C. Ultrafast cardiac magnetic resonance imaging of infants <6 months of age without sedation or cardiac anesthesia in <5 minutes: competition for computerized tomography? J Am Coll Cardiol. 2008;51(No 10, suppl A):A86–7 (abstract 1011–117).

18. Nayak KS, Hargreaves BA, Hu BS, Nishimura DG, Pauly JM, Meyer CH. Spiral balanced steady-state free precession cardiac imaging. Magn Reson Med. 2005;53:1468–73.

19. Scheffler K, Lehnhardt S. Principles and applications of balanced SSFP techniques. Eur Radiol. 2003;13:2409–18.

20. Lorenz CH, Walker ES, Morgan VL, Klein SS, Graham Jr TP. Normal human right and left ventricular mass, systolic function, and gender differences by cine magnetic resonance imaging. J Cardiovasc Magn Reson. 1999;1:7–21.

21. Marcus JT, DeWaal LK, Götte MJ, van der Geest RJ, Heethaar RM, Van Rossum AC. MRI-derived left ventricular function parameters and mass in healthy young adults: relation with gender and body size. Int J Card Imaging. 1999;15:411–9.

22. Sandstede J, Lipke C, Beer M, Hofmann S, Pabst T, Kenn W, Neubauer S, Hahn D. Age- and gender-specific differences in left and right ventricular cardiac function and mass determined by cine magnetic resonance imaging. Eur Radiol. 2000;10:438–42.

23. Mostbeck GH, Caputo GR, Higgins CB. MR measurement of blood flow in the cardiovascular system. AJR Am J Roentgenol. 1992;159:453–61.

24. Chatzimavroudis GP, Oshinski JN, Franch RH, Walker PG, Yoganathan AP, Pettigrew RI. Evaluation of the precision of magnetic resonance phase velocity mapping for blood flow measurements. J Cardiovasc Magn Reson. 2001;3:11–9.

25. Brenner LD, Caputo GR, Mostbeck G, et al. Quantification of left-to-right atrial shunts with velocity-encoded cine nuclear magnetic resonance imaging. J Am Coll Cardiol. 1992;20:1246–50.

26. Rebergen SA, Niezen RA, Helbing WA, et al. Cine gradient-echo MR imaging and MR velocity mapping in the evaluation of congenital heart disease. Radiographics. 1996;16:467–81.

27. John AS, Dill T, Brandt RR, Rau M, Ricken W, Bachmann G, Hamm CW. Magnetic resonance to assess the aortic valve area in aortic stenosis: how does it compare to current diagnostic standards? J Am Coll Cardiol. 2003;42:519–26.

28. Schlosser T, Malyar N, Jochims M, Breuckmann F, Hunold P, Bruder O, Erbel R, Barkhausen J. Quantification of aortic valve stenosis in MRI-comparison of steady-state free precession and fast low-angle shot sequences. Eur Radiol. 2007;17:1284–90.

29. Westenberg JJ, Roes SD, Ajmone Marsan N, Binnendijk NM, Doornbos J, Bax JJ, Reiber JH, de Roos A, van der Geest RJ. Mitral valve and tricuspid valve blood flow: accurate quantification with 3D velocity-encoded MR imaging with retrospective valve tracking. Radiology. 2008;249:792–800.

30. Firmin DN, Nayler GL, Klipstein RH, Underwood SR, Rees RS, Longmore DB. In vivo validation of MR velocity imaging. J Comput Assist Tomogr. 1987;11:751–6.

31. Caputo GR, Kondo C, Masui T, Geraci SJ, Foster E, O'Sullivan MM, Higgins CB. Right and left lung perfusion: *in vitro* and *in vivo* validation with oblique-angle, velocity-encoded cine MR imaging. Radiology. 1991;180:693–8.

32. Rebergen SA, Chin JGJ, Ottenkamp J, van der Wall EE, de Roos A. Pulmonary regurgitation in the late postoperative follow-up of tetralogy of Fallot: volumetric quantification by MR velocity mapping. Circulation. 1993;88:2257–66.

33. Beerbaum P, Korperich H, Barth P, et al. Non-invasive quantification of left-to-right shunt in pediatric patients. Phase-contrast cine magnetic resonance imaging compared with invasive oximetry. Circulation. 2001;103:2476–82.

34. Harris MA, Weinberg PM, Whitehead KK, Fogel MA. Usefulness of branch pulmonary artery regurgitant fraction to estimate the relative right and left pulmonary vascular resistances in congenital heart disease. Am J Cardiol. 2005;95:1514–7.

35. Steffens JC, Bourne MW, Sakuma H, O'Sullivan M, Higgins CB. Quantification of collateral blood flow in coarctation of the aorta by velocity encoded cine magnetic resonance imaging. Circulation. 1994;90(2):937–43.

36. Whitehead KK, Gillespie MJ, Harris MA, Fogel MA, Rome JJ. Noninvasive quantification of systemic to pulmonary collateral flow: a major source of inefficiency in patients with superior cavopulmonary connections. Circ Cardiovasc Imaging. 2009;2:405–11. Epub 2009 Jul 8. 2009.

37. Tzemos N, Therrien J, Yip J, Thanassoulis G, Tremblay S, Jamorski MT, Webb GD, Siu SC. Outcomes in adults with bicuspid aortic valves. JAMA. 2008;300:1317–25.

38. Gleeson TG, Mwangi I, Horgan SJ, Cradock A, Fitzpatrick P, Murray JG. Steady-state free-precession (SSFP) cine MRI in distinguishing normal and bicuspid aortic valves. J Magn Reson Imaging. 2008;28:873–8.

39. Thomson LE, Kim RJ, Judd RM. Magnetic resonance imaging for the assessment of myocardial viability. J Magn Reson Imaging. 2004;19:771–88.

40. Kwong RY, Korlakunta H. Diagnostic and prognostic value of cardiac magnetic resonance imaging in assessing myocardial viability. Top Magn Reson Imaging. 2008;19:15–24.

41. Kim RJ, Wu E, Rafael A, et al. The use of contrast-enhanced magnetic resonance imaging to identify reversible myocardial dysfunction. N Engl J Med. 2000;343:1445–53.

42. Wu E, Judd RM, Vargas JD, Klocke FJ, Bonow RO, Kim RJ. Visualisation of presence, location, and transmural extent of healed Q-wave and non-Q-wave myocardial infarction. Lancet. 2001;357:21–8.

43. Simonetti OP, Kim RJ, Fieno DS, et al. An improved MR imaging technique for the visualization of myocardial infarction. Radiology. 2001;218:215–23.

44. Moon JC, Reed E, Sheppard MN, et al. The histologic basis of late gadolinium enhancement cardiovascular magnetic resonance in hypertrophic cardiomyopathy. J Am Coll Cardiol. 2004;43:2260–4.

45. Babu-Narayan SV, Goktekin O, Moon JC, et al. Late gadolinium enhancement cardiovascular magnetic resonance of the systemic right ventricle in adults with previous atrial redirection surgery for transposition of the great arteries. Circulation. 2005;111:2091–8.

46. Babu-Narayan SV, Kilner PJ, Li W, et al. Ventricular fibrosis suggested by cardiovascular magnetic resonance in adults with repaired tetralogy of fallot and its relationship to adverse markers of clinical outcome. Circulation. 2006;113:405–13.

47. Wald RM, Haber I, Wald R, Valente AM, Powell AJ, Geva T. Effects of regional dysfunction and late gadolinium enhancement on global right ventricular function and exercise capacity in patients with repaired tetralogy of Fallot. Circulation. 2009;119:1370–7.

48. Choudhury L, Mahrholdt G, Wagner A, et al. Myocardial scarring in asymptomatic or mildly symptomatic patients with hypertrophic cardiomyopathy. J Am Coll Cardiol. 2002;40:2156–64.

49. Teraoka K, Hirano M, Ookubo H, et al. Delayed contrast enhancement of MRI in hypertrophic cardiomyopathy. Magn Reson Imaging. 2004;22:155–61.

50. Moon J, McKenna W, McCrohon JA, Elliott PM, Smith GC, Pennell DJ. Toward clinical risk assessment in hypertrophic cardiomyopathy with gadolinium cardiovascular magnetic resonance. J Am Coll Cardiol. 2003;41:1561–7.

51. Danias PG, Stuber M, Botnar RM, Kissinger KV, Edelman RR, Manning WJ. Relationship between motion of coronary arteries and diaphragm during free breathing: lessons from real-time MR imaging. AJR Am J Roentgenol. 1999;172:1061–5.

52. Oncel D, Oncel G, Türko lu I. Accuracy of MR coronary angiography in the evaluation of coronary artery stenosis. Diagn Interv Radiol. 2008;14:153–8.

53. Donofrio MT, Clark BJ, Ramaciotti C, Jacobs ML, Fellows KE, Weinberg PM, Fogel MA. Regional wall motion and strain of transplanted hearts in pediatric patients using magnetic resonance tagging. Am J Physiol. 1999;277:R1481–7.

54. Fogel MA, Gupta K, Baxter MS, Weinberg PM, Haselgrove J, Hoffman EA. Biomechanics of the deconditioned left ventricle. Am J Physiol. 1996;40:H1193–206.

55. Fogel MA, Gupta KB, Weinberg PW, Hoffman EA. Regional wall motion and strain analysis across stages of Fontan reconstruction by magnetic resonance tagging. Am J Physiol. 1995;38:H1132–52.

56. Fogel MA, Weinberg PM, Fellows KE, Hoffman EA. A study in ventricular – ventricular interaction: single right ventricles compared with systemic right ventricles in a dual chambered circulation. Circulation. 1995;92:219–30.

57. Beyer R, Sideman S. A computer study of left ventricular performance based on fiber structure, sarcomere dynamics, and transmural electrical propagation velocity. Circ Res. 1984;55:358–75.

58. Young AA, Axel L, Dougherty L, et al. Validation of tagging with MR imaging to estimate material deformation. Radiology. 1993;188:101–8.

59. Waldman LK, Fung YC, Covell JW. Transmural myocardial deformation in the canine left ventricle. Circ Res. 1985;57:152–63.

60. Garot J, Bluemke DA, Osman NF, Rochitte CE, McVeigh ER, Zerhouni EA, Prince JL, Lima JAC. Fast determination of regional myocardial strain fields from tagged cardiac images using harmonic phase MRI. Circulation. 2000;101:981–8.

61. Osman NF, Prince JL. Regenerating MR tagged images using harmonic phase (HARP) methods. IEEE Trans Biomed Eng. 2004;51:1428–33.

62. Osman NF, Prince JL. Visualizing myocardial function using HARP MRI. Phys Med Biol. 2000;45:1665–82.

63. Menteer J, Weinberg PM, Fogel MA. Quantifying regional right ventricular function in tetralogy of Fallot. J Cardiovasc Magn Reson. 2005;7:753–61.

Roger Luechinger

2.1 Introduction

Magnetic resonance imaging (MRI) is a safe diagnostic tool and over 600 million diagnostic studies have been performed safely up to now. However, there have been at least 15 published cases of patient deaths associated with MRI scanning; 10 cases with implanted pacemakers [1–5], 2 patients with an insulin pump [3], 1 patient with a neuro-stimulator, 1 patient with an aneurysm clip [6], and 1 child killed by an oxygen tank [7]. Additionally, hundreds of severe burns [8] or injuries due to ferromagnetic projectiles have also been reported. The loud noises (up to 120 dBA) induced by the fast switching gradient fields make ear protections mandatory for all patient. The sources of all these risks are the electromagnetic fields of the MRI scanner.

Medications or contrast agents used during CMR imaging may also pose significant risks. During the last 10 years, over 600 cases of Nephrogenic Systemic Fibrosis (NFS) associated with linear Gadolinium-based contrast media (GBCM) have been reported in patients with severe renal impairment [9].

Besides these known and preventable risks, there are no known short or long-term side effects attributed to the MRI magnetic field strengths currently used in clinical practice. It should be noted that MRI like ultrasound, does not use any ionizing radiation, thus avoiding the risk of carcinogenesis.

2.2 Safety Risks from MRI Scanner

MRI uses three electromagnetic fields to acquire the images. A strong static magnetic field also called $B_0 \sim 30,000$ (1.5 T scanner) to 60,000 (3 T scanner) times the earth magnetic field (0.05 mT), is used to align the spins of the proton of the hydrogen atom. For the spacial localization of the signal, fast switching magnetic fields, so called gradient fields, are used. The non-ionizing radiofrequency (RF) field also called B_1 field is used to excite the hydrogen protons. The frequency of the RF field depends upon the main magnetic field (B_0) and is of the order of those used by common radio waves. However, the used power is much stronger and need to be controlled to avoid any negative effects on the patient.

Each of these three electromagnetic fields may pose safety risk. The risk may significantly increase if implants are present and this applies to any non MR safe device/equipment entering the MR area. Possible interactions are summarized in Table 2.1.

2.3 Force and Torque Effects

Active shielded magnets (the commonly used magnets) have a fast increasing magnetic field. Ferromagnetic materials can be brought close to the magnet without any noticeable force. However, moving them by less than a meter further in the direction of the magnet may induce magnetic forces more than 100× the weight of the device turning ferromagnetic devices into projectiles with speeds of over 50 km/h over a distance of 2–3 m! Therefore, it is absolutely essential that no ferromagnetic devices be moved into the scanner room (Fig. 2.1), preferable not even into the MRI center. Monitoring devices, IV poles etc. have to be tested and labeled as MR safe or MR conditional before use in the MR room.

Some medical devices, like infusion pumps, are only allowed to enter limited magnetic fields. To avoid these devices from becoming projectiles, they should be stored in a special container, preferable with continuous monitoring of the magnetic field strength and acoustic alarm.

Patients have to be very carefully screened to exclude ferromagnetic implants or ferromagnetic foreign bodies. Two cases of fatal accidents associated with magnetic force and torque effects have been reported to date. In 2001, a 6-year-old boy was killed by a projectile ferromagnetic oxygen tank. In 1992 a patient with a ferromagnetic aneurysm clip died

R. Luechinger, Ph.D.
Institute for Biomedical Engineering, University and ETH Zurich,
Raemistrasse 100, Zurich 8091, Switzerland
e-mail: luechinger@biomed.ee.ethz.ch

M.A. Syed, R.H. Mohiaddin (eds.), *Magnetic Resonance Imaging of Congenital Heart Disease*,
DOI 10.1007/978-1-4471-4267-6_2, © Springer-Verlag London 2012

6. Klucznik RP, et al. Placement of a ferromagnetic intracerebral aneurysm clip in a magnetic field with a fatal outcome. Radiology. 1993;187(3):855–6.

7. Boy, 6, Dies of skull injury during M.R.I. The New York Times, 31 July 2001.

8. Hardy 2nd PT, Weil KM. A review of thermal MR injuries. Radiol Technol. 2010;81(6):606–9.

9. ACR. ACR manual on contrast media (Version 8), American College of Radiology, Editor; 2012. Available from: http://www.acr.org/Quality-Safety/Resources/Contrast-Manual. Accessed on 9, 2012).

10. Chakeres DW, et al. Effect of static magnetic field exposure of up to 8 Tesla on sequential human vital sign measurements. J Magn Reson Imaging. 2003;18(3):346–52.

11. Price DL, et al. Investigation of acoustic noise on 15 MRI scanners from 0.2 T to 3 T. J Magn Reson Imaging. 2001;13(2):288–93.

12. Kugel H, et al. Hazardous situation in the MR bore: induction in ECG leads causes fire. Eur Radiol. 2003;13(4):690–4.

13. Patel MR, et al. Acute myocardial infarction: safety of cardiac MR imaging after percutaneous revascularization with stents. Radiology. 2006;240(3):674–80.

14. Shellock FG. Reference manual for magnetic resonance safety, implants, and devices, 2011 edition. Los Angeles: Biomedical Research Publishing Group; 2011.

15. Levine GN, et al. Safety of magnetic resonance imaging in patients with cardiovascular devices: an American heart association scientific statement from the committee on diagnostic and interventional cardiac catheterization, council on clinical cardiology, and the council on cardiovascular radiology and intervention: endorsed by the American college of cardiology foundation, the North American society for cardiac imaging, and the society for cardiovascular magnetic resonance. Circulation. 2007;116(24):2878–91.

16. Wilkoff BL, et al. Magnetic resonance imaging in patients with a pacemaker system designed for the magnetic resonance environment. Heart Rhythm. 2011;8(1):65–73.

17. Sommer T, et al. Strategy for safe performance of extrathoracic magnetic resonance imaging at 1.5 Tesla in the presence of cardiac pacemakers in non-pacemaker-dependent patients: a prospective study with 115 examinations. Circulation. 2006;114(12):1285–92.

18. Shinbane JS, Colletti PM, Shellock FG. MR in patients with pacemakers and ICDs: defining the issues. J Cardiovasc Magn Reson. 2007;9(1):5–13.

19. Naehle CP, et al. Safety, feasibility, and diagnostic value of cardiac magnetic resonance imaging in patients with cardiac pacemakers and implantable cardioverters/defibrillators at 1.5 T. Am Heart J. 2011;161(6):1096–105.

20. Luechinger R. In vivo heating of pacemaker leads during magnetic resonance imaging. Eur Heart J. 2005;26(4):376–83. discussion 325–7.

21. Luechinger R, et al. Safety considerations for magnetic resonance imaging of pacemaker and ICD patients. Herzschr Elektrophys. 2004;15(1):73–81.

22. Roguin A, et al. Magnetic resonance imaging in individuals with cardiovascular implantable electronic devices. Europace. 2008; 10:336–743.

23. Kanal E, et al. ACR guidance document for safe MR practices: 2007. AJR Am J Roentgenol. 2007;188(6):1447–74.

24. Cowper SE, et al. Scleromyxoedema-like cutaneous diseases in renal-dialysis patients. Lancet. 2000;356(9234):1000–1.

25. Grobner T. Gadolinium – a specific trigger for the development of nephrogenic fibrosing dermopathy and nephrogenic systemic fibrosis? Nephrol Dial Transplant. 2006;21(4):1104–8.

26. FDA. FDA drug safety communication: new warnings for using gadolinium-based contrast agents in patients with kidney dysfunction. 2010. Available from: http://www.fda.gov/Drugs/DrugSafety/ucm223966.htm. Accessed on 9, 2012.

27. Wahl A, et al. Safety and feasibility of high-dose dobutamine-atropine stress cardiovascular magnetic resonance for diagnosis of myocardial ischaemia: experience in 1000 consecutive cases. Eur Heart J. 2004;25(14):1230–6.

28. Karamitsos TD, et al. Feasibility and safety of high-dose adenosine perfusion cardiovascular magnetic resonance. J Cardiovasc Magn Reson. 2010;12:66.

29. Kramer CM, et al. Standardized cardiovascular magnetic resonance imaging (CMR) protocols, society for cardiovascular magnetic resonance: board of trustees task force on standardized protocols. J Cardiovasc Magn Reson. 2008;10:35.

Introduction to Congenital Heart Disease Anatomy

3

Pierangelo Renella and J. Paul Finn

3.1 Introduction

Imaging of the complex anatomy associated with many forms of congenital heart disease (CHD) requires knowledge of the morphology of the various cardiac chambers and extra-cardiac vessels. For the cardiac diagnostician, assembling together the pieces of disordered anatomy is best done with the so-called "segmental approach." This approach breaks down the cardiovascular anatomy sequentially, considering first the position of the abdominal viscera, next the cardiac atria, then the looping pattern of the ventricles, and finally, the position of the semilunar valves and great arteries. In this manner, the various forms of CHD may be precisely identified and the proper management applied by the clinician. The large unrestricted field of view, coupled with three-dimensional multiplanar reconstruction and volume rendering capability, as well as the lack of ionizing radiation exposure to the patient, make cardiac magnetic resonance (CMR) the ideal imaging modality for the initial evaluation and serial follow-up of patients with CHD. This holds particularly true for adult and post-operative patients who may have suboptimal echocardiographic imaging windows. This chapter introduces the segmental approach to the diagnosis of CHD. Each "segment" of the cardiovascular system is described with particular attention paid to the distinguishing features of normal structures so that abnormal features may be more clearly identified. Salient examples of pathology in each segment are also presented with their relevant clinical features.

3.2 Viscero-Atrial Anatomy and Morphology

The specific arrangement of the various thoraco-abdominal organs is commonly described as the viscero-atrial "situs." Situs may be classified as solitus (normal arrangement), inversus, or ambiguous (Fig. 3.1) [1]. In viscero-atrial situs "solitus," the abdominal and thoracic organs are arranged in the normal fashion, with the liver on the right side, and the spleen and stomach on the left. In addition, the right-sided lung is trilobed with an eparterial bronchus, while the left-sided lung has two lobes and a hyparterial bronchus. In viscero-atrial situs solitus, the morphologically left atrium is left-sided and posterior of the morphologically right atrium. Conversely, the morphologically right atrium resides rightward and anterior of the morphologically left atrium. Morphologically features of left and right atria are presented in Table 3.1. Situs "inversus" refers to the mirror image of the normal arrangement. The third category, in which elements of both situs solitus and inversus co-exist in the same patient, is termed situs ambiguous (Fig. 3.1). Several different permutations of the thoracic and abdominal organ locations are possible in situs ambiguous, including the presence

P. Renella, M.D. (✉)
Department of Radiology Sciences,
David Geffen School of Medicine, Ronald Reagan
UCLA Medical Center, Los Angeles, CA, USA

Department of Pediatric Cardiology, UC-Irvine College
of Medicine, Children's Hospital Orange County,
200 S. Main Street, Suite 200, Orange, CA 92868, USA

University of California Los Angeles (UCLA),
Peter V. Ueberroth Building, Suite 3371, 10945 Le Conte Avenue,
Los Angeles, CA 90095-7206, USA
e-mail: prenella@mednet.ucla.edu

J.P. Finn, M.D.
Department of Radiology Sciences,
David Geffen School of Medicine, Ronald Reagan
UCLA Medical Center, Los Angeles, CA, USA

University of California Los Angeles (UCLA),
Peter V. Ueberroth Building, Suite 3371, 10945 Le Conte Avenue,
Los Angeles, CA 90095-7206, USA

Department of Radiology, Diagnostic Cardiovascular
Imaging Section, UCLA, Ueberroth Building,
10945 Le Conte Avenue, Los Angeles, CA 90095 USA
e-mail: pfinn@mednet.ucla.edu

Electronic supplementary material
The online version of this chapter (doi:10.1007/978-1-4471-4267-6_3) contains supplementary material, which is available to authorized users.

Fig. 3.1 Types of viscero-atrial situs [40]. Shown are the three types of spatial arrangement of the visceral organs and the cardiac atria. Situs "solitus" is the normal configuration with the stomach and spleen on the left side of the body and the liver on the right. Situs "inversus" is the mirror image of situs solitus. The term situs "ambiguous" is applied when there is ambiguity with respect to the specific sidedness of the organs and the atrial morphology cannot be precisely determined. *RA* right atrium, *LA* left atrium

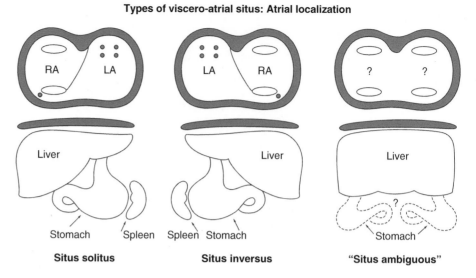

Types of viscero-atrial situs: Atrial localization

Situs solitus   Situs inversus   "Situs ambiguous"

Table 3.1 Morphologically features of the atria

Left atrium	Right atrium
Thin "finger-like" appendage	Broad pyramidal shaped appendage
Smooth wall	Pectinate muscles
Pulmonary venous connections	Crista terminalis
Ostium secundum	Coronary sinus ostium
	Connection of the inferior vena cava
	Connection of the superior vena cava

of two morphologically left or right atria and/or two morphologically left or right bronchi. The liver may be either on the left side or transverse in location. The stomach may be found on either side of the abdominal cavity [2, 3].

3.2.1 Heterotaxy Syndrome

In the heterotaxy syndrome, significant aberrations of thoraco-abdominal organ right-left orientation may be seen (Fig. 3.2). There exist several published definitions of heterotaxy. A unified definition was proposed by The International Nomenclature Committee for Pediatric and Congenital Heart Disease Nomenclature Working Group [3]. According to this definition, heterotaxy is "…an abnormality where the internal thoraco-abdominal organs demonstrate abnormal arrangement across the left-right axis of the body." This definition excludes patients with pure situs inversus and includes all patients with situs ambiguous. Heterotaxy may be associated with either the absence of a spleen (asplenia) or with multiple spleens (polysplenia). Asplenia has also been labelled "bilateral right-sidedness" and polysplenia has been referred to as "bilateral left-sidedness." For example, a patient with heterotaxy and asplenia (i.e. bilateral right-sidedness) may have bilateral morpho-

logically right-sided bronchi and atria, while in heterotaxy with polysplenia, there may be bilateral morphologically left-sided bronchi and atria.

Heterotaxy syndrome is uncommon, occurring in only approximately 1% of patients with congenital heart disease (CHD) [4]. However, when present it is often associated with severe cardiac abnormalities (Table 3.2). The 1-year survival without surgical intervention is poor (<15 % in asplenia and <50 % in polysplenia) [5, 6]. In spite of specialized palliative medical and surgical strategies, approximately one-half of patients will die within 15 years of surgery (usually some time after the Fontan operation) [7].

Transthoracic echocardiography and cardiac catheterization have long been routinely and successfully utilized in patients with heterotaxy syndrome. Cardiac magnetic resonance imaging (CMR) has been also been shown to be of value in this patient population and, in fact, may be superior with respect to the precise characterization of the position of the thoraco-abdominal organs, bronchial anatomy, cardiac chamber morphology, as well as the pulmonary and systemic venous anomalies often encountered [8, 9].

3.3 Veno-Atrial Connections

Two different venous systems connect to the cardiac atria: the *systemic* veins (inferior vena cava, superior vena cava, hepatic veins, coronary sinus) and the *pulmonary* veins (Fig. 3.3). Normally, the systemic veins carry deoxygenated blood to the morphologically right atrium. Conversely, the pulmonary veins normally carry oxygenated blood to the morphologically left atrium. In fact, as already reviewed above, the very connections of the coronary sinus (CS) and inferior vena cava (IVC) to the right atrium help precisely define it as the morphologically right atrium (Table 3.1). Similarly, the

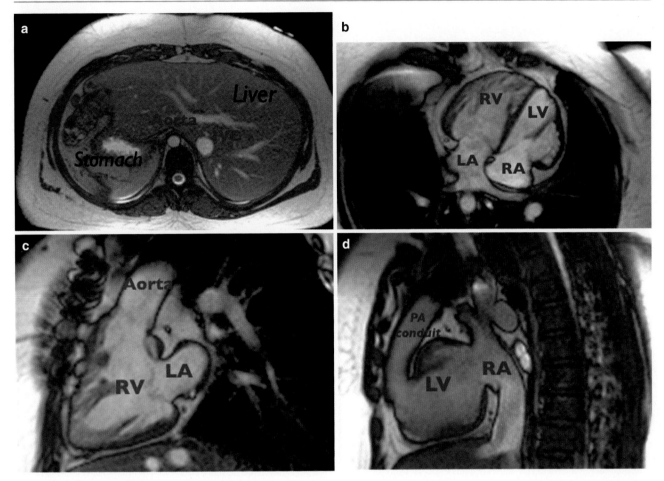

Fig. 3.2 Heterotaxy syndrome with viscero-atrial situs inversus (MR steady state free precession imaging). (**a**) SSFP image in the axial plane through abdomen demonstrating visceral situs "inversus" (left-sided liver and right-sided stomach). Note also that the IVC is on the left and the aorta is on the right. (**b**) SSFP image of atrio-ventricular discordance in a patient with l-loop transposition of the great arteries. In this patient, there is viscero-atrial situs inversus with discordant connections of the atrial to their respective ventricles. (**c**) Same patient as in (**b**) depicting the atrio-ventricular and ventriculo-arterial discordance ("double discordance"). The RV connects to the anteriorly and leftward positioned (l-malposed) aorta. (**d**) Same patient as in (**b**). This patient has undergone surgical LV to PA conduit placement to bypass native sub-pulmonary stenosis. *IVC* inferior vena cava, *LV* left ventricle, *RV* right ventricle, *LA* left atrium, *RA* right atrium, *PA* pulmonary artery

Table 3.2 Cardiac malformations associated with heterotaxy syndrome

Anatomic feature	Asplenia ("bilateral right-sidedness")	Polysplenia ("bilateral left-sidedness")
Liver position	Transverse (76–91 %)	Transverse (50–67 %)
Lung lobes	Bilaterally trilobed (81–93 %)	Bilaterally bilobed (72–88 %)
Bronchial morphology	Bilaterally eparterial (95 %)	Bilaterally hyparterial (68–88 %)
Superior vena cava	Bilateral (46–71 %)	Bilateral (33–50 %)
Inferior vena cava	Interrupted with azygos continuation (rare)	Interrupted with azygos continuation (58–100 %)
Pulmonary veins	Total anomalous connection (64–72 %)	Anomalous drainage (normal connection) due to atrial septal malalignment (37–50)
Atrial morphology	Common atrium (57 %)	Common atrium (25–30 %)
Cardiac crux	AV canal defects (84–92 %)	AV canal defects (80 %)
Ventricles	Functional single ventricle (44–55 %)	Functional single ventricle (37 %)
Cardiac position	Dextrocardia (36–41 %)	Dextrocardia (33–42 %)
Ventriculo-arterial connection	Double outlet right ventricle (82 %); Transposition of the great arteries (9 %)	Double outlet right ventricle (17–37 %)

Adapted from Bartram et al. [4]

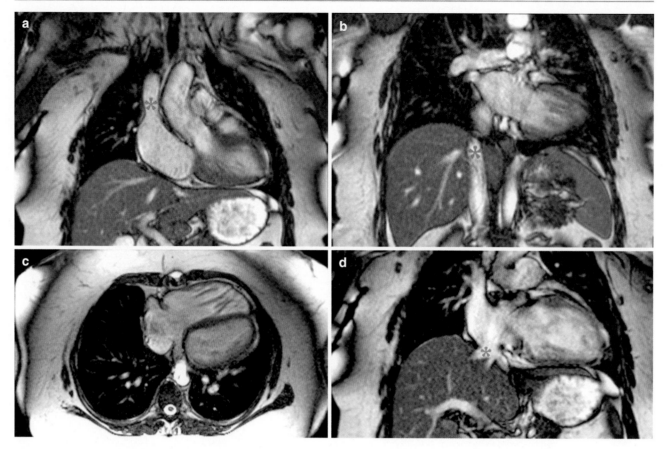

Fig. 3.3 Normal systemic and pulmonary veno-atrial connections. (**a**) The superior vena cava (*SVC*) carries venous drainage from the upper body to the morphologically right atrium (*asterisk*). (**b**) The inferior vena cava (*IVC*) carries lower body venous drainage to the morphologically right atrium (*RA*), and indeed, this IVC connection is one of the defining features of an RA (*asterisk*). (**c**) The coronary sinus (*CS*) ostium is likewise a defining feature of a morphologically RA. It carries the coronary venous blood (*asterisk*). (**d**) The hepatic veins either connect to the IVC and/or directly to the floor of the RA (*asterisk*)

connections of the pulmonary veins to the left atrium are a distinguishing feature of a morphologically left atrium.

3.3.1 Systemic Venous Connections

The superior vena cava (SVC) forms from both brachiocephalic (inominate) veins. There is usually a single right SVC, although it is possible to have a single left SVC (with an absent right SVC) or bilateral SVC's (with or without a bridging vein). The right SVC normally courses anterior to the right pulmonary artery and against the posterolateral aspect of the ascending aorta before connects to the roof of the morphologically right atrium (Fig. 3.3a) [10].

The IVC receives systemic venous drainage from the lower body, including the retroperitoneum, portal circulation, and lower extremities (Fig. 3.3b). After traversing superiorly, it courses within the liver and through the diaphragmatic hiatus to reach the floor of the right atrium [10]. This normally occurs on the right side of the body, but may be on the left or even midline, depending on the atrial situs. In atrial situs inversus, for example, the IVC may connect to a morphologically right atrium located on the left side of midline (Fig. 3.3). The intrahepatic portion of the IVC may be absent (interrupted) as a normal variant or in the heterotaxy syndrome, particularly the polysplenia subtype (as described above). In this case, the IVC blood would continue to the SVC via the azyous vein [11, 12].

The coronary sinus (CS) is the confluence of the majority of the coronary venous drainage and opens normally to the morphologically right atrium (Fig. 3.3c). It may also receive a persistent left superior vena cava (LSVC) or an anomalously connected pulmonary vein or veins. In rare instances, the CS may be "unroofed" and thus open directly into the morphologically left atrium, resulting in a right-to-left shunt. Complete atresia of the CS ostium has also been reported [10].

The hepatic veins typically drain to the IVC directly and/or the floor of the morphologically right atrium (Fig. 3.3d). In the case of an interrupted IVC with azygous continuation, the hepatic veins will connect directly to the floor of the morphologically right atrium. Naturally, when there is viscero-atrial situs inversus the hepatic veins may be found left of midline. If there is situs ambiguous, the hepatic veins may drain in the midline to a common atrium of indeterminate morphology.

3.3.1.1 Total Anomalous Systemic Venous Connection

Very rarely all the systemic veins may connect anomalously to the morphologically left atrium. This is known as total anomalous systemic venous connection. In this lesion, there is usually a single left SVC connecting to an unroofed CS, such that venous drainage from the upper body drains directly to the left atrium. In addition, the IVC is interrupted with continuation via the azygous vein to the left SVC. Finally, the hepatic veins also anomalously connect to the floor of the left atrium. Most often, this occurs in the setting of heterotaxy and complex CHD [11]. In isolation, this defect would be expected to cause profound arterial desaturation and cyanosis. However, arterial saturation may be somewhat improved by a bidirectional atrial level shunt (in the setting of a common atrium, for example). Surgical repair may consist of a intra-atrial baffle constructed to direct the IVC, SVC, and CS flow to the right atrium [11].

3.3.2 Pulmonary Venous Connections

In the normal heart, the venous drainage from the lungs returns via the pulmonary veins to the morphologically left atrium. In the normal configuration, two pulmonary veins (one upper and one lower) from each lung course to the morphologically left atrium. The right upper and lower pulmonary veins course posteriorly to the right atrium and SVC, while the left- upper and lower pulmonary veins course just anterior to the descending thoracic aorta. The right upper pulmonary vein is usually formed by branches from the right upper and right middle lobes of the lung. The right upper and right middle pulmonary veins typically join together prior to connecting to the left atrium. However, as a normal variant, the right middle branch may enter the left atrium separately. In addition, it is not uncommon for the two left-sided pulmonary veins to join the atrium as a single common vein [13]. Of clinical interest, the cardiac end of the pulmonary veins contain myocardial cells rather than smooth muscle cells [13]. This area of the pulmonary veins has been implicated as being part of abnormal electrical circuits which predispose patients to atrial fibrillation. As such, the proximal pulmonary veins are potential targets of transcatheter radiofrequency ablation therapy for atrial fibrillation [14].

During the embryological development of the pulmonary veins, there exist connections between the primitive pulmonary and splanchnic plexi of veins. The persistence of these connections, due to the failure of the common pulmonary vein to connect to the morphologically left atrium, results in anomalous pulmonary venous connections of various types [15]. In the case of total anomalous pulmonary venous connection (TAPVC), all the pulmonary veins retain their embryonic connections to the systemic venous system and do not connect to the morphologically left atrium. These connections may become obstructed and present either at birth or within the first part of infancy with rapid clinical deterioration. In fact, "obstructed TAPVC" is one of the few surgical emergencies in pediatric cardiology. With partial anomalous pulmonary venous connection (PAPVC), at least one, but not all, of the pulmonary veins connect abnormally.

Three general categories of TAPVC are described based on which systemic veins the anomalous pulmonary veins maintain an embryonic connection to (Fig. 3.4). In decreasing order of frequency these are: (1) supracardiac, (2) cardiac, and (3) infradiaphragmatic. When the pulmonary venous connections consist of some combination of these categories, then the designation of "mixed" TAPVC is given. The "mixed" form of TAPVC is the least common, occurring in only 8 % of patients [16]. "Supracardiac" TAPVC occurs in approximately 50 % of the cases and consists of pulmonary venous blood being redirected to usually the inominate vein on its way to the right SVC, or to a left SVC directly [15]. The "cardiac" form of the disease typically involves drainage of the pulmonary veins directly to the coronary sinus. The "infradiaphragmatic" form of TAPVC is described below.

3.3.2.1 Infradiaphragmatic Total Anomalous Pulmonary Venous Connection (TAPVC)

Although a relatively uncommon form of TAPVC, when the connection of the pulmonary venous confluence to the systemic circulation is via an infradiaphragmatic route, the risk of obstruction and subsequent clinical deterioration is relatively high. In infradiaphragmatic TAPVC, the pulmonary venous return courses via a vertical vein running parallel to the aorta, through the diaphragm (at the esophageal hiatus), connects to the portal vein, and then into the the hepatic circulation (via the ductus venosus), on its way to the right atrium (Fig. 3.5). This roundabout pathway back to the heart creates multi-level resistance to blood flow. In particular, the more common sites of obstruction are at the level of the vertical vein as it passes through the diaphragm, from closure of the ductus venosus, and/or due to high resistance intra-hepatic connections [15].

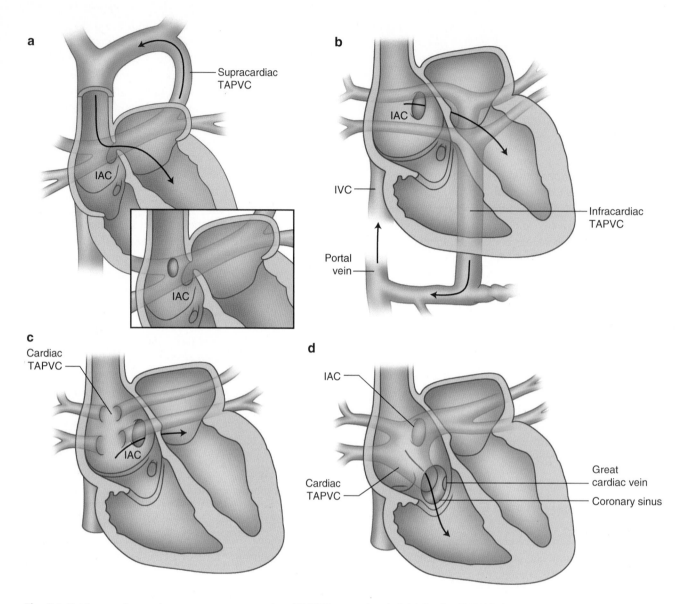

Fig. 3.4 Total anomalous pulmonary venous connection (TAPVC) [41]. This diagram depicts the three general categories of TAPVC. (**a**) Supracardiac TAPVC: the pulmonary venous blood returns to the heart via a vertical vein and ultimately to the SVC and right atrium. (**b**) Infracardiac (infradiaphragmatic) TAPVC: a particularly insidious subtype of TAPVC due to its relatively higher propensity for pulmonary venous obstruction and clinical deterioration in the neo-

natal period. (**c**) Cardiac TAPVC shown with direct pulmonary venous connections to the right atrium (**d**) and with the more common scenario involving drainage to the right atrium via direct connection of the pulmonary vein confluence with the coronary sinus. *IAC* inter-atrial communication, *TAPVC* total anomalous pulmonary venous connection. Copyright 1985 by the Texas Heart Institute, Houston. Illustration by Bill Andrews

3.4 Atrio-Ventricular Connections and Ventricular Morphology

The accurate diagnosis of certain forms of complex CHD depends on distinguishing the morphology and position within the chest of the heart chambers, as well as the specific atrio-ventricular connections and alignments. The morphologically components of the right and left atria are reviewed above (Table 3.1). Like the atria, the left and right ventricles each have distinguishing morphologically

features (Table 3.3). Notably, the shape of the morphologically left ventricle (LV) resembles a prolate ellipsoid (Fig. 3.6a). It has a smooth basal septal surface and the mitral valve apparatus attaches to the free wall rather than the ventricular septum ("septophobic" attachments). The shape of the morphologically right ventricle (RV) is a complex pyramidal shape [17, 18]. It has three distinct parts: (1) inflow portion, (2) body, and an (3) outflow or "infundibulum." There is a moderator band toward the apex and the tricuspid valve apparatus attaches to both the ventricular

Fig. 3.5 Infradiaphragmatic TAPVC. Infant boy with infradiagphagmatic TAVPC. The *left* panel is a coronal projection of a high resolution contrast enhanced MR angiogram showing all four pulmonary veins joining a confluence and coursing via a (*asterisk*) caudally towards the liver to eventually drain to the portal circulation and subsequently back to the IVC The vertical vein is indicated by the asterisk. The panel on the *right* is a posterior projection of a volume rendered image of the MR angiogram

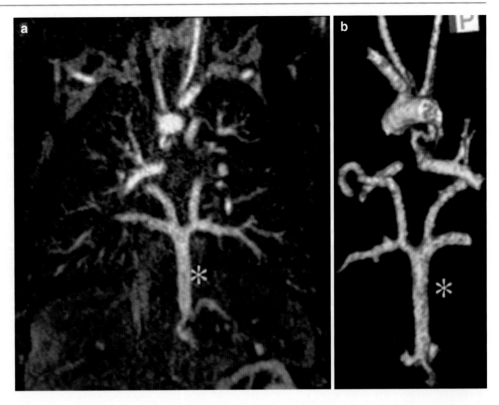

Table 3.3 Morphological features of the ventricles

Left ventricle	Right ventricle
Smooth basal septal surface	Muscular infundibulum (outflow tract)
Fine trabeculations	Coarse trabeculations
Guarded by mitral valve	Guarded by tricuspid valve
Prolate ellipsoid shape	Complex pyramidal shape
	Moderator band
	Relatively thin free wall

septum ("septophillic" attachments) and the RV free wall (Fig. 3.6b–d).

After establishing the morphology of the atria and ventricles, attention can then be directed to how the chambers connect. In the normal configuration, a given ventricle typically receives inflow of blood only from its respective atrium via one of the two atrioventricular (AV) valves, the mitral or tricuspid valve. Normally, the left atrium connects to the LV via the mitral valve and the right atrium connects to the RV via the tricuspid valve. The various permutations of these connections are the basis of some forms of CHD. For example, in double inlet left ventricle (DILV), both atrioventricular valves connect to the single morphologically left ventricle (see below). This ventricle would then give off either the aorta or the pulmonary artery. In these cases, there also exists a small outflow chamber that receives blood via the single left ventricle (via a bulboventricular foramen) that then connects to the other great artery. This outflow chamber does not have a direct atrio-ventricular connection (see below), and thus is not a true ventricle in the strict sense.

In the very rare case of a double inlet right ventricle (DIRV), the opposite applies. That is, the single morphologically RV receives the inflow of both the left ("mitral") and right ("tricuspid") AV valves, and connects to one of the great arteries. Just as in the case of DILV, in DIRV there also exists a diminutive outflow chamber that connects to the other great artery. DILV and DIRV have also been referred to as types of "univentricular atrioventricular connections." Conversely, in the case of complete atrioventricular canal defect (AVCD), there are two distinct ventricles with one common AV valve, rather than separate mitral and tricuspid valves (see below). The common AV valve may either direct blood equally to the two ventricles, in which case it is referred to as a "balanced" AVCD. This results in both ventricles being of adequate size. In "unbalanced" AVCD, however, the common AV valve orifice is directed preferentially toward one ventricle, causing the other ventricle to become hypoplastic and often not able to handle a full cardiac output. Thus, most patients with unbalanced AVCD may not be candidates for standard closure of the defect and may in fact require "single ventricle" surgical palliation [19].

3.4.1 Unbalanced Right-Dominant Complete Atrioventricular Canal Defect (AVCD)

As described above, the complete form of the atrioventricular canal defect (AVCD), also known as "atrioventricular canal" or "atrioventricular septal defect," arises from the incomplete differentiation of the crux of the heart. This

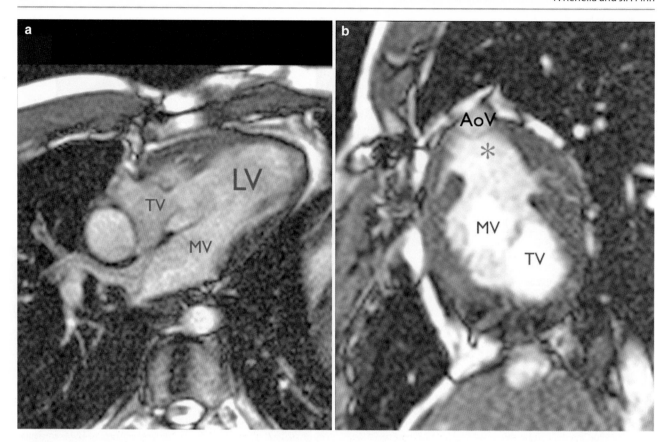

Fig. 3.9 Double inlet left ventricle (DILV) [26]. (**a**) SSFP MR imaging in the horizontal long axis ("four chamber") view of a patient with DILV. Both the mitral (*MV*) and tricuspid valves (*TV*) are aligned with the single left ventricle (*LV*). (**b**) SSFP MR imaging in the short axis plane. Note that both atrioventricular valves are clearly aligned with the left ventricle (*LV*). The aortic valve (*AoV*) arises from the anterior and leftward diminutive "outflow chamber" (*asterisk*), as there is no true right ventricle in this lesion

3.4.2 Double Inlet Left Ventricle (DILV)

Double inlet Left Ventricle (DILV) is the most common form of "single ventricle" and occurs due to the persistence of the primitive state of the bulboventricular loop and a failure of the atria to properly align themselves with the AV valves [25]. This results in the morphologically left ventricle receiving the inflow of both atria. In the majority of cases, the outflow of the left ventricle usually occurs via a transposed pulmonary artery and the aorta arises from a rudimentary outflow chamber positioned anterior and leftward of the left ventricle (Fig. 3.9) [26]. In approximately 15 % of cases, the great arteries arise in a normal orientation (the so-called "Holmes heart"). The great artery arising from the smaller outflow chamber is prone to obstruction, in the sub-valvar, valvar, and supra-valvar areas, as well as distally along length of the vessel. For example, in cases where the aorta arises from the diminutive outflow chamber, there is a higher chance of associated coarctation. It is also possible to encounter a double inlet right ventricle (DIRV), but this lesion is considerably rarer.

Physiologically, all types of "functionally single ventricle" exhibit total mixing of venous and arterial blood at the atrial and/or ventricular levels. Depending on the balance of pulmonary versus systemic blood flow, the patient may be deeply cyanotic, less cyanotic but in congestive heart failure from a large left-to-right shunting, or relatively well-balanced (mildly cyanotic and not in significant heart failure).

3.5 Ventriculo-Arterial Connections

Embryologically, both the aortic and pulmonary valves become associated with a "pedestal" of tissue known as the conus arteriosus overlying the morphologically RV. According to one popular theory, beginning at approximately 30–34 days of gestation, the conus under the aortic valve begins to resorb. This allows for the aortic valve to move into its conventional position posterior and rightward of the pulmonary valve. When the sub-aortic conus persists and the sub-pulmonary conus resorbs instead, the aortic valve position is *anterior* and rightward of the pulmonary valve and becomes associated with the RV, leaving the pulmonary valve to connect to the LV. If the ventricles are normally looped, this "dextro-transposition" of the aortic valve may lead to a condition known as d-loop or complete transposition of the great arteries (TGA) (see below) [27]. Alternatively, when both sides of the conus fail to resorb, association of both the aortic and pulmonary valves to the RV occurs (i.e. "double outlet right ventricle").

3.5.1 D-Loop Transposition of the Great Arteries (d-Loop TGA, Complete TGA)

In d-loop TGA, the most common form of transposition, the aorta is positioned anterior and rightward of the pulmonary artery and is connected to the morphologically RV. It is the most commonly encountered type of "discordance" of the ventriculo-arterial connections, occurring in approximately 2.4 in 10,000 live births [28]. D-loop TGA is often found in isolation with no other associated cardiac or extracardiac pathology. The most common subtype is "simple" d-loop TGA. That is, the ventricles have normal looping and there are no associated ventricular septal defects (VSD) or other cardiac abnormalities. A VSD may be present in approximately one-half of patients, and has been termed "complex" d-loop TGA. With a VSD present, there may be associated pulmonary valve stenosis/atresia, subvalvar pulmonary stenosis, or coarctation of the aorta [29].

Physiologically, de-oxygenated blood from the RV is directly distributed to the systemic circulation via the transposed aorta. Oxygenated blood is sent back to the lungs, resulting in inefficient gas exchange. As a result, profound cyanosis may occur, particularly in the absence of an adequate inter-mixing of the two circulations. Mixing usually occurs via an atrial septal defect, VSD, or patent ductus arteriosus. Inadequate mixing will eventually lead to death if not promptly addressed.

3.5.2 L-Loop Transposition of the Great Arteries ("Congenitally Corrected" Transposition)

In contrast to d-loop TGA, the l-loop variety is considerably more rare, occurring in approximately 2–7 in 100,000 live births, or 0.5 % of all CHD [28, 30]. L-loop TGA is characterized by "doubly discordant" atrio-ventricular and ventriculo-arterial connections. In contrast to d-loop TGA, the ventricles are l-looped. This allows for the alignment of the morphologically right ventricle with the morphologically left atrium, and vice versa for the right atrium and left ventricle. The aortic valve is most often positioned anterior and leftward of the pulmonary valve and is connected to the right ventricle. As such, patients are not typically cyanotic since oxygenated blood from the left atrium courses to the aorta, albeit via a "systemic" right ventricle. It is for this reason that l-loop TGA has been referred to as "congenitally corrected" or "physiologically corrected" transposition.

The vast majority of l-loop TGA patients have associated cardiac structural abnormalities. These include VSD, left ventricular outflow tract (sub-pulmonary) stenosis, Ebstein's malformation of the tricuspid valve, mitral valve dysplasia, and a 2% per year incidence of spontaneous complete heart block [30]. In addition, dextrocardia or mesocardia may be seen in association with l-loop TGA [31].

3.6 Arterial Malformations (Vascular "Rings" and "Slings")

A variety of malformations of the aorta and pulmonary arteries (vascular rings and slings) that may cause tracheal and/or esophageal compression have been described [32]. The most common types are presented in Table 3.4. A complete vascular "ring" occurs when various components of the aortic arch and ligamentum arteriosum completely encircle the trachea and esophagus often compressing these structures. With incomplete vascular rings, and in the case of a vascular "sling," tracheal and/or esophageal compression can occur, but the involved vascular components do not completely encircle the trachea and esophagus.

Vascular rings and slings arise form aberrations in the complex sequence of formation and regression of the six pairs of embryonic aortic arches that connect the truncus arteriosus and aortic sac with the paired dorsal aortae. This process has been well described elsewhere [32, 33]. Edwards proposed a simplified model of the various types of vascular rings and slings via the conceptualization of a "hypothetical double arch with bilateral ductus arteriosus" (Fig. 3.10) [34]. The Edwards model may be further simplified into a series of line drawings, as shown in Fig. 3.11 [32]. By imagining the regression of specific segments of this double arch, one may arrive at the various types of existing aortic arch anomalies.

Although aortic arch anomalies consist of less than 1 % of all CHD, they may cause varying degrees of tracheal and/or esophageal compression, particularly in children. In the child with significant wheezing, stridor, feeding intolerance, and/or recurrent airway obstruction, it is important to

Table 3.4 Most common vascular malformations causing tracheal and/or esophageal compression

Left aortic arch with aberrant right subclavian artery incomplete ring
Double aortic arch (vascular ring)
Right aortic arch with aberrant left subclavian artery (from a diverticulum of Kommerell) and left ligamentum arteriosum (vascular ring)
Left pulmonary artery sling (vascular sling)

Adapted from Kussman et al. [35]

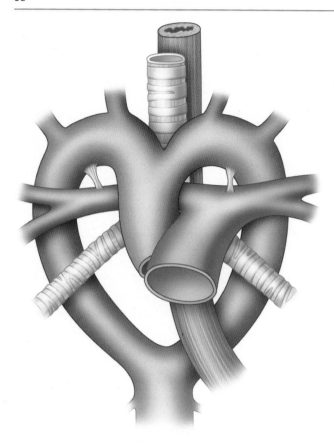

Fig. 3.10 Edwards' hypothetical "double aortic arch with bilateral ductus ateriosus" model [32]

maintain a high index of suspicion for vascular malformations, particularly when other more common causes have been ruled out [35].

3.6.1 Complete Vascular Rings

The most common complete vascular ring is the double aortic arch. In this lesion, the two aortic arches persist and surround the trachea and esophagus (Fig. 3.11a). Rarely are both arches patent, however (only approximately 5 % of cases). In up to 80 % of the time the right arch is patent ("dominant") and the left arch is atretic. The left arch is patent and the right arch atretic in the remainder of cases [36]. It is important to remember that atretic arch segments are not usually visualized by imaging techniques and must be inferred based upon the appearance of vascular outpouchings or based on knowledge of their typical location. This also holds true for the ductus arteriosus portion of vascular rings.

The second most common complete vascular ring is formed by a right aortic arch with aberrant left subclavian artery and a left ductus arteriosus (Fig. 3.11c and Movie 3.2). In this lesion, the ring is formed by the left

common carotid artery, the transverse aortic arch, a posterior aberrant left subclavian artery, and the left-sided ductus arteriosus. The left subclavian artery arises from a remnant of the left fourth arch called the diverticulum of Kommerell, which encircles the esophagus posteriorly [36].

3.6.2 Incomplete Vascular Ring

A left aortic arch with an aberrant right subclavian artery is the most common aortic arch variant with an incidence of approximately 0.5 % in the general population (Fig. 3.11b) [37]. This variation of aorta anatomy forms an incomplete vascular ring as the aberrant right subclavian compresses the esophagus posteriorly as it traverses towards the right arm. This anatomic variant only rarely has any clinical consequences.

3.6.3 Left Pulmonary Sling

In left pulmonary artery sling, the left branch pulmonary artery arises more distally than normal off of the right pulmonary artery. The left pulmonary artery then courses around the right bronchus and then between the trachea and esophagus in order to reach the left lung hilum (Fig. 3.12). Approximately half of patients may have associated "complete" tracheal rings, rather than the normal "C" shaped tracheal rings. Posterior tracheal compression from the left pulmonary artery in conjunction with tracheal luminal narrowing by the complete tracheal rings often manifests as stridor, wheezing, and recurrent pneumonia in the neonatal period [38].

3.6.4 Corctation of the Aorta

In addition to the anatomic aberrancies of the aortic arch reviewed above, the aorta and its branches may have a normal configuration but be discretely narrowed. This is termed "coarctation" of the aorta and occurs in 6–8 % of infants born with CHD [39]. Severe coarctation most often presents in the first 1–2 weeks of life as circulatory shock, as the patent ductus arteriosus closes thus eliminating adequate blood flow to the lower body. The usual location is "juxtaductal," which is the area of the aortic isthmus opposite the insertion of the ductus arteriosus into the descending thoracic aorta (Fig. 3.13 and Movie 3.3). There is often an associated long-segment narrowing of the transverse aortic arch proximal to the area of coarctation. Other associated defects include bicuspid aortic valve, ventricular septal defects, and mitral valve abnormalities.

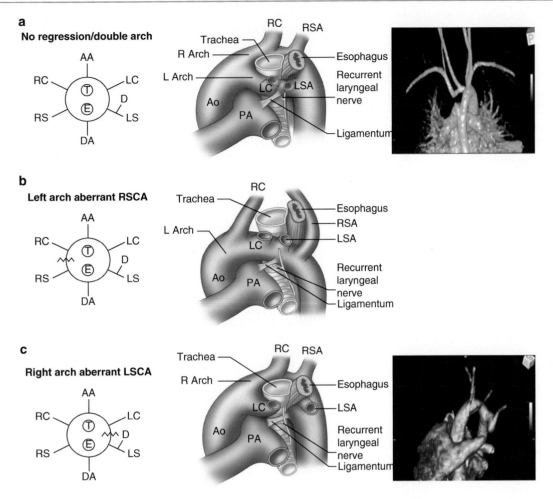

Fig. 3.11 Vascular rings [32, 36]. Line diagram illustrating the origin of various types of vascular rings and slings (derived from Edwards' double arch model in Fig. 3.10). (a) The double aortic arch is the most common type of vascular ring. In this lesion, neither of the dorsal aortae regresses. The *right most* panel is a 3D volume rendered MR angiogram of a double aortic arch with an atretic left arch. The atretic arch does not fill with contrast and thus its presence must be inferred. (b) Left aortic arch with aberrant right subclavian artery is an incomplete ring and, as such, infrequently causes symptoms. (c) Right aortic arch with aberrant left subclavian artery is the second most common type of vascular ring. The *right most* panel is a 3D volume rendered MR angiogram of this lesion

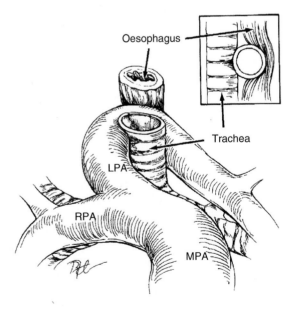

Fig. 3.12 Left pulmonary artery sling [36]. The left pulmonary artery arises more distally off the right pulmonary artery and makes an acute turn, coursing in between the trachea and esophagus to reach the left lung hilum. This causes the classic anterior compression of the esophagus seen on conventional upper GI imaging

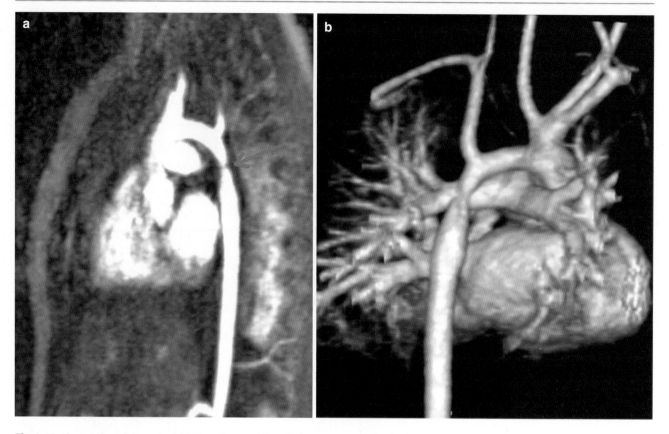

Fig. 3.13 Coarctation of the aorta. (**a**) MR angiogram 3D multiplanar reconstruction in the sagittal plane demonstrating a juxtaductal coarctation of the aorta (*red arrow*) in an newborn boy. (**b**) 3D volume rendered MR angiogram of the same (posterior projection)

Conclusion

CMR imaging is ideally suited for the characterization of congenital anatomic and physiologic aberrations of the cardiovascular system. The advantages of CMR over other imaging modalities include its non-invasive nature, absence of ionizing radiation, use of a non-iodinated contrast agent, comprehensive view of both the intra-cardiac structures and extra-cardiac vasculature, and the quantification of blood flow. Further technical developments will ensure CMR's integral role in the comprehensive assessment of patients with congenital heart disease.

3.8   Practical Pearls

- CMR imaging allows for a comprehensive assessment of intra-cardiac structures, extra-cardiac vasculature, and blood flow.
- The non-invasive nature of CMR, and the lack of ionizing radiation and iodinated contrast, make CMR imaging advantageous in the population of congenital heart disease patients who require serial life-long imaging studies.
- In the initial diagnosis and serial evaluation of congenital heart disease patients, CMR imaging should be

considered complimentary to other traditional imaging techniques such as echocardiography and cardiac catheterization.
- CMR in congenital heart disease is ideally performed and interpreted in concert with specially trained Radiologists, Cardiologists, and Cardiothoracic Surgeons.

References

1. VanPraagh R. Segmental approach to diagnosis. In: Keane JE, Lock JE, Flyer DC, editors. Nadas' pediatric cardiology. 2nd ed. Philadelphia: Saunders Elsevier; 2006. p. 39–46.
2. Cohen MS, Anderson RH, Cohen MI, Atz AM, Fogel M, Gruber PJ, Lopez L, Rome JJ, Weinberg PM. Controversies, genetics, diagnostic assessment, and outcomes relating to the heterotaxy syndrome. Cardiol Young. 2007;17 Suppl 2:29–43.
3. Jacobs JP, Anderson RH, Weinberg PM, Walters 3rd HL, Tchervenkov CI, Del Duca D, Franklin RC, Aiello VD, Beland MJ, Colan SD, Gaynor JW, Krogmann ON, Kurosawa H, Maruszewski B, Stellin G, Elliott MJ. The nomenclature, definition and classification of cardiac structures in the setting of heterotaxy. Cardiol Young. 2007;17 Suppl 2:1–28.
4. Bartram U, Wirbelauer J, Speer CP. Heterotaxy syndrome – asplenia and polysplenia as indicators of visceral malposition and complex congenital heart disease. Biol Neonate. 2005;88(4): 278–90.

5. Van Mierop L, Gessner IH, Schiebler GL. Asplenia and polysplenia syndrome. Birth Defects. 1972;8:74–84.
6. Peoples WM, Moller JH, Edwards JE. Polysplenia: a review of 146 cases. Pediatr Cardiol. 1983;4(2):129–37.
7. Bartz PJ, Driscoll DJ, Dearani JA, Puga FJ, Danielson GK, O'Leary PW, Earing MG, Warnes CA, Hodge DO, Cetta F. Early and late results of the modified fontan operation for heterotaxy syndrome 30 years of experience in 142 patients. J Am Coll Cardiol. 2006;48(11):2301–5.
8. Geva T, Vick 3rd GW, Wendt RE, Rokey R. Role of spin echo and cine magnetic resonance imaging in presurgical planning of heterotaxy syndrome. Comparison with echocardiography and catheterization. Circulation. 1994;90(1):348–56.
9. Hong YK, Park YW, Ryu SJ, Won JW, Choi JY, Sul JH, Lee SK, Cho BK, Choe KO. Efficacy of MRI in complicated congenital heart disease with visceral heterotaxy syndrome. J Comput Assist Tomogr. 2000;24(5):671–82.
10. Edwards WD. Cardiac anatomy and examination of cardiac specimens. In: Allen HD, Driscoll DJ, Shaddy RE, Feltes TF, editors. Moss and Adams' heart disease in infants, children, and adolescents, vol. 1. Philadelphia: Lippincott, Williams, and Wilkins; 2007. p. 5–8.
11. Mazzucco A, Bortolotti U, Stellin G, Gallucci V. Anomalies of the systemic venous return: a review. J Card Surg. 1990;5(2):122–33.
12. Celentano C, Malinger G, Rotmensch S, Gerboni S, Wolman Y, Glezerman M. Prenatal diagnosis of interrupted inferior vena cava as an isolated finding: a benign vascular malformation. Ultrasound Obstet Gynecol. 1999;14(3):215–8.
13. Edwards WD. Cardiac anatomy and examination of cardiac specimens. In: Allen HD, Driscoll DJ, Shaddy RE, Feltes TF, editors. Moss and Adams' heart disease in infants, children, and adolescents, vol. 1. 7th ed. Philadelphia: Lippincott Williams & Wilkins; 2008. p. 2–33.
14. Pappone C, Rosanio S, Oreto G, Tocchi M, Gugliotta F, Vicedomini G, Salvati A, Dicandia C, Mazzone P, Santinelli V, Gulletta S, Chierchia S. Circumferential radiofrequency ablation of pulmonary vein ostia: a new anatomic approach for curing atrial fibrillation. Circulation. 2000;102(21):2619–28.
15. Stein P. Total anomalous pulmonary venous connection. AORN J. 2007;85(3):509–20; quiz 521–504.
16. Keane JF, Flyer DC. Total anomalous pulmonary venous return. In: Keane JF, Lock JE, Flyer DC, editors. Nadas' pediatric cardiology. 2nd ed. Philadelphia: Saunders Elsevier; 2006. p. 773–81.
17. Dorosz JL, Bolson EL, Waiss MS, Sheehan FH. Three-dimensional visual guidance improves the accuracy of calculating right ventricular volume with two-dimensional echocardiography. J Am Soc Echocardiogr. 2003;16(6):675–81.
18. Kuhl HP, Schreckenberg M, Rulands D, Katoh M, Schafer W, Schummers G, Bucker A, Hanrath P, Franke A. High-resolution transthoracic real-time three-dimensional echocardiography: quantitation of cardiac volumes and function using semi-automatic border detection and comparison with cardiac magnetic resonance imaging. J Am Coll Cardiol. 2004;43(11):2083–90.
19. Owens GE, Gomez-Fifer C, Gelehrter S, Owens ST. Outcomes for patients with unbalanced atrioventricular septal defects. Pediatr Cardiol. 2009;30(4):431–5.
20. Rogers HM, Edwards JE. Incomplete division of the atrioventricular canal with patent inter-atrial foramen primum, persistent common atrioventricular ostium; report of five cases and review of the literature. Am Heart J. 1948;36(1):28–54.
21. Dunlop KA, Mulholland HC, Casey FA, Craig B, Gladstone DJ. A ten year review of atrioventricular septal defects. Cardiol Young. 2004;14(1):15–23.
22. Geva T, Ayres NA, Pignatelli RH, Gajarski RJ. Echocardiographic evaluation of common atrioventricular canal defects: a study of 206 consecutive patients. Echocardiography. 1996;13(4):387–400.
23. Laursen HB. Congenital heart disease in Down's syndrome. Br Heart J. 1976;38(1):32–8.
24. Cetta F, Minich L, Edwards WD, Dearani JA, Puga FJ. Atrioventricular septal defects. In: Allen HD, Driscoll DJ, Shaddy RE, Feltes TF, editors. Moss and Adams' heart disease in infants, children, and adolescents, vol. 1. 7th ed. Philadelphia: Lippincott Williams & Wilkins; 2008. p. 647–67.
25. Lev M, Liberthson RR, Kirkpatrick JR, Eckner FA, Arcilla RA. Single (primitive) ventricle. Circulation. 1969;39(5):577–91.
26. Keane JF, Flyer DC. Single ventricle. In: Keane JF, Lock JE, Flyer DC, editors. Nadas' pediatric cardiology. 2nd ed. Philadelphia: Saunders Elsevier; 2006. p. 743–51.
27. Fulton DR, Flyer DC. D-transposition of the great arteries. In: Keane JF, Lock JE, Flyer DC, editors. Nadas' pediatric cardiology. 2nd ed. Philadelphia: Saunders Elsevier; 2006. p. 645–61.
28. Botto LD, Correa A, Erickson JD. Racial and temporal variations in the prevalence of heart defects. Pediatrics. 2001;107(3):E32.
29. Blume ED, Altmann K, Mayer JE, Colan SD, Gauvreau K, Geva T. Evolution of risk factors influencing early mortality of the arterial switch operation. J Am Coll Cardiol. 1999;33(6):1702–9.
30. Hornung TS, Calder L. Congenitally corrected transposition of the great arteries. Heart. 2010;96(14):1154–61.
31. Van Praagh R, Van Praagh S. Anatomically corrected transposition of the great arteries. Br Heart J. 1967;29(1):112–9.
32. Powell AJ, Mandell VS. Vascular rings and slings. In: Keane JF, Lock JE, Flyer DC, editors. Nadas' pediatric cardiology. 2nd ed. Philadelphia: Saunders Elsevier; 2006. p. 811–23.
33. Kellenberger CJ. Aortic arch malformations. Pediatr Radiol. 2010;40(6):876–84.
34. Edwards JE. Anomalies of the derivatives of the aortic arch system. Med Clin North Am. 1948;32:925–49.
35. Kussman BD, Geva T, McGowan FX. Cardiovascular causes of airway compression. Paediatr Anaesth. 2004;14(1):60–74.
36. Dodge-Khatami A, Tulevski II, Hitchcock JF, de Mol BA, Bennink GB. Vascular rings and pulmonary arterial sling: from respiratory collapse to surgical cure, with emphasis on judicious imaging in the hi-tech era. Cardiol Young. 2002;12(2):96–104.
37. Edwards JE. Malformations of the aortic arch system manifested as vascular rings. Lab Invest. 1953;2(1):56–75.
38. Fiore AC, Brown JW, Weber TR, Turrentine MW. Surgical treatment of pulmonary artery sling and tracheal stenosis. Ann Thorac Surg. 2005;79(1):38–46; discussion 38–46.
39. Beekman RH. Coarctation of the aorta. In: Allen HD, Driscoll DJ, Shaddy RE, Feltes TF, editors. Moss and Adams' heart disease in infants, children, and adolescents, vol. 2. 7th ed. Philadelphia: Lippincott Williams & Wilkins; 2008. p. 987–1005.
40. Praagh RV, Praagh SV. Morphologic anatomy. In: Keane JF, Lock JE, Flyer DC, editors. Nadas' pediatric cardiology. 2nd ed. Philadelphia: Saunders Elsevier; 2006. p. 27–37.
41. Reardon MJ, Cooley DA, Kubrusly L, Ott DA, Johnson W, Kay GL, Sweeney MS. Total anomalous pulmonary venous return: report of 201 patients treated surgically. Tex Heart Inst J. 1985 Jun;12(2):131–41.

Venoatrial Abnormalities

4

Henryk Kafka and Raad H. Mohiaddin

4.1 Introduction

Congenital venous anomalies of the thorax may be encountered in patients with documented congenital heart disease, those patients with abnormal echocardiographic findings (dilated right ventricle or pulmonary hypertension, for example), or unexpectedly, in patients having CT scan or magnetic resonance examination of the thorax for other reasons. These anomalies can range from the clinically important (partial anomalous pulmonary venous connection) to the clinically inconsequential (persistent left superior vena cava) and it is essential for the reading physician to be able to identify these anomalies and associated intracardiac or extracardiac defects in order to decide whether further imaging and investigation is warranted.

Cardiac magnetic resonance imaging can detect both simple and complex thoracic venous anomalies. It has the advantages of wide field-of-view, multiplanar capability without being restricted by anatomic limitations, ability to assess structure and function, ability to reliably measure flow through the use of phase-contrast mapping, ability to rapidly acquire 3-D imaging with MR angiography [17], and lack of ionizing radiation. There are some disadvantages of cardiac magnetic resonance imaging to consider and these include metal related artifact (an important factor in patients with treated congenital heart disease), the amount of time required for imaging, the cost of cardiac magnetic resonance imaging, concerns about claustrophobia and patient sedation. In the past 5 years, there have also been concerns about the use of

gadolinium and nephrogenic systemic sclerosis, but gadolinium enhanced MR angiography may not be necessary in all cases. Adequate visualization of anomalous veins has been demonstrated to be possible without the use of gadolinium [9] and there have been recent reports of successful steady-state free precession (SSFP) magnetic resonance angiography without the use of intravenous contrast agent for visualizing the pulmonary veins [12].

Congenital thoracic venous anomalies are classified as pulmonary venoatrial anomalies (Table 4.1) or systemic venous anomalies (Table 4.2). The pulmonary venoatrial anomalies are more likely to be of clinical significance and to have associated cardiac defects. It is, nevertheless, still important to identify the systemic venous anomalies because they may be confused with more important pulmonary venous anomalies and may lead to unnecessary further imaging and investigation.

4.2 Pulmonary Venoatrial Anomalies

4.2.1 Pulmonary Vein Development and Anatomy

In humans, the lungs, larynx and tracheobronchial tree are derived from the foregut. In early stages of development, the lungs are enmeshed by the splanchnic plexus. As pulmonary differentiation progresses, part of the splanchnic plexus forms the pulmonary vascular bed. Initially, there is no direct connection between the heart and the pulmonary vascular bed, with the pulmonary vascular bed draining through the splanchnic plexus via the umbilicovitelline and cardinal system of veins. Eventually, the pulmonary veins connect with the left atrium by establishing connection with the common

H. Kafka, M.D., FRCPC, FACC (✉)
Departments of Cardiology and Radiology, Queen's University,
Kingston General Hospital,
76 Stuart Street, Kingston, ON, K7L2V7, Canada
e-mail: kafkamd@usa.net

R.H. Mohiaddin, M.D., Ph.D., FRCR, FRCP, FESC
Cardiovascular Magnetic Resonance Unit, Royal Brompton Hospital
and National Heart and Lung Institute, Imperial College London,
Sydney Street, London, SW3 6NP, UK

Electronic supplementary material The online version of this chapter (doi:10.1007/978-1-4471-4267-6_4) contains supplementary material, which is available to authorized users.

Table 4.1 Pulmonary veno atrial anomalies

1. Partial anomalous pulmonary venous connection
   1.1. Right sided veins
       1.1.1. Superior vena cava or right atrium
       1.1.2. Scimitar
       1.1.3. Azygos
   1.2. Left sided veins
       1.2.1. Left innominate
       1.2.2. Inferior vena cava, superior vena cava, azygos
2. Total anomalous pulmonary venous connection
   2.1. Supracardiac
       2.1.1. Left innominate vein
       2.1.2. Right atrium/right superior vena cava
       2.1.3. Coronary sinus
   2.2. Infradiaphragmatic
       2.2.1. Portal vein
       2.2.2. Inferior vena cava
3. Pulmonary vein number anomalies
4. Cor triatriatum
   4.1. Classic
   4.2. Subtotal
5. Central and peripheral pulmonary vein stenosis
   5.1. Central
   5.2. Peripheral

Table 4.2 Anomalies of systemic thoracic veins

1. Superior vena cava
   1.1. Persistent left superior vena cava
   1.2. Absent right superior vena cava
   1.3. Superior vena cava to left atrium
2. Inferior vena cava
   2.1. Interrupted inferior vena cava
   2.2. Duplicate inferior vena cava
   2.3. Inferior vena cava to left atrium
3. Anomalous left innominate vein
   3.1. Retroaortic
   3.2. Duplicated
4. Azygos system
   4.1. Absent azygos vein
   4.2. Azygos lobe

pulmonary vein which arises from the left atrium whilst the initial connection between the pulmonary portion of the splanchnic plexus and the cardinal and umbilicovitelline systems involutes. The pulmonary vascular bed then drains by four individual major pulmonary veins into the common pulmonary vein which drains into the left atrium. Eventually the common pulmonary vein becomes part of the left atrium resulting in the anatomic arrangement that we recognize with four individual pulmonary veins connected directly to the left atrium. Defects in the development of the common pulmonary vein provide the basis for most anomalies of the pulmonary veins [7]. Pulmonary venous anomalies can be classified as anomalies in the number of pulmonary veins;

anomalies in the connections of the pulmonary veins; and stenotic pulmonary vein connections. Atresia of the common pulmonary vein, whilst the pulmonary to systemic venous connections are still present, can give rise to total anomalous pulmonary venous connection or partial anomalous pulmonary venous connections. Stenosis of the common pulmonary vein would result in cor triatriatum, whereas abnormal absorption of the common pulmonary vein into the left atrium will give rise to stenosis of the individual pulmonary veins or lead to an abnormal number of pulmonary veins [7].

4.2.2 Partial Anomalous Pulmonary Venous Connection (PAPVC)

Partial anomalous pulmonary venous connection involves one or more of the pulmonary veins (but not all) connected to a systemic vein. The common types of PAPVC are: right-sided pulmonary veins to the superior vena cava and/or right atrium; right sided pulmonary veins to the inferior vena cava; and left-sided pulmonary veins to the left innominate vein (Fig. 4.1). There have been reports of unusual sites of connection, such as to the azygos vein or the coronary sinus [2, 7, 13]. Patients may even have combinations of connections with a right pulmonary vein to the right superior vena cava and the left pulmonary vein to the left innominate [9]. PAPVC results in a left to right shunt with volume loading of the right ventricle. The hemodynamic importance of any PAPVC is linked to the amount of lung draining anomalously into the systemic venous circulation. Patients with a small shunt may never develop symptoms or any hemodynamic consequence. Patients with larger shunts may present with dyspnea and echocardiographic evidence of a dilated right ventricle and pulmonary hypertension. MRI is ideally suited to assess right ventricular size and function with SSFP cine imaging and to provide a reliable measure of the left to right shunting through the use of phase contrast mapping.

4.2.2.1 Right PAPVC to the Superior Vena Cava or Right Atrium

The most common type of partial anomalous pulmonary venous connection encountered clinically is that of one or more pulmonary veins from the right lung draining into the superior vena cava and/or the right atrium. This type of PAPVC is frequently associated with the sinus venosus defect (see Chap. 5), reported in 42–87 % of patients with right PAPVC [1, 2, 8, 9]. The sinus venosus defect is an interatrial communication due to the unroofing of the common wall between the right superior vena cava and the right upper pulmonary vein (Fig. 4.2). Patients with sinus venosus defect have been reported to have as high as a 95 % prevalence of PAPVC of the right pulmonary vein [9]. The relationship

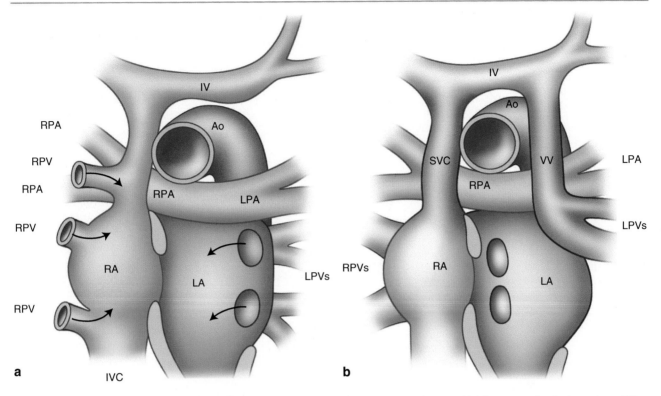

Fig. 4.1 Partial anomalous pulmonary vein connections. (**a**) Depicts the commonest locations of anomalous right pulmonary vein (*RPV*) connections into the superior vena cava (*SVC*), right atrium (*RA*) or inferior vena cava (*IVC*). (**b**) Demonstrates the commonest type of anomalous left pulmonary vein (*LPV*) connection with the LPV drain-ing to a vertical vein (*VV*) which is connected to the innominate (*IV*) or brachiocephalic vein and thence to the SVC. *Ao* aorta, *LA* left atrium, *LPA* left pulmonary artery, *RPA* right pulmonary artery (From Ammash et al. [2], with permission)

between sinus venosus defects and PAPVC from the right lung is so strong that the finding of one on echocardiography, transesophageal echocardiography, CT or MRI mandates a careful search for the other. Although sinus venosus defect is the most common association with PAPVC, secundum atrial septal defect has been described with PAPVC as well [9]. Less frequent associated anomalies include tetralogy of Fallot and double outlet right ventricle.

4.2.2.2 Scimitar Syndrome

There may be anomalous connection of the pulmonary veins from the right lung (occasionally just those from right middle lobe and right lower lobe) into the inferior vena cava, above or below the diaphragm. Connections into the hepatic vein have been described. The drainage pattern of the pulmonary veins in the right lung is changed and has been described as having a "fir tree" configuration [7]. This anomalous right pulmonary venous connection is referred to as the scimitar syndrome (Fig. 4.3) and is associated with other anomalies: hypoplasia of the right lung; anoma-lies of the bronchial system; anomalous arterial connection to the right lung; hypoplasia of the right pulmonary artery; and pulmonary sequestration. There is no association with sinus venosus defect and the atrial septum is frequently

intact. Unlike the other previously described PAPVC, the scimitar syndrome more likely represents developmental abnormality of the right lung [7]. A pseudoscimitar syn-drome has been described where there is a single pulmo-nary vein, draining the entire right lung that follows a meandering course towards the diaphragm but then turns cephalad and connects to the left atrium. Although the course is aberrant, there is an appropriate connection back to the left atrium, and so there is no clinical consequence to this lesion. There may be lung hypoplasia with this pseudo-scimitar syndrome as well [5]. The significance of the pseudoscimitar syndrome lies in its differentiation from a true anomalous connection, and avoidance of additional imaging and intervention.

4.2.2.3 Azygos Vein

Anomalous connection of a right pulmonary vein to the azy-gos vein has been described [7, 13] and is uncommonly seen (Fig. 4.4). Even anomalous connection of an upper left pul-monary vein to the azygos vein has been reported. These reports stress the importance of imaging the more cephalad aspect of the SVC to avoid missing an anomalous connection to the azygos vein or a high connection to the SVC in the region of the azygos [16].

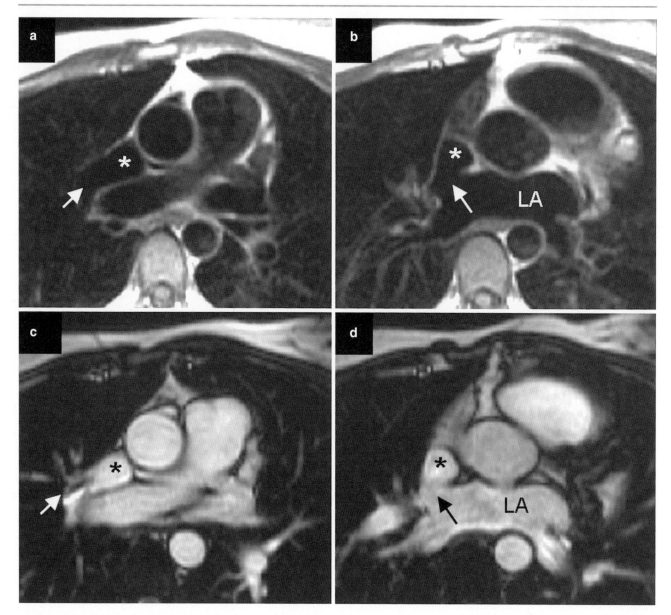

Fig. 4.2 PAPVC with sinus venosus defect. Forty-six-year-old woman with partial anomalous pulmonary venous connection and sinus venosus defect. *LA* left atrium, *asterisk* indicates superior vena cava (*SVC*). (**a**) Turbo spin-echo image shows connection of right upper pulmonary vein (*arrow*) to SVC. (**b**) Slice 20 mm caudad to (**a**) clearly shows sinus venosus defect (*arrow*). (**c** and **d**) Steady-state free precession cine still images at same levels as (**a** and **b**) also show sinus venosus defect (*arrow*, **d**). *Arrow* in (**c**) indicates anomalous connection of upper pulmonary vein to the SVC (Reprinted with permission from Kafka and Mohiaddin [9])

4.2.2.4 Left Pulmonary Vein Anomalous Connection

The partial anomalous connection of left pulmonary veins, the vein from the left upper lobe or from the entire left lung, is usually through a vertical vein up to the left innominate vein (Figs. 4.1 and 4.3). The left PAPVC has been reported less commonly in the clinical situation but may be more common in the asymptomatic adult. A recent retrospective review of 45,538 MDCT in adults, with no previous history of PAPVC or sinus venosus defect, demonstrated PAPVC in 47 patients (0.1 % prevalence) with left upper lobe veins involved in 24 patients and right upper lobe veins in 19 patients [8]. This surprising result may simply reflect the fact that patients with left PAPVC tend to have a smaller hemodynamic burden from the left to right shunting and are less likely to present clinically. Left PAPVC is not associated with sinus venosus defects but secundum atrial septal defects are frequently seen [9]. Left PAPVC can be an isolated incidental finding [8] and if the anomalous drainage involves just the left upper lobe, there may not be enough of a left to right shunt to be of any clinical significance and no treatment would be required. Less frequent sites of left PAPVC are to

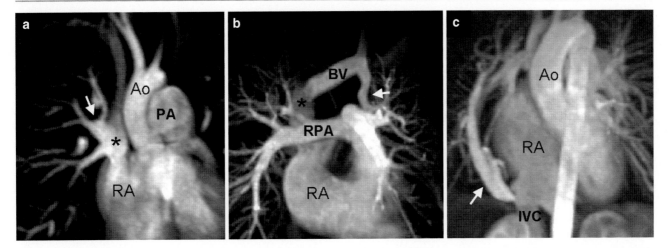

Fig. 4.3 PAPVC CE-MRA. Contrast-enhanced MR angiography maximum-intensity-projection coronal images in three patients with partial anomalous pulmonary venous connection. *Ao* aorta, *RA* right atrium. (**a**) Eighteen-year-old woman with anomalous connection of right pulmonary vein (*arrow*) to superior vena cava (*SVC*) (*asterisk*). *PA* pulmonary artery. (**b**) Sixty-three-year-old woman with anomalous connection of left upper pulmonary vein to vertical vein (*arrow*) that drains into brachiocephalic vein (*BV*) and from there into SVC (*asterisk*). *RPA* right pulmonary artery. (**c**) Forty-five-year-old woman with anomalous scimitar vein. Image shows that all right pulmonary veins are connected to an anomalous vein (*arrow*) that, in turn, drains into inferior vena cava (*IVC*) (Reprinted with permission from Kafka and Mohiaddin [9])

the coronary sinus, inferior vena cava, right superior vena cava, left subclavian vein and azygos vein [7].

4.2.2.5 Imaging for PAPVC

Transthoracic echocardiography can detect sinus venosus defect and anomalous pulmonary venous connections in the young. However in the older patient, transthoracic echocardiography cannot reliably detect sinus venosus defect or anomalous pulmonary venous connections. Transesophageal echocardiography is better capable of detecting the sinus venosus defect and most of the anomalous venous connections. Even so, several reports have indicated that even in the best of hands, transesophageal echocardiography may not detect all the anomalous pulmonary venous connections that were noted at surgery [2, 16]. Cardiac magnetic resonance imaging enjoys the advantage of a wide field of view that allows it to detect anomalous connections in the upper superior vena cava that may not be visible by transesophageal echocardiography. Furthermore, the cardiac magnetic resonance imaging is not limited to any prespecified imaging planes, allowing it to detect anomalous connections above and below the diaphragm and follow these connections along their course. In addition to the spin echo images, SSFP cine imaging produces better delineation of blood-tissue borders (Fig. 4.2) and is able to demonstrate turbulent flow. Contrast-enhanced magnetic resonance angiography provides a rapid 3D image of the anomalous veins (Fig. 4.4). Phase-contrast mapping provides reproducible measurement of systemic and pulmonary flow, as well as measurement of differential flow to the lungs. These significant advantages of cardiac magnetic resonance imaging make it the preferred imaging modality in these patients [6, 9, 19]. Multislice CT with contrast

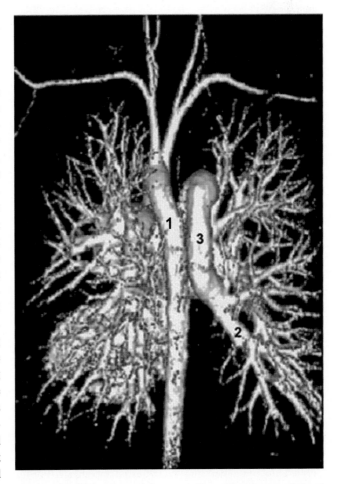

Fig. 4.4 PAPVC azygos vein connection. 3D contrast-enhanced MRA. Surface rendered image in the posteroanterior view. (*1*) Descending thoracic aorta. (*2*) Anomalous right middle and lower pulmonary vein. (*3*) Dilated azygos vein (Adapted from Locca et al. [13])

will demonstrate the anomalous pulmonary venous connections [8] but it does not provide the same functional information available from cardiac magnetic resonance imaging and it does require the use of radiation and iodinated contrast.

4.2.2.6 Image Guided Management Decision Making in Patients with PAPVC

The management of patients with these partial anomalous pulmonary venous connections depends primarily on the symptoms, the presence of associated defects and the degree of hemodynamic consequence of the shunts, both those arising from the anomalous pulmonary venous connection and those due to associated sinus venosus defects or atrial septal defects. Imaging will help determine the presence of associated defects and can assess the presence of right ventricular volume overload with a dilated right ventricle and abnormal interventricular septal motion. Specifically phase-contrast MR mapping will be able to accurately calculate the flow through the pulmonary artery and the aorta in order to determine the degree of shunting. In the patient with scimitar syndrome and no interatrial connection, phase-contrast MR mapping will be able to determine the relative pulmonary blood flow to each lung in order to determine the hemodynamic consequence of the anomalous pulmonary venous connection. Often, the flow to the right lung may represent only a quarter or third of total pulmonary blood flow because of the other associated pulmonary defects [7].

The only definitive therapy for clinically significant PAPVC is surgical repair. The type of repair depends on the anatomy of the connection [1]. For the right PAPVC to the superior vena cava with sinus venosus defect, the superior vena cava is divided above the anomalous pulmonary vein(s) and the tip of the right atrial appendage is anastomosed to the superior vena cava. A pericardial patch is sutured to the margin of the sinus venosus defect in order to channel blood flow from the anomalous pulmonary vein(s) into the left atrium through the sinus venosus defect. The sinus venosus defect may need to be enlarged in order to accommodate the pulmonary venous flow. Another approach is to make an incision into the superior vena cava over the insertion of the anomalous pulmonary veins and to create an atrial septal defect, if none is already present. A pericardial patch is used to baffle the blood from the anomalous pulmonary veins into the left atrium through the sinus venosus defect or newly created atrial septal defect. The superior vena cava incision is repaired with a patch of pericardium in order to minimize the superior vena cava narrowing at that site [1]. For the patient with a left PAPVC requiring surgery, the vertical vein between the innominate vein and the pulmonary vein is divided and implanted into the left atrial appendage. For the patient with the scimitar type of right PAPVC to the inferior vena cava, the surgery is more complex. An atrial septal defect is created, and a long baffle of pericardium is placed into the lumen of the inferior vena cava to channel the flow from the anomalous pulmonary vein to the right atrium and through the new atrial septal defect into the left atrium. Often it is necessary to enlarge the inferior vena cava with a pericardial patch in an effort to prevent vena cava obstruction [1]. These operations can be carried out with very low mortality and morbidity risks and good long-term outlook [1, 3]. However the repair of the anomalous pulmonary venous connection in scimitar syndrome is associated with a high incidence of late postoperative pulmonary venous obstruction. The value of MR imaging post operatively is to look for stenotic lesions at anastomosis sites, assess for narrowing in the superior vena cava or inferior vena cava and to rule out any baffle leaks or residual interatrial communication. Cardiac magnetic resonance imaging will be especially valuable in the assessment of obstruction along the extensive baffle used in scimitar syndrome repair.

4.2.3 Total Anomalous Pulmonary Venous Connection (TAPVC)

In total anomalous pulmonary venous connection, the pulmonary veins have no direct connection with the left atrium. The pulmonary veins connect to a systemic vein and, therefore, an interatrial communication is mandatory in order to maintain life. Usually TAPVC is an isolated anomaly but it has been associated with other defects, such as tetralogy of Fallot, transposition of the great arteries, truncus arteriosus and tricuspid atresia. Patients with asplenia have a high incidence of TAPVC.

4.2.3.1 Supracardiac and Infradiaphragmatic TAPVC

The anomalous connections can be generally classified as those which are supracardiac (left innominate vein, right superior vena cava, coronary sinus, right atrium) without pulmonary venous obstruction and those which are infradiaphragmatic (to portal vein or IVC) with pulmonary venous obstruction (Fig. 4.5) and those which are mixed with pulmonary veins draining to at least two different locations [6]. The most common site of connection is to the left innominate vein. In this situation, the pulmonary veins from both lungs connect into a pulmonary venous confluence that is posterior to the left atrium. A vertical vein from this chamber courses cephalad, passing anterior to the aortic arch and joins the left innominate vein which continues in its usual course to the right-sided superior vena cava. In another supracardiac variant, the anomalous vessel arises from the right side of the pulmonary venous confluence and passes cephalad to enter the superior vena cava posteriorly. There can also be a direct connection between the pulmonary venous confluence and the coronary sinus which will be significantly dilated because

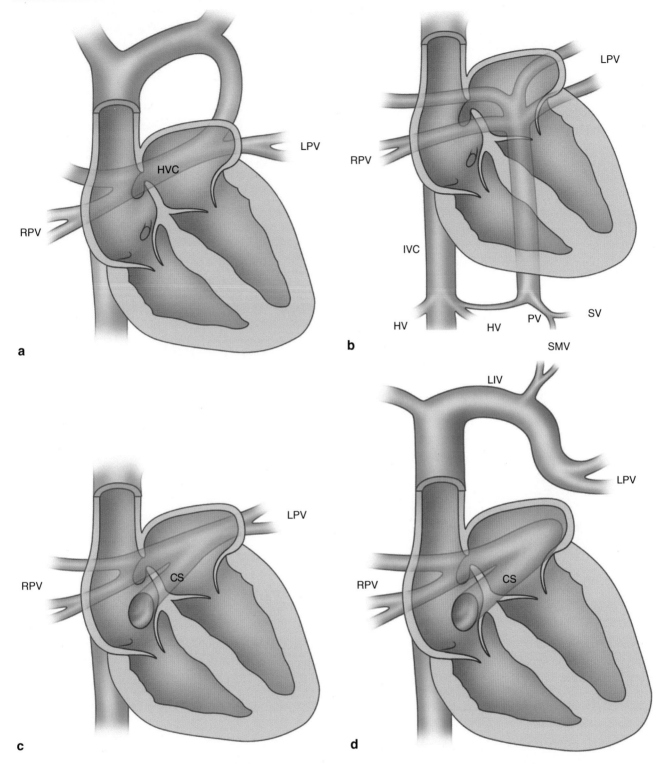

Fig. 4.5 Diagram of common types of totally anomalous pulmonary venous connection (*TAPVC*). (**a**) Supracardiac TAPVC to the left innominate vein. The individual pulmonary veins form a horizontal pulmonary venous confluence (*HVC*) that connects to the left innominate vein by way of a vertical vein. (**b**) Infradiaphragmatic TAPVC to the portal vein. The pulmonary veins form a vertical confluence that descends below the diaphragm and typically joins the portal vein (*PV*). Pulmonary venous blood then drains into the inferior vena cava (*IVC*) via the ductus venosus or the hepatic sinusoids. The individual pulmonary veins may join the vertical vein at different levels. (**c**) TAPVC to the coronary sinus (*CS*). (**d**) Mixed-type TAPVC. In the example shown, the left pulmonary veins (*LPV*) connect to the left innominate vein (*LIV*), and the right pulmonary veins (*RPV*) connect with the CS. *HV* hepatic vein, *LA* left atrium, *RA* right atrium, *SMV* superior mesenteric vein, *SV* splenic vein (Adapted with permission from Chap. 37 (Fig. 37.15) Geva and Van Praagh [7])

of the increased flow, or a direct connection to the right atrium [6]. Infradiaphragmatic anomalous connections involve the vein from the common vessel posterior to the left atrium descending through the diaphragm and then connecting to the portal vein. It may connect to a hepatic vein or connect directly to the inferior vena cava. Such infradiaphragmatic connections usually have some component of obstruction [7].

4.2.3.2 Management of Patients with TAPVC

Total anomalous pulmonary venous connection will result in significant right ventricular volume overload with signs and symptoms related to that, and the imaging needs to differentiate it from other causes of right heart overload such as atrial septal defect and PAPVC. There will be decreased left ventricular volume and decreased systemic output. In the cases with pulmonary venous obstruction (usually subdiaphragmatic) the elevated pulmonary venous pressure may lead to pulmonary edema. Diagnosis is usually made in the first months of life. The only long term effective therapy for TAPVC involves a surgical repair. Essentially, a side-to-side anastomosis is made between the pulmonary venous confluence and the left atrium. The anomalous connection is then closed, as is the interatrial connection. Postoperative complications have involved the late stenosis of the left atrial-pulmonary venous confluence anastomosis and residual patch leaks.

4.2.3.3 Imaging for TAPVC

In these patients, echocardiography will show features of right ventricular volume overload and there will be difficulty in demonstrating the pulmonary veins. The pulmonary venous confluence can be identified as a chamber posterior to the small left atrium and the course of the pulmonary veins should be tracked.

Cardiac magnetic resonance imaging has the advantage of the wider field-of-view and can provide a comprehensive assessment of the pulmonary venous confluence and its connections (Fig. 4.6). It is especially of benefit to define the level of obstruction in patients with infradiaphragmatic connection. However in infants, the windows available to echocardiography are such that a comprehensive and diagnostic study can usually be undertaken in TAPVC. The major role of MRI in total anomalous pulmonary venous connection is to assess the patient following surgical repair for followup, assess for associated conditions and to rule out late complications (Fig. 4.7). SSFP imaging can track the connections as well as quantifying chamber size and ventricular performance, assessing the dimensions of the orifice connecting the left atrium to the pulmonary venous confluence, and detecting any residual patch leaks. Phase-contrast mapping can help in the search for evidence of any persistent shunting.

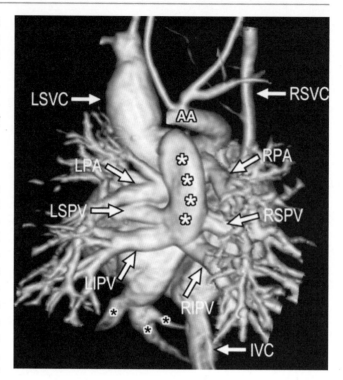

Fig. 4.6 One-month-old girl with total anomalous pulmonary venous connection, asplenia, complete atrioventricular septal defect, double-outlet right ventricle, and bilateral superior venae cavae. Contrast-enhanced volume-rendered MR image in posterior view confirms drainage of all pulmonary veins into a common pulmonary vein (*white asterisks*) that drains into a markedly dilated left superior vena cava (*LSVC*). Small right superior vena cava (*RSVC*) and inferior vena cava (*IVC*) drain into right atrium. Note portions of distal aortic arch and descending thoracic aorta have been removed on posterior image. *Black asterisks* show hepatic veins. *LSVC* left superior vena cava, *LSPV* left superior pulmonary vein, *RSPV* right superior pulmonary vein, *RIPV* right inferior pulmonary vein, *LIPV* left inferior pulmonary vein, *RPA* right pulmonary artery, *LPA* left pulmonary artery, *AA* aortic arch (Reprinted with permission from Dillman et al. [6])

4.2.4 Variation in the Number of Pulmonary Veins

The normal distribution of pulmonary veins is to have two pulmonary veins on the right and two pulmonary veins on the left. Recently, because of increased imaging by cardiac magnetic resonance imaging and CT angiography in preparation for radiofrequency ablation, significant variations in pulmonary vein number and course have been noted. In a recent study, 68 % of the patients had two ostia on the right side, one each for upper and lower lobe veins, with the middle lobe vein joining the upper lobe vein [14]. The most common variation on the right was the middle lobe vein connected directly to the left atrium and was seen in 26 % of the patients and 2 % had a single pulmonary venous ostium on the right side. Another 4 % had four or five atrial ostia on the right. There was less anatomic variability seen with the left pulmonary venous connection patterns. Two ostia, one for each of

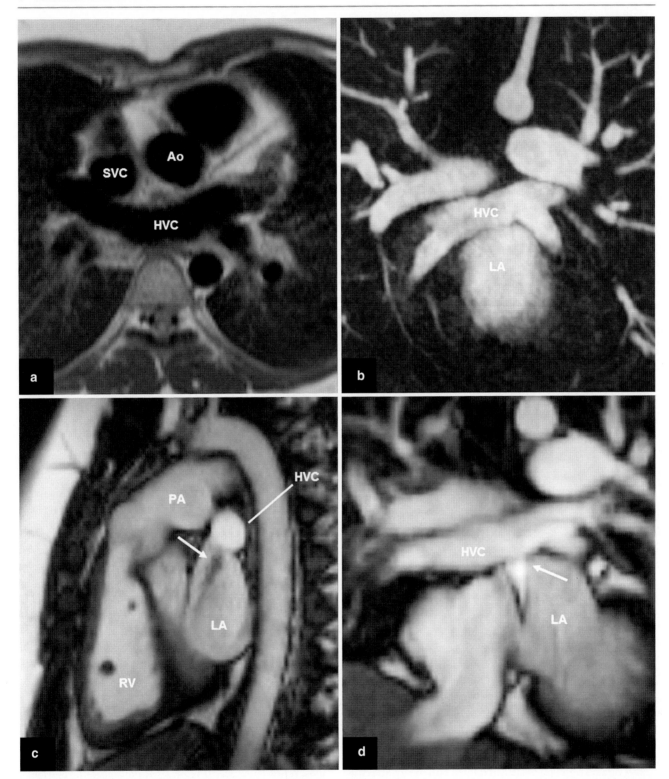

Fig. 4.7 Twenty-year old woman who had repair of a supracardiac TAPVC in infancy and is assessed for increasing dyspnea and Xray evidence of heart failure. (**a**) Single shot turbo spin echo axial image demonstrating the posterior location of the horizontal pulmonary venous confluence (*HVC*). (**b**) Contrast-enhanced Magnetic Resonance Angiography: Maximum intensity projection (*mip*) coronal image. This demonstrates the connections of the four pulmonary veins into the HVC. (**c**) Sagittal still image from SSFP cine confirming the superior location of the HVC and stenosis of the orifice between the HVC and the left atrium (*LA*). Note the hypertrophied right ventricle (*RV*). (**d**) Coronal still image from SSFP cine demonstrating the stenotic orifice and the turbulent flow into the LA (*arrow*) from the HVC. SSFP cines for (**c** and **d**) are available as Movies 4.1 and 4.2

the upper and lower lobe veins, were seen in 86 % of the patients and a common trunk forming a single ostium into the left atrium was seen in the remaining 14 %. Although abnormal number of pulmonary veins and variations of connection to the left atrium should not lead to any hemodynamic impairment, variations in the anatomy are important to document in preparation for pulmonary vein isolation procedures in the treatment of atrial fibrillation.

4.2.5 Cor Triatriatum

4.2.5.1 Cor Triatriatum and Subtotal Cor Triatriatum

Failure of incorporation of the common pulmonary vein into the left atrium will give rise to cor triatriatum. In the classic form of cor triatriatum, all the pulmonary veins enter an accessory atrial chamber that is attached to the left atrium through a narrowed orifice. There are variants where the accessory chamber receives all the pulmonary veins and does not communicate with the left atrium. In that case, there may be total anomalous pulmonary venous connection or an anomalous connection directly to the right atrium. In subtotal cor triatriatum, the accessory atrial chamber does not receive all of the pulmonary veins. The other pulmonary veins either connect normally or there is a partial anomalous pulmonary venous connection [7, 13].

4.2.5.2 Management of Patients with Cor Triatriatum

Cor triatriatum will give rise to pulmonary venous hypertension because of the obstruction to the pulmonary venous flow and patient presentation will mimic that of mitral stenosis with symptoms of dyspnea and evidence of pulmonary hypertension or even pulmonary edema. The only treatment for clinically significant cor triatriatum involves surgical excision of the left atrial membrane. This is done through a right atrial approach with a high success rate and there have been no reports of recurrence of the left atrial membrane after successful surgical excision.

4.2.5.3 Imaging for Cor Triatriatum

Expected findings associated with cor triatriatum would include right ventricular hypertrophy and dilatation, as well as right atrial enlargement. Echocardiography will be able to detect dilated right ventricle and dilated pulmonary artery as well as right ventricular hypertrophy. The apical four-chamber view may be able to delineate the cor triatriatum membrane and transesophageal echocardiography should be able to clearly demonstrate the membrane and the orifice size.

Cardiac magnetic resonance imaging will be able to demonstrate the membrane, the size of the orifice, and right sided consequences of the stenosis within that membrane leading to right ventricular hypertrophy and a dilated right atrium.

SSFP cine imaging will demonstrate the membrane and can be used to assess right-sided hypertrophy and dilatation (Fig. 4.8). SSFP cine imaging will detect the jet through the membrane and phase-contrast mapping can be used to better delineate the stenosis and gradient. Magnetic resonance angiography will confirm pulmonary venous connections and rule out anomalous connections.

4.2.6 Pulmonary Vein Stenosis

Stenosis in the pulmonary veins at their junction with the left atrium may be a consequence of abnormal incorporation of the common pulmonary vein. Congenital pulmonary vein stenosis is of two general types: a localized stenosis where the pulmonary vein has a narrowing at its junction with the left atrium; or a diffuse narrowing of the lumen of the pulmonary vein for some distance. This latter more peripheral stenosis can be considered a hypoplasia of the pulmonary vein [7]. Pulmonary vein stenosis, depending on the amount of lung drained by the stenotic vein(s), can give rise to pulmonary hypertension. Echocardiography will be useful to document the pulmonary hypertension but may have difficulty in adequately characterizing the region of stenosis. Cardiac magnetic resonance imaging and MR angiography, as well as CT angiography, will be able to localize the stenosis and allow careful measurement of the residual lumen (Fig. 4.9). In the adult patient, pulmonary vein stenosis is more likely to be an acquired lesion, as a late complication of repair of PAPVC with stenosis at the site of pulmonary vein re-implantation or due to scarring at the site of radiofrequency ablation used for pulmonary vein isolation in the treatment of atrial fibrillation.

4.2.7 CMR Sequences and Protocols for Pulmonary Venous Imaging

Our standard approach to the imaging of thoracic venous anomalies has been previously described [9]. We use multislice single shot spin-echo images (HASTE) in three orthogonal planes to define the cardiac anatomy, and supplement this with SSFP multislice images that provide a better definition of the blood-tissue borders. Turbo spin-echo imaging can often better delineate edges of atrial septal defects or sinus venosus defects (Fig. 4.2). Right and left ventricular volumes and systolic function are evaluated by using ECG-gated SSFP cine images. These SSFP cine images also can demonstrate turbulent flow and help better focus the next imaging plane. The cine phase-contrast velocity flow maps are used to enhance and define the anomalous flow patterns (Fig. 4.10) and provide the calculation of differential flows and the pulmonary to systemic blood flow ratio. Contrast-enhanced MR angiography is obtained in the coronal plane

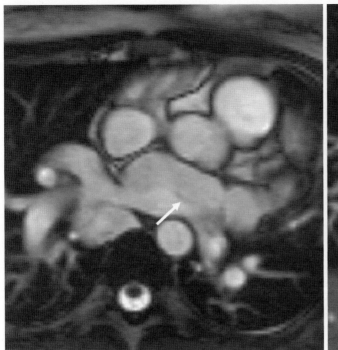 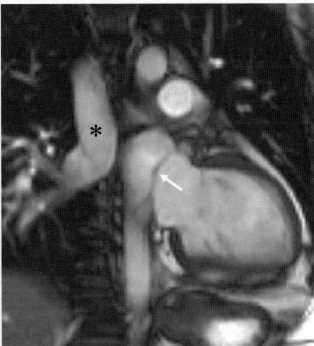

Fig. 4.8 Cor triatriatum. Cine MRI images (balanced steady state free precession sequences) acquired in transaxial plane through the left atrium (*left*) and in the left ventricular outflow tract (*right*). *Arrow* indicates cor triatriatum membrane. Note the anomalous right pulmonary venous connection to the azygos vein (*asterisk*). The movement of the membrane and the flow through the membrane can be better appreciated in the cine loops, Movies 4.3 and 4.4. (Adapted from Locca et al. [13])

during breath-hold at end inspiration before and after the IV administration of gadolinium. We time the bolus to the arrival of the contrast agent in the ascending aorta. Our standard imaging parameters for the protocol are summarized in Table 4.3.

Transverse imaging is well suited to detect the connections between anomalous pulmonary veins and the right atrium, the superior vena cava or the inferior vena cava, because of the excellent cross-sectional visualization of the caval veins and the right atrium. The ascending vein of a left PAPVC or supracardiac TAPVC will be identified in the axial view. Once these have been identified, optimal imaging planes can be selected and enhanced with cine SSFP imaging, in order to better visualize the actual areas of connection. Contrast-enhanced magnetic resonance angiography can be used to confirm the course and connections of the anomalous veins. Finally cine phase-contrast velocity flow mapping allows the calculation of the pulmonary systemic shunt ratio (Qp:Qs). Once the presence of an anomalous pulmonary venous connection is established, it is necessary to perform complete cardiac imaging, not only to assess the hemodynamic burden on the right ventricle, but also to look for associated defects, especially the sinus venosus defect. The best views for the sinus venosus defect are transverse and sagittal planes because they are perpendicular to the border between the superior vena cava and the left atrium.

Specifically SSFP cine imaging in these planes will provide a better delineation of blood tissue borders (Fig. 4.11).

4.3 Thoracic Systemic Vein Anomalies

4.3.1 Thoracic Systemic Vein Development and Anatomy

The superior vena cava (SVC) courses from the junction of the right and left innominate veins to the right atrium. It is developed from the most proximal portion of the right anterior cardinal vein and the right common cardinal vein. The left innominate vein develops at the seventh week of gestation, with the involution of the left superior vena cava [7]. The left horn of the sinus venosus and the adjacent part of the left common cardiac vein go on to form the coronary sinus. The right posterior cardinal vein gives rise to the root of the azygos vein [15].

The azygos vein is formed by the suprarenal segment of the right supracardinal vein and the cephalic remnant of the right posterior cardinal vein [7]. The azygos and hemiazygos systems can be thought of as forming an H shaped network of veins, with the azygos providing the right-sided aspect of the H while the hemiazygos provides the left lower segment and the accessory hemiazygos provides the left upper segment [15].

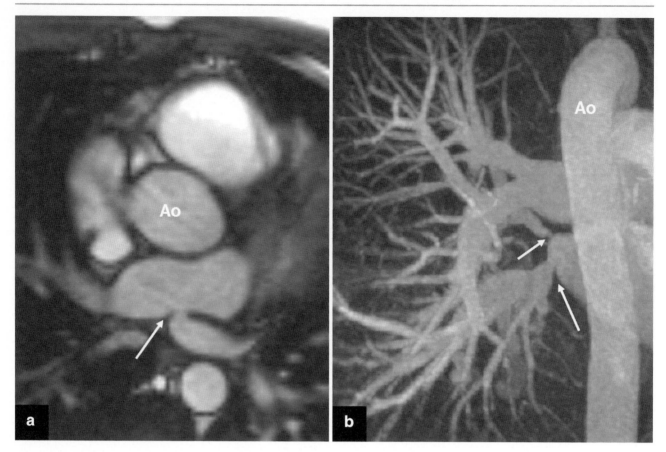

Fig. 4.9 Pulmonary vein stenosis. (**a**) Twenty-five year old woman with dyspnea. Still axial image from a SSFP cine demonstrates stenosis (*arrow*) at the connection of the left lower pulmonary vein to the left atrium. This can be better appreciated on the SSFP cine and corresponding phase contrast flow study study in Movies 4.5 and 4.6. (**b**) Thirty-four year old woman with dyspnea and dilated pulmonary artery on echocardiography. Contrast-enhanced MR angiography coronal image. *Arrows* point to the stenoses of the right lower and right upper pulmonary veins at the left atrium. *Ao* aorta

The azygos vein starts in the right lumbar region and passes through the aortic opening of the diaphragm to enter the thorax on the right of the aorta as it continues to receive drainage from the right lower ten intercostal veins. At the level of T4 it passes anteriorly to form a right sided arch that joins to the posterior aspect of the SVC. The hemiazygos vein starts at the left lumbar region and ascends along the left side of the spine to the level of T8. Then, turning right, it passes behind the aorta, and terminates in the azygos vein. The accessory hemiazygos (left upper hemiazygos) collects the left intercostal veins that did not drain into the left superior intercostal vein and either connects to the lower hemiazygos or crosses over to the right to join the azygos vein. Where there is no connection to the hemiazygos or to the azygos vein, the accessory hemiazygos may connect directly to the left innominate vein.

The inferior vena cava (IVC) is the largest vein in the body. The inferior vena cava starts at the junction of the common iliac veins (the infrarenal IVC) and travels cephalad, receiving the drainage from the renal veins, and courses posterior to the liver (hepatic IVC) where the hepatic veins join to form the suprahepatic IVC with direct drainage into the right atrium. The development of the IVC is a complex process of five venous systems involving the posterior cardinals, the right supracardinals, the subcardinals, the hepatic segment of the inferior vena cava and the hepatic veins [15].

In the normal systemic venous system, all systemic venous blood enters the right atrium via the right sided inferior vena cava and the right-sided superior vena cava which are connected to the left side by the left common iliac vein, the left renal vein, the hemiazygos vein, and the left innominate vein. In general, the anomalies of the systemic thoracic veins are unlikely to be of hemodynamic consequence. However, their identification is important because of associated cardiac and noncardiac anomalies and to differentiate the systemic venous anomalies from the more important pulmonary venous anomalies that may require more imaging and investigation.

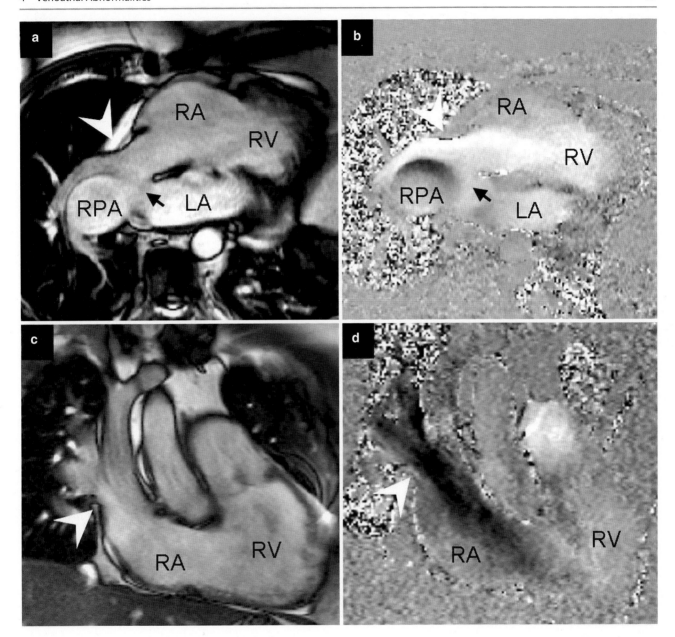

Fig. 4.10 PAPVC flow studies. Fifty-seven-year-old man with sinus venosus defect and right partial anomalous pulmonary venous connection. *LA* left atrium, *RA* right atrium, *RPA* right pulmonary artery, *RV* right ventricle. (**a** and **b**) Oblique axial steady-state free precession cine image (a) shows anomalous connection of right upper pulmonary vein (*arrowhead*). Sinus venosus defect (*arrow*) is also evident at this level. Bright white signal in this velocity flow map (**b**) confirms flow from pulmonary vein into RA. (**c** and **d**) Coronal steady-state free precession cine image (**c**) shows connection of right pulmonary vein to RA–superior vena cava junction (*arrowhead*). Dark signal in this velocity flow map (**d**) shows flow (*arrowhead*) from anomalous pulmonary vein into RA. The cines corresponding to the stills in (**c**) and (**d**) can be viewed as Movies 4.7 and 4.8 (Reprinted with permission from Kafka and Mohiaddin [9])

4.3.2 Superior Vena Cava

4.3.2.1 Persistent Left Superior Vena Cava

A persistent left superior vena cava results from the failure of the involution of the left anterior and left common cardinal veins. In the vast majority of cases, the persistent left superior vena cava drains into the right atrium through the coronary sinus. In a small number, it may drain into the left atrium by means of an unroofed coronary sinus. In many cases, the left innominate vein may still be present to connect the left superior vena cava to the right superior vena cava [7]. The size of the left superior vena cava has been noted to vary greatly and

Table 4.3 Imaging parameters

	TE (ms)	TR (R-R) (ms)	FOV (mm)	Pixel size (mm)	Slice thickness (mm)
HASTE	42	700–1,000	340–400	2.7 × 1.7	6.0
SSFP	1.13	40	340–400	1.7 × 1.7	7.0
TSE	29	700–1,000	340–400	2.2 × 1.3	6.0
CE-MRA	1.19	2.85	360–400	1.1 × 0.9	1.3
Phase contrast velocity flow mapping	3.9	75	340–400	2.5 × 1.3	6.0

SSFP steady-state free precession, *TSE* turbo spin echo, *CE-MRA* contrast enhanced magnetic resonance angiography

appears to be related to the presence and size of the left innominate vein. The left superior vena cava is commonly found in conjunction with other defects such as tetralogy of Fallot and atrioventricular septal defects but can be often present as an isolated finding. The left superior vena cava descends anterior to the aortic arch and to the left pulmonary artery, running along the posterior wall of the left atrium and into the left atrioventricular groove to drain through the coronary sinus and into the right atrium. Because of its drainage through the coronary sinus into the right atrium, there is enlargement of the coronary sinus. In fact, the echocardiographic finding of a dilated coronary sinus may often be the first indication of a persistent left superior vena cava and can be confirmed with an injection of agitated saline into the left arm to demonstrate bubble contrast in the dilated coronary sinus on echocardiography. No treatment is necessary for persistent left superior vena cava but, once identified, it will be necessary to ensure that there are no other associated defects and that there is clear documentation of a left superior vena cava. This will have future implications for the patient if consideration is ever given to insertion of a pacemaker or ablation catheter through the left subclavian vein [11].

Cardiac MRI can quickly identify the presence and the course of the left superior vena cava (Fig. 4.12). On axial imaging, a persistent left superior vena cava can be confused with an anomalous left pulmonary vein (Fig. 4.13). Phase-contrast velocity flow maps will demonstrate that the flow is directed caudad with a persistent left superior vena cava and cephalad with an anomalous left pulmonary vein draining into the left innominate vein. The simple presence of a left superior vena cava cannot account for a dilated right ventricle or other features of right-sided volume overload. In such a situation, it is important to seek out associated defects and especially to rule out the presence of an unroofed coronary sinus.

4.3.2.2 Absent Right Superior Vena Cava

This is a rare anomaly and has been reported with equal frequency in the presence of associated cardiac defects or with a normal heart. The right innominate vein drains, via the left innominate vein, to the left superior vena cava and the azygos vein is connected to the left superior vena cava. There is no clinical consequence to this finding but it is important to document the absent right superior vena cava in order to prevent problems at cardiac catheterization or with central line placement.

4.3.2.3 Superior Vena Cava to Left Atrium

There have been rare reports of the right superior vena cava draining to the left atrium [7] that can be a cause of unexplained cyanosis, with right to left shunting. This connection is due to a sinus venosus defect in conjunction with atresia of the superior vena cava orifice. If there is a patent but stenotic SVC orifice, then the superior vena cava would drain into both the right atrium and the left atrium. The standard imaging approach used to detect sinus venosus defect will demonstrate the sinus venosus defect and the SVC stenosis or atresia in this situation.

4.3.2.4 Inferior Vena Cava

Interrupted Inferior Vena Cava

The term interrupted inferior vena cava usually refers to the situation with absence of the hepatic segment of the inferior vena cava. The infrahepatic venous drainage continues via

Fig. 4.11 Sinus venosus defect with PAPVC – velocity flow maps. (**a** and **b**) Transverse images in 32-year-old man with sinus venosus defect. Steady-state free precession cine image (**a**) shows sinus venosus defect (*black arrow*) between left atrium (*LA*) and superior vena cava (*SVC*) (*asterisk*). Corresponding in-plane velocity flow map (**b**) shows dark inflow from pulmonary vein (*white arrow*) into LA crossing sinus venosus defect and entering the SVC. (**c** and **d**) Sagittal images in 35-year-old woman with sinus venosus defect. Steady-state free precession cine frame (**c**) shows superior nature of sinus venosus defect (*arrow*) between LA and SVC (*asterisk*). Corresponding in-plane velocity flow map (**d**) shows dark inflow from LA across sinus venosus defect (*arrow*) into right atrium (*RA*). (**e** and **f**) Coronal images in 18-year-old woman with sinus venosus defect. FLASH image (**e**) shows bright flow disturbance in SVC (*asterisk*) related to flow through sinus venosus defect. Through-plane velocity flow map (**f**) in same position as (**e**) shows sinus venosus defect as dark region of flow (*arrow*) from LA. *Ao* aorta. (**f**) This can be better appreciated in Movie 4.9 (Reprinted with permission from Kafka and Mohiaddin [9])

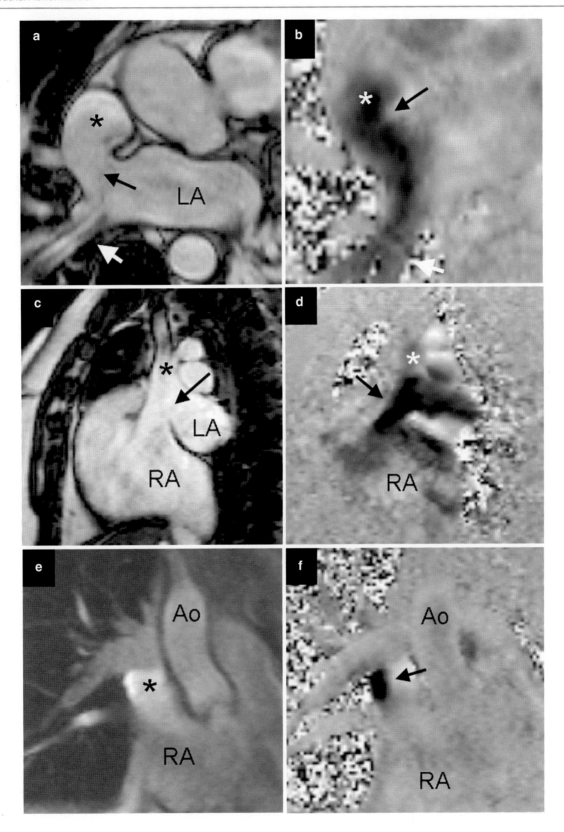

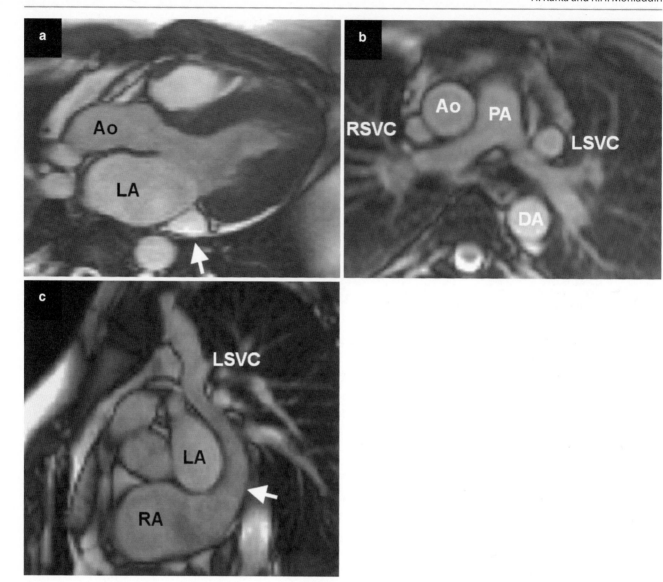

Fig. 4.12 Left superior vena cava. Still image from SSFP cine LVOT view demonstrating dilated coronary sinus (*white arrow*) posterior to the left atrium (*LA*). (**a**) Still image from SSFP cine LVOT view demonstrating dilated coronary sinus (*white arrow*) posterior to the left atrium (*LA*). (**b**) Still image from SSFP cine transverse view. The left superior vena cava (*LSVC*) is seen anterior to the left pulmonary artery. (**c**) Still image from SSFP cine sagittal oblique demonstrates the LSVC entering the dilated coronary sinus (*white arrow*) and flowing into the right atrium (*RA*). The cine from which this still is derived is available as Movie 4.10. Ao ascending aorta, DA descending aorta, RSVC right superior vena cava, PA main pulmonary artery

the azygos vein and drains into the superior vena cava, either right or left sided. The hepatic veins drain separately into the right atrium. Rarely, the IVC may continue to bilateral superior venae cavae through bilateral azygos veins [4, 7]. Another variant may involve atresia of the suprahepatic vena cava. In that case, the hepatic veins must drain into the hepatic inferior vena cava and up through the azygos system. Interrupted left sided IVC has been described with a dilated hemi-azygos vein draining normally into the azygos at T8, or draining into a persistent left superior vena cava, or draining to the upper hemiazygos vein and from there into the left innominate vein following its usual course to the right superior vena cava [5]. Interrupted IVC will not result in any

physiologic abnormality because abdominal venous return is assured. Its significance lies in its frequent association with other findings such as persistent left SVC, but especially with the heterotaxy syndrome and polysplenia. In fact, interrupted IVC is considered one of the features of the polysplenia syndrome. It may be found in the absence of other anomalies [4] and it may complicate cardiac catheterization via the route from the femoral veins. Obviously, this anomalous anatomy will have an effect on cardiac interventions such as Fontan procedure that involves surgical diversion of IVC flow [7].

Cardiac magnetic resonance imaging will reveal that the intrahepatic segment of the IVC is absent but there may be hepatic veins attached to the suprahepatic IVC, draining into

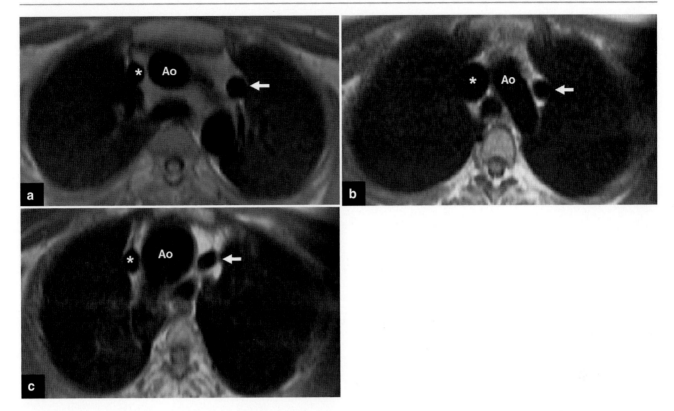

Fig. 4.13 Left sided vertical vein. Single shot turbo spin echo axial images from three different patients illustrating three different causes of a left sided vein (*arrow*). (**a**) Persistent left superior vena cava is the cause of the left sided vein in this patient –see Fig. 4.12. (**b**) Partial anomalous pulmonary venous connection with a vertical vein (*arrow*) connecting upper left pulmonary vein with the innominate vein. Note the large size of the SVC (*) – see Fig. 4.3. (**c**) Retroaortic innominate vein (*arrow*) along its vertical course before crossing under the aortic arch to join the superior vena cava. Note the right aortic arch. – see Fig. 4.16. *Ao* aorta, * superior vena cava

the right atrium. The most striking feature will be that of the markedly dilated azygos vein and the appearance of two vascular arches, the aortic arch and the azygos arch (Fig. 4.14). The finding of an interrupted IVC requires careful scrutiny to detect associated cardiac and extracardiac lesions.

Duplicated IVC

As previously postulated by Geva, the bilateral nature of the development of the IVC with five venous systems that contribute to the formation of the IVC can explain the presence of bilateral inferior venae cavae above and below the liver [7]. Bilateral suprahepatic inferior venae cavae can be frequently found in cases of visceral heterotaxy with asplenia (Fig. 4.15). There is no clinical significance to this finding, except for its association with other defects.

Inferior Vena Cava Connection to the Left Atrium

Although cases of IVC connection to the left atrium have been reported in previous reviews [18, 20], the IVC probably was connected to a left sided, but morphologically right, atrium with absence of the septum secundum, resulting in drainage of the inferior vena cava into the pulmonary veins [7]. This right to left shunting gives rise to cyanosis and to the risk of paradoxical embolization. Treatment requires surgical diversion of the inferior vena caval blood into the right atrium.

4.3.3 Azygos Vein Anomalies

Absence of the azygos vein is rare [5] and has been described with the hemiazygos vein draining most of the right and left intercostal veins. The most common congenital lesion directly affecting the azygos vein is the azygos lobe. The azygos lobe is a small accessory lobe above the hilum of the right lung. This occurs due to failure of the azygos vein to migrate over the apex of the lung during embryologic development. It is present in 1 % of people and results in no venous impairment. Its only significance is to identify it as a normal variant and to not proceed to further imaging when it is detected [5]. The most striking congenital anomalies affecting the azygos vein are linked to interrupted IVC (see above). More commonly, in the patient with congenital heart disease, the finding of a dilated azygos vein will be due to impaired drainage through the inferior vena cava or superior vena cava as a result of dilated pulmonary artery [10] or postoperative

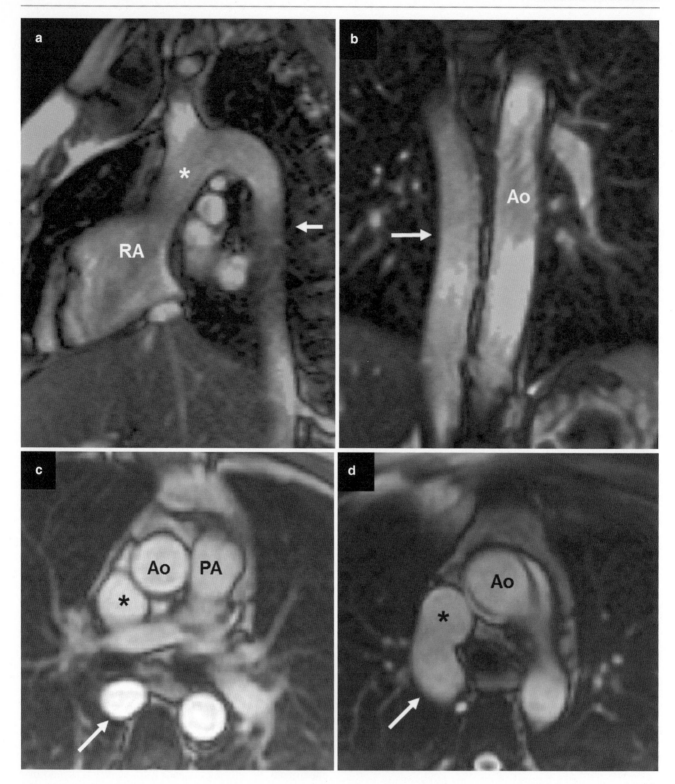

Fig. 4.14 Interrupted IVC with azygos continuation. Adult female presented with PSVT. She was referred for ablation but the right atrium could not be accessed via the femoral vein route. On MR imaging she was found to have an interrupted IVC with azygos continuation. (**a**) SSFP bright blood sagittal image demonstrating the dilated azygos vein (*arrow*) and azygos arch connecting to the superior vena cava (*). Note absence of the intrahepatic IVC. (**b**) SSFP bright blood coronal image demonstrating the double arch appearance with the dilated azygos vein (*arrow*) on the right of the aorta (*Ao*). (**c**) SSFP bright blood axial image at the level of the pulmonary artery (*PA*) bifurcation demonstrating the dilated azygos vein (*arrow*) and superior vena cava (*). (**d**) SSFP bright blood axial image caudal to plane of (**c**) demonstrating the azygos arch and the aortic arch. The *SSFP* sagittal plane cine (a) is available for viewing as Movie 4.11

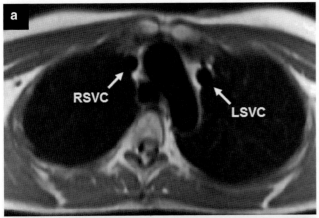

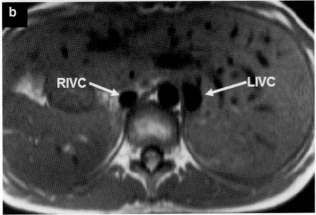

Fig. 4.15 Duplicated IVC. Sixteen year old woman with double outlet right ventricle, right atrial isomerism and asplenia. (**a**) Single shot turbo spin echo axial image at the level of the aortic arch demonstrating both a right superior vena cava (*RSVC*) and a persistent left superior vena cava (*LSVC*). (**b**) Single shot turbo spin echo axial image below the diaphragm demonstrating both a right inferior vena cava (*RIVC*) and a left inferior vena cava (*LIVC*). Note the liver on the left extending across the abdomen

complications following Mustard repair, Fontan procedure, or repair of PAPVC.

4.3.4 Anomalous Course of the Left Innominate Vein

The normal left innominate vein courses from left to right, anterior to the aortic arch, joining the right innominate to form the superior vena cava. In retroaortic innominate vein, after the left subclavian and left common jugular veins form the innominate vein, it turns to run inferiorly and then makes a right turn behind the ascending aorta and reaches the superior vena cava below the insertion of the azygos vein (Fig. 4.16). This is a rare anomaly and has no direct clinical consequence, but is usually associated with cardiac defects such as tetralogy of Fallot, atrioventricular septal defect and

coarctation of the aorta [7]. It is important to identify a retroaortic innominate vein in these patients because it may interfere with planned surgery for correction of the other defects. Care needs to be taken not to confuse the appearance of a persistent left SVC or anomalous connection of the pulmonary vein to the left innominate vein with that of a retroaortic innominate vein (Fig. 4.13). A duplicated innominate vein has been described. This has both an anterior and a retroaortic component and forms a ring that encircles the aorta [7].

4.3.5 CMR Sequences and Protocols for Thoracic Systemic Vein Imaging

The approach and imaging parameters described in 4.2.7 for pulmonary venous imaging apply equally to CMR imaging of thoracic systemic veins. Careful attention to the initial transverse images will provide clues to anomalies of the SVC, IVC, innominate vein and azygos vein. Those transverse images can then be used for choosing the optimal planes for better visualization of the identified anomalies, and to instigate a search for associated anomalies.

> **Conclusion**
>
> Veno atrial anomalies comprise a diverse set of abnormalities affecting both the pulmonary venous and the systemic thoracic venous systems. One standard cardiac magnetic resonance imaging approach (4.2.7) can be used for the evaluation of these anomalies and has the additional advantage of being able, not only, to assess for associated intracardiac and extracardiac anomalies, but also, to provide physiologic information about cardiac function and the extent of intravascular shunting, all during one cardiovascular examination. Although echocardiography still forms the basis of imaging in congenital heart disease, cardiac magnetic resonance imaging is especially of value in the imaging of these venous anomalies because the anatomic constraints of echocardiography do not apply to MR imaging and its ability to encompass a wide field of view and visualize venous structures and their course in multiple planes.

4.4 Practical Pearls

1. Every patient with unexplained pulmonary hypertension or dilated right ventricle needs to have cardiac magnetic resonance imaging to rule out PAPVC, sinus venosus defect, unroofed coronary sinus, cor triatriatum, pulmonary vein stenosis.

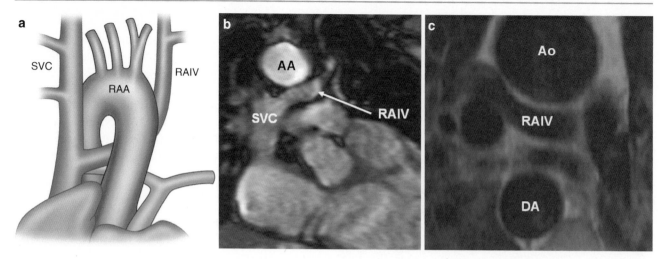

Fig. 4.16 Retroaortic innominate vein. (**a**) Diagram showing a retroaortic innominate vein (*RAIV*) associated with a right aortic arch (*RAA*). (**b**) Coronal view demonstrating the RAIV passing under the aortic arch (*AA*) to connect to the superior vena cava (*SVC*). (**c**) Axial single shot turbo spin echo showing the RAIV posterior to the ascending aorta (*Ao*). Note the descending aorta (*DA*) on the right. ((**a**) is adapted with permission from Chap. 38 (Fig. 38.15) Geva and Van Praagh [7])

2. Every patient with a right-sided PAPVC needs careful evaluation for sinus venosus defect. Every patient with sinus venosus defect needs careful evaluation for PAPVC.
3. A persistent left SVC will cause a dilated coronary sinus, but not a dilated right ventricle. The presence of a dilated right ventricle in the setting of a persistent left SVC, requires a careful search for an unroofed coronary sinus, or other source of right ventricular volume overload.
4. A left-sided vertical vein is not always a persistent left SVC. The presence of a left-sided vertical vein requires sufficient imaging to differentiate it from a left PAPVC.

References

1. Alsoufi B, Cai S, Van Arsdell GS, Williams WG, Caldarone CA, Coles JG. Outcomes after surgical treatment of children with partial anomalous pulmonary venous connection. Ann Thorac Surg. 2007;84:2020–6.
2. Ammash NM, Seward JB, Warnes CA, Connolly HM, O'Leary PW, Danielson GK. Partial anomalous pulmonary venous connection: diagnosis by transesophageal echocardiography. J Am Coll Cardiol. 1997;29:1351–8.
3. Attenhofer Jost CH, Connolly HM, Danielson GK, Bailey KR, Schaff HV, Shen W-K, Warnes CA, Seward JB, Puga FJ, Tajik AJ. Sinus venosus atrial septal defect: long-term postoperative outcome for 115 patients. Circulation. 2005;112:1953–8.
4. Bartram U, Fischer G, Kramer HH. Congenitally interrupted inferior vena cava without other features of the heterotaxy syndrome: report of five cases and characterization of a rare entity. Pediatr Dev Pathol. 2008;11:266–73.
5. Demos TC, Posniak HV, Pierce KL, Olson MC, Muscato M. Venous anomalies of the thorax. AJR Am J Roentgenol. 2004; 182:1139–50.
6. Dillman JR, Yarram SG, Hernandez RJ. Imaging of pulmonary venous developmental anomalies. AJR Am J Roentgenol. 2009; 192:1272–85.
7. Geva T, Van Praagh S. Anomalies of the pulmonary veins. Abnormal systemic venous connections. In: Allen HD, Gutgesell HP, Clark EB, Driscoll DJ, editors. Moss and Adams' heart disease in infants, children and adolescents. 7th ed. Philadelphia: Lippincott Williams & Wilkins; 2008. p. 761–817.
8. Ho ML, Bhalla S, Bierhals A, Gutierrez F. MDCT of partial anomalous pulmonary venous return (PAPVR) in adults. J Thorac Imaging. 2009;24:89–95.
9. Kafka H, Mohiaddin RH. Cardiac MRI and pulmonary MR angiography of sinus venosus defect and partial anomalous pulmonary venous connection in cause of right undiagnosed ventricular enlargement. AJR Am J Roentgenol. 2009;192:259–66.
10. Kafka H, Gatzoulis MA, Rubens MB. Superior vena cava obstruction due to markedly enlarged right pulmonary artery in Eisenmenger syndrome. Eur Heart J. 2007;28:1404.
11. Keeble W, Mohiaddin R. Technical failure to perform cardiac resynchronization therapy: use of cardiac magnetic resonance imaging techniques to clarify a left-sided superior vena cava and coronary sinus morphology. Can J Cardiol. 2008;24:589–90.
12. Krishnam MS, Tomasian A, Malik S, Singhal A, Sassani A, Laub G, Finn JP, Ruehm S. Three-dimensional imaging of pulmonary veins by a novel steady-state free-precession magnetic resonance angiography technique without the use of intravenous contrast agent: initial experience. Invest Radiol. 2009;44:447–53.
13. Locca D, Hughes M, Mohiaddin R. Cardiovascular magnetic resonance diagnosis of a previously unreported association: cor triatriatum with right partial anomalous pulmonary venous return to the azygos vein. Int J Cardiol. 2009;135:e80–2.
14. Marom EM, Herndon JE, Kim YH, McAdams HP. Variations in pulmonary venous drainage to the left atrium: implications for radiofrequency ablation. Radiology. 2004;230:824–9.
15. Mozes G, Gloviczki P. Venous embryology and anatomy. In: Bergan JJ, editor. The Vein Book. Oxford: Elsevier; 2007. p. 15–26.
16. Pascoe RD, Oh JK, Warnes CA, Danielson GK, Tajik AJ, Seward JB. Diagnosis of sinus venosus atrial septal defect with transesophageal echocardiography. Circulation. 1996;94:1049–55.

17. Prasad SK, Soukias N, Hornung T, Khan M, Pennell DJ, Gatzoulis MA, Mohiaddin RH. Role of magnetic resonance angiography in the diagnosis of major aortopulmonary collateral arteries and partial anomalous pulmonary venous drainage. Circulation. 2004;109:207–14.

18. Rahmani N, White CS. MR imaging of thoracic veins. Magn Reson Imaging Clin N Am. 2008;16:249–62.

19. Valente AM, Sena L, Powell AJ, del Nido PJ, Geva T. Cardiac magnetic resonance imaging evaluation of sinus venosus defects: comparison to surgical findings. Pediatr Cardiol. 2007;28:51–6.

20. White CS, Baffa JM, Haney PJ, Pace ME, Campbell AB. MR imaging of congenital anomalies of thoracic veins. Radiographics. 1997;17:595–608.

Septal Defects

5

Sharon L. Roble and Subha V. Raman

5.1 Introduction

Atrial and ventricular septal defects are some of the most common congenital heart lesions seen in patients today [1, 2]. Standard imaging used to consist primarily of echocardiography with catheterization to quantify the degree of shunting and potential need for repair. However, with the advent of high-resolution, volumetric techniques optimized for imaging cardiac anatomy and physiology, cardiovascular magnetic resonance (CMR) now plays a major role in the treatment and evaluation of children and adults with septal defects. CMR can provide structural as well as functional information which reduces the need for invasive procedures such as cardiac catheterizations. This chapter focuses on CMR of atrial and ventricular septal defects.

5.2 Definition

Atrial septal defects are defects located within the interatrial septum and are due to both anomalies of septation and venous development. Atrial septal defects are the most common congenital heart disease detected in adulthood, accounting for one-third of cases. Overall, atrial septal defects account for 7–11 % of all congenital heart disease.

Ventricular septal defects are any defects within the interventricular septum and are the most common congenital heart disease at birth [2]. VSDs can occur in isolation or with other associated anomalies.

5.3 Morphology

There are five types of atrial septal defects (Fig. 5.1):
1. Secundum defects are the most common (75 %) and are due to an absence of tissue at the fossa ovalis (Fig. 5.2).
2. Primum defects occur in the inlet portion of the atrial septum and are a form of endocardial cushion (atrioventricular) defect.
3. Sinus venosus defects account for 5–10 % of ASDs and are found high in the septum where the superior vena cava enters the right atrium.
4. Coronary sinus defects are rare (<1 % of cases) and usually associated with other congenital anomalies.
5. Patent foramen ovale is actually a failure of closure of the physiologic fossa ovalis, and occurs in 25–30 % of the general population.

The ventricular septum is made up of four components:
- *Inlet septum*: separates the mitral and tricuspid valves and has also been called AV canal septum.
- *Trabecular (muscular) septum*: extends from the attachments of the tricuspid leaflets outward toward the apex and upward to the crista supraventricularis.
- *Outlet (infundibular) septum*: is a smooth walled structure, extends from the crista supraventricularis to the pulmonic valve.
- *Membranous septum*: lies between the anterior and septal leaflets of tricuspid valve just below the aortic valve.

Ventricular septal defects are classified as *perimembranous*, *outlet*, *inlet*, or *muscular* (Fig. 5.1). Perimembranous defects involve the membranous portion of the septum and extend into the adjacent inlet, outlet, or muscular septum. This is the most common defect, accounting for 70–80 % of all cases. Perimembranous VSDs may also be called infracristal or membranous defects.

S.L. Roble, M.D.
Department of Cardiology, The Ohio State University,
473 West 12th Avenue, 200 DHLRI, Columbus, OH 43210, USA
e-mail: sharon.roble@osumc.edu

S.V. Raman, M.D., MSEE (✉)
CMR/CT, The Ohio State University,
473 West 12th Avenue, Suite 200, Columbus, OH 43210, USA
e-mail: raman.1@osu.edu

Electronic supplementary material The online version of this chapter (doi:10.1007/978-1-4471-4267-6_5) contains supplementary material, which is available to authorized users.

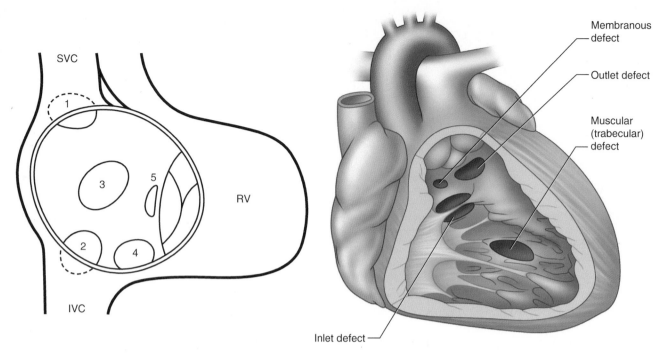

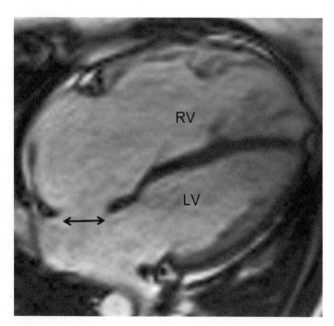

Fig. 5.1 Types of atrial (*left*) and ventricular (*right*) septal defects. Atrial septal defect types include *1* and *2* sinus venosus, *3* secundum, *4* coronary sinus, and *5* primum. *SVC* superior vena cava, *IVC* inferior vena cava, *RV* right ventricle (Figure on *right* reproduced with permission from Wolters Kluwer Health, Inc. – Lippincott Williams & Wilkins)

Fig. 5.2 Still frame from a horizontal long-axis cine acquisition depicts a large secundum atrial septal defect with the *arrow* along the length of the defect. Note relative enlargement of the right ventricle (*RV*) compared to the left ventricle (*LV*)

Outlet ventricular septal defects account for 5–7 % of all ventricular septal defects and are found within the right ventricular outflow tract. These defects are also known as supracristal,

infundibular, conal, or subpulmonary defects. Inlet defects are found posterior and inferior to the membranous septum beneath the septal leaflet of the tricuspid valve and account for 5–8 % of all ventricular defects. Muscular septal defects account for 5–20 % of all ventricular septal defects (Fig. 5.3, Movie 5.1). Muscular defects can occur in any portion of the septum and multiple defects occur frequently giving the appearance of "swiss cheese". Seventy-five to eighty percent of ventricular septal defects close spontaneously before adolescence.

5.4   Associated Anomalies

5.4.1   Atrial Septal Defects

- Secundum defects are often found in isolation; however, they may also be seen with complex congenital heart disease or with syndromes such as Holt-Oram (secundum ASD, upper limb abnormalities), Noonan Syndrome (secundum ASD, pulmonic valve stenosis, typical facies) or Lutembacher Syndrome (secundum ASD and mitral stenosis).
- Cleft mitral valve (Fig. 5.4, Movie 5.2) and mitral regurgitation are seen with primum atrial septal defects and are part of the spectrum of AV canal or endocardial cushion defects.

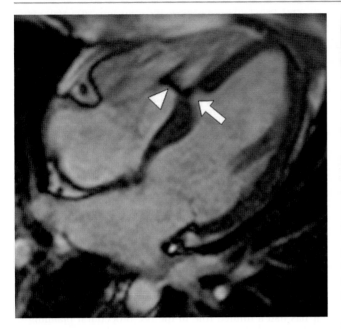

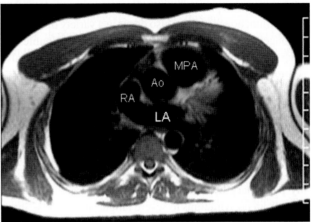

Fig. 5.5 Dark blood axial turbo spin echo image demonstrates a sinus venosus atrial septal defect at the superior aspect of the interatrial septum. *RA* right atrium, *LA* left atrium, *Ao* aorta, *MPA* main pulmonary artery

Fig. 5.3 A muscular ventricular septal defect is evident (*arrow*) on this systolic frame from a horizontal long axis cine acquisition. Also note the turbulent flow into the right ventricle through the defect (*arrowhead*)

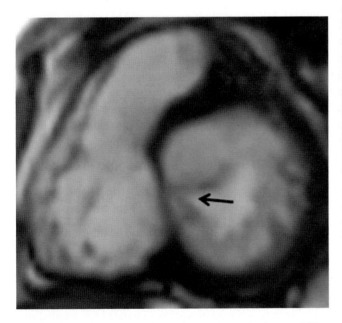

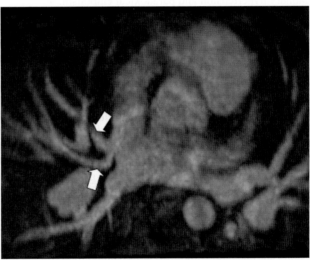

Fig. 5.6 Contrast-enhanced 3D magnetic resonance angiogram rendered as a maximum intensity projection in an oblique axial plane shows several pulmonary veins (*arrows*) draining in an anomalous fashion in association with a sinus venosus atrial septal defect

5.4.2 Ventricular Septal Defects

- Perimembranous ventricular septal defects are frequently associated with minor abnormalities of the tricuspid valve. These tricuspid valve anomalies include extra septal leaflet tissue or pouches (ventricular septal aneurysms) that may partially or completely occlude the defect.
- Aortic regurgitation may occur with perimembranous or outlet defects due to prolapse of an aortic valve cusp into the defect. Prolapse of the aortic valve may result in partial or complete closure of the septal defect over time with resultant aortic regurgitation.

Fig. 5.4 This basal short axis frame from a short-axis cine acquisition demonstrates a cleft mitral valve (*arrow*) that occurred in association with an ostium primum atrial septal defect

- Sinus venosus ASDs are often associated with anomalous pulmonary venous return (Figs. 5.5 and 5.6). The most common pulmonary venous anomaly involves drainage of the right pulmonary veins into the right atrium through the defect.

of large unrepaired ventricular septal defects in which there is equalization of right and left ventricular pressures and, in turn, equalization of stroke volume. As with any volumetric technique, accurate assessment of the endocardial borders is crucial to obtain correct measurements which impact clinical decision making.

Once the planes have been prescribed, the next step involves setting the appropriate VENC which should be slightly above the maximal expected velocity to avoid aliasing. Excessively high VENC settings for the expected peak velocity will adversely affect precision in measurement. When calculating Qp:Qs using planes through the aortic root and pulmonary artery, initial VENC settings of 150–200 cm/s are reasonable. Associated stenotic valvular or sub/supravalvular disease may further increase the systolic velocities in the aorta or pulmonary arteries, and the VENC setting can be incrementally advanced until aliasing is eliminated.

In-plane imaging for septal defects can also be performed and give valuable information about the degree and direction of shunting. For atrial septal defects with low flows, the VENC should be set at 50–100 cm/s. For large ventricular septal defects, VENC is set at 150 cm/s. For small, restrictive ventricular septal defects, VENC may need to be set considerably higher due to the marked pressure gradient between left and right ventricles. Note that once right ventricular systolic pressures start to increase due to development of pulmonary hypertension, the peak velocity decreases due to diminished LV-RV gradient and shunt flow may diminish or even reverse (Eisenmenger physiology).

For atrial septal defects, systematic prescription of in-plane and finally through-plane velocity-encoded cines can yield an *en face* view of flow through the defect (Fig. 5.7). This, in turn, allows planimetric measurement of the defect and aids in planning percutaneous transcatheter closure, particularly of secundum defects.

5.6.2.3 Contrast Angiography (MRA)

Dynamic or first-pass contrast-enhanced MR angiography is a useful, qualitative way to evaluate for intracardiac shunting (Fig. 5.8, Movie 5.5), although small defects with minimal shunting may be missed with this technique. One clue to an intracardiac shunt may come from inspecting signal intensity-vs.-time curves that simultaneously display contrast transit through right vs. left heart chambers; for instance, an early recirculation secondary peak in the right heart curve may indicate left-to-right shunting.

Three-dimensional contrast-enhanced MR angiography may also be useful in detecting concomitant pulmonary vein anomalies that may occur with atrial septal defects, classically abnormal drainage of right pulmonary veins in sinus venosus ASDs or persistent left-sided superior vena cava draining into the coronary sinus [8]. Missing pulmonary venous anomalies may result in poor outcomes when referring

patients for transcatheter or surgical repair due to the unaddressed defects. Angiography may also be useful to further assess the aortic size when indicated, such as in the patient with tetralogy of Fallot who requires surgical repair for aortic root enlargement and residual VSD. Finally, noncontrast whole-heart MRA techniques are now widely available, and may be of particular appeal in the patient for whom gadolinium-based contrast administration may be contraindicated, such as the pregnant female who requires CMR-based assessment of congenital heart disease or in patients with advanced renal dysfunction.

5.6.2.4 Late Gadolinium Enhancement CMR (LGE-CMR)

LGE-CMR has become a relied-upon technique to noninvasively delineate ventricular myocardial scar of various etiologies, but may also highlight defects of the ventricular septum (Fig. 5.9). Although not an essential acquisition in all cases of septal defects, LGE-CMR may in some instances add valuable information. In a patient whose prior congenital heart disease and surgical history is not available, demonstration of an apical scar in an otherwise normal-functioning left ventricle suggests prior apical venting that has been used in the past to approach various lesions. There may be an occasional patient who has previously undergone VSD surgical repair may develop arrhythmias related to scar at the repair site, and LGE-CMR may aid in planning ablative procedures by localizing regions of scar. Right ventricular scar has been described in various congenital defects, most notably repaired Tetrology of Fallot. If including LGE in the CMR protocol, standard acquisition planes should be included i.e. long axis planes, outflow tract views, and a stack of short axis planes, all with inversion time optimally selected to null normal myocardium. Imaging atrial scar, which holds particular appeal given frequency of atrial arrhythmias in patients with congenital heart disease, remains a technique in development.

Typical CMR protocol elements in assessing septal defects are summarized in Table 5.1.

5.7 Discussion

CMR has become an invaluable noninvasive imaging modality in the evaluation of congenital heart disease, including septal defects. With CMR, intracardiac and extracardiac structures can be imaged in any plane or volume to yield detailed anatomic information about the intracardiac septae. Just as valuable, particularly in patients for whom presence of a defect has already been established, is the physiological information yielded by CMR – need for parameters such as RV ejection fraction and Qp:Qs remains a leading CMR referral indication. Adult patients with congenital heart disease

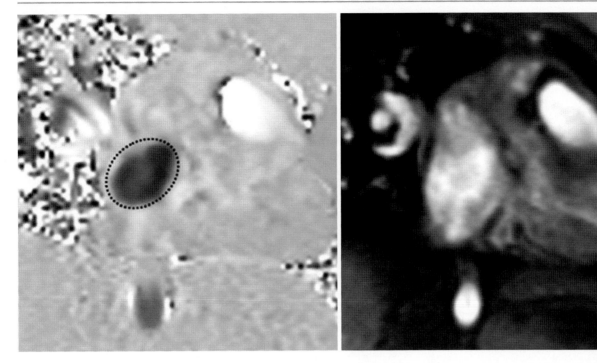

Fig. 5.7 Through-plane velocity-encoded cine acquisition prescribed after several iterations of in-plane and through-plane imaging demonstrates an *en face* view of a large secundum atrial septal defect, encircled on the velocity-encoded image on the *left*. The *right* image is the corresponding reference image that helps delineate the anatomy corresponding to sites of flow

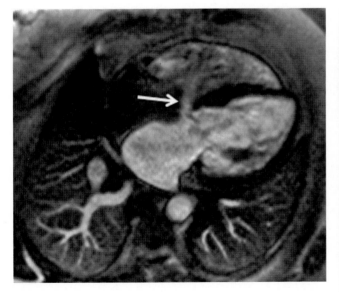

Fig. 5.8 A frame from a first-pass contrast enhancement acquisition in the horizontal long-axis plane demonstrates intracardiac shunt flow (*arrow*) in a patient with a primum atrial septal defect

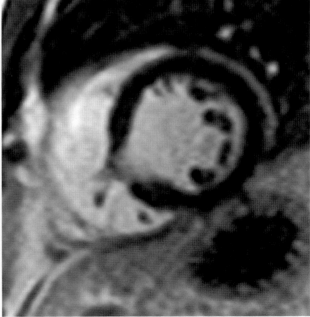

Fig. 5.9 Late post-gadolinium enhancement imaging demonstrates a discontinuity in the interventricular septum in a patient with a muscular ventricular septal defect

have often undergone surgical procedures resulting in scar tissue and other artifacts which impair echocardiographic windows and deliver limited transthoracic echo-based information. Echocardiography also provides incomplete visualization of vasculature and associated anomalies. This is especially problematic in patients with unrepaired defects,

when planning requires recognition of concomitant anomalous pulmonary venous drainage as the approach may be modified by recognition of altered pulmonary artery architecture due to

Table 5.1 Sample CMR protocol for septal defect assessment

Scan	Plane/volume of acquisition
Localizer scans	Axial, sagittal, coronal; cardiac planes
Dark blood imaging e.g. HASTE or TSE	Axial, sagittal and coronal stacks; additional planes of interest
Cine imaging	HLA, VLA, three-chamber, left ventricular outflow, right ventricular outflow; SAX stack, may include atria and pulmonary veins; additional planes of interest e.g. horizontal long axis stack to localize defect(s)
Phase contrast imaging	Through-plane flow measurement through aortic root and main pulmonary artery; serial in-plane velocity-encoded and through plane velocity-encoded acquisitions along regions of interest to localize defects and quantify size and flow
First-pass perfusion imaging	Planes of interest e.g. HLA, 3-chamber
Whole-heart navigator or contrast-enhanced magnetic resonance angiogram	Coronal or appropriate volume for pulmonary vein or other vascular assessment
Late gadolinium enhancement imaging	Typically in the same planes as cine imaging

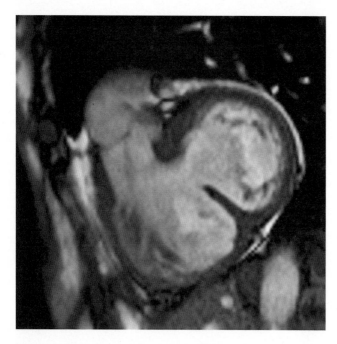

Fig. 5.10 Basal short axis frame demonstrates a large ventricular septal defect that was unrepaired in a patient who presented with Eisenmenger physiology

long-standing right heart volume overload. CMR does not require an 'acoustic window', as the signal emanates from abundant protons throughout all tissues and is generally unaffected by changes in body habitus over time, presuming the patient can fit in the MR scanner. Most surgical repairs do not impair MR-based imaging, save the occasional embolization coil or other implanted material that produces widespread susceptibility artifact.

CMR may be the ideal modality for noninvasive pulmonary and systemic blood flow measurement, the ratio of which provides insight into the hemodynamic significance of septal defects. As previously described, there have been several small studies which have demonstrated good agreement between phase contrast CMR and invasive oximetry evaluation of pulmonary and systemic blood flow both in children and adults with congenital heart disease. However, echo is more sensitive in detecting small defects that may have minimal hemodynamic effect but still have clinical sequelae, such as a portal for paradoxical embolism. Also, shunt flow may be minimal in the patient who has developed Eisenmenger physiology; a large septal defect evident on anatomic imaging (Figs. 5.10 and 5.11) without corresponding appreciable shunt flow should raise suspicion of such.

With the development of multi-slice scanners with electrocardiographic gating, computed tomography (CT) has increasingly become a useful modality for congenital heart disease imaging [9]. CT can be used to evaluate both the interatrial and interventricular septae in patients with any of the standard contraindications to magnetic resonance (e.g. presence of ferromagnetic foreign bodies or active implants such as pacemakers) who also have poor echo windows. In instances where implanted material may be MR-compatible but susceptibility artifact limits utility of CMR, cardiovascular computed tomography (CCT) may be an alternative modality for imaging heart and vascular structures, albeit without delivering as much physiological and hemodynamic information. With its requirement for ionizing radiation exposure to produce images, CCT is almost never the first imaging modality chosen in children, and this limitation is increasingly part of the decision-making process when choosing among various imaging modalities for adult patients with CHD.

5.8 Limitations and Pitfalls

Limitations of magnetic resonance imaging in evaluating the atrial and ventricular septum can be minimized by selecting the appropriate patients for imaging, obtaining and reviewing patients previous imaging studies and adjusting

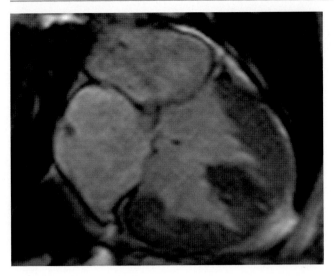

Fig. 5.11 Horizontal long-axis cine frame demonstrates a large unrepaired ventricular septal defect in a patient with Eisenmenger physiology

protocols as needed during image acquistion to optimize image quality and accuracy of data. While several studies have shown good correlation between phase contrast CMR and invasive oximetry in the assessment of pulmonary and systemic blood flows, there may be variable results when assessing shunt calculations with through-plane imaging directly through the defects. In very young patients, sedation or anesthesia with ventilatory support may be necessary to complete CMR examination; as these may also be needed with invasive catheterization, the elimination of radiation exposure and arterial/venous cannulation may make CMR the more appealing modality for diagnosis.

Conclusions

Atrial and ventricular septal defects are some of the most common congenital heart lesions in both children and adults. Because of its accuracy and reproducibility, plus high spatial and temporal resolution for delivery of anatomical and physiological information, CMR has become an invaluable non-invasive technique for evaluating patients with septal defects. As the number of adults with congenital heart disease continue to increase, it will be imperative that physicians performing and interpreting CMR have an understanding of the techniques necessary for imaging patients with congenital heart disease [10]. Close interaction with the referring cardiologist both before and after the examination and use of structured reporting in accordance with societal guidelines [11] will insure that a high quality service is provided with the greatest value to individual patient care.

5.9 Practical Pearls

- The patient referred for CMR to evaluate septal defects has almost always first undergone evaluation with transthoracic echocardiography. Results of such should always be reviewed in planning the CMR examination.
- Delineation of atrial septal defect(s) by CMR requires careful, serial examination of the interatrial septum with both in-plane as well as through-plane and ultimately *en face* velocity-encoded acquisitions.
- Shunt fraction can be readily estimated by obtaining the ratio of pulmonary to aortic flow via through-plane velocity-encoded cines through the proximal main pulmonary artery and aortic root.
- Ventricular septal defects may have complex three-dimensional anatomy, particularly those involving the perimembranous septum. Demonstration of not only the defect but also any associated valvular abnormalities is important in pre-repair planning.
- Anomalous pulmonary venous return can usually be identified by contiguous, single heartbeat dark blood imaging covering the chest. Occasionally, additional 3D MRA is needed to precisely define the number and locations of pulmonary veins. This can be done either with or without contrast.
- Communicating with the referring physician before and after the procedure helps maximize utility of the CMR examination in guiding patient care.

References

1. Warnes CA. ACC/AHA 2008 guidelines for the management of adults with congenital heart disease: a report of the American college of cardiology/American heart association task force on practice guidelines (writing committee to develop guidelines on the management of adults with congenital heart disease). developed in collaboration with the American society of echocardiography, heart rhythm society, international society for adult congenital heart disease, society for cardiovascular angiography and interventions, and society of thoracic surgeons. J Am Coll Cardiol. 2008; 52(23):e1–121.
2. Hoffman JI, Kaplan S. The incidence of congenital heart disease. J Am Coll Cardiol. 2002;39(12):1890–900.
3. Teo KSL, et al. Assessment of atrial septal defects in adults comparing cardiovascular magnetic resonance with transesophageal echocardiography. J Cardiovasc Magn Reson. 2010;12:44.
4. McCarthy KP, Ching Leung PK, Ho SY. Perimembranous and muscular ventricular septal defects--morphology revisited in the era of device closure. J Interv Cardiol. 2005;18(6):507–13.
5. Thomson LE, et al. Direct en face imaging of secundum atrial septal defects by velocity-encoded cardiovascular magnetic resonance in patients evaluated for possible transcatheter closure. Circ Cardiovasc Imaging. 2008;1(1):31–40.
6. Beerbaum P, et al. Noninvasive quantification of left-to-right shunt in pediatric patients: phase-contrast cine magnetic resonance imaging

compared with invasive oximetry. Circulation. 2001; 103(20):2476–82.

7. Debl K, et al. Quantification of left-to-right shunting in adult congenital heart disease: phase-contrast cine MRI compared with invasive oximetry. Br J Radiol. 2009;82(977):386–91.

8. Kafka H, Mohiaddin RH. Cardiac MRI and pulmonary MR angiography of sinus venosus defect and partial anomalous pulmonary venous connection in cause of right undiagnosed ventricular enlargement. AJR Am J Roentgenol. 2009;192(1):259–66.

9. Cook SC, Raman SV. Multidetector computed tomography in the adolescent and young adult with congenital heart disease. J Cardiovasc Comput Tomogr. 2008;2(1):36–49.

10. Kilner PJ, et al. Recommendations for cardiovascular magnetic resonance in adults with congenital heart disease from the respective working groups of the European Society of Cardiology. Eur Heart J. 2010;31(7):794–805.

11. Hundley WG, et al. Society for cardiovascular magnetic resonance guidelines for reporting cardiovascular magnetic resonance examinations. J Cardiovasc Magn Reson. 2009;11:5.

Right Ventricular Anomalies

Frédérique Bailliard and Marina L. Hughes

6.1 Introduction

The advantages of cardiovascular magnetic resonance (CMR) imaging for static and dynamic characterization of the right ventricle are increasingly being realized. The advantages are even more pronounced when imaging the right ventricle affected by congenital malformation, in every age group.

The right ventricle (RV) has notoriously been difficult to image by two-dimensional echocardiography as well as cardiac catheterization for multiple reasons:

- The anterior position of the RV in the chest can result in poor acoustic echocardiographic windows, preventing accurate assessments of the RV free wall, or of an unusually positioned outflow tract.
- The right ventricular outflow tract (RVOT) formed by the outlet septum, the ventriculo-infundibular fold and the septomarginal trabeculations can be difficult to conceptualize, particularly when malformed, and even more so when the great arteries are malpositioned.
- The complex anatomy of the RV cavity precludes simple mathematical models for providing quantitative functional data.

In congenital heart disease, the RV therefore becomes more challenging to image, while simultaneously playing a disproportionately important role in the pathophysiology. CMR imaging, not limited by the location of the RV in the chest, has the ability to provide high-resolution anatomical and functional data for morphologically abnormal right ventricles, or those affected by abnormal loading conditions.

In this chapter we will provide an overview of CMR imaging of the abnormal right ventricle, with reference to specific lesions. We will provide a methodical, fundamental imaging protocol (Table 6.1), with appropriate modifications guided by the pathophysiology and surgical techniques for individual lesions. We will discuss four principal subtypes of "abnormal RV":

- The RV with abnormal great artery position: double outlet RV
- The RV with abnormal division of the trabeculations: double-chambered RV
- The RV with abnormal pulmonary outlet: pulmonary atresia with intact ventricular septum
- The RV with abnormal afterload: pulmonary arterial hypertension and Eisenmenger syndrome

6.2 Right Ventricular Imaging and Analysis

As discussed in other chapters, with any anatomic or functional assessment, the accuracy of CMR imaging of the heart with an abnormal RV critically depends on image position, the technical quality of the images (temporal and spatial resolution) and the post-processing techniques. Much subjectivity, and therefore poor reproducibility, can be introduced by imprecise or non-systematic methods of post-processing and measurement, even in the setting of excellent image quality.

Planning the slice positions for acquisition of a short axis stack of images to cover the RV, requires more attention than an axial stack, and begins with careful acquisition of long-axis images utilized to plan the stack. The RV long axis view must transect the right-sided atrioventricular valve (AVV) and the RV apex. The short axis stack is subsequently planned

F. Bailliard, M.D., M.S. (✉)
Centre for Cardiovascular Imaging, Great Ormond Street Hospital for Children NHS Trust, London, UK

Bailliard Henry Pediatric Cardiology,
2304 Wesvill Court, Raleigh, NC 27607, USA
e-mail: fredebailliard@gmail.com

M.L. Hughes, DPhil, MRCP, FRACP
Centre for Cardiovascular Imaging, Great Ormond Street Hospital for Children NHS Trust, London, UK

Cardiorespiratory Unit, Great Ormond Street Hospital for Children Foundation Trust, Great Ormond Street, London WC1N 3JH, UK
e-mail: marina.hughes@gosh.nhs.uk

Electronic supplementary material The online version of this chapter (doi:10.1007/978-1-4471-4267-6_6) contains supplementary material, which is available to authorized users.

Table 6.1 Example of the standard sequences and views of a routine congenital cardiac scan with additional images (marked with an asterisk) to complete a comprehensive 'RV assessment', in the order of workflow

	Sequence	Planning	1° purpose	2° purpose
Scout	Single shot bSSFP images.	Contiguous slices in all three radiological planes covering all relevant anatomy.	Isocentering of the heart in the scanner.	Preview of thoracic anatomy. May be used for planning should other images be unable to be obtained.
Axial stack	Respiratory-navigated, ECG-gated, 'black-blood' images (HASTE or TSE). Contiguous axial slices.	Coverage from liver to neck Include aortic arch and proximal head and neck vessels. Include systemic and pulmonary veins.	Planning subsequent cine imaging planes.	Provides a map of thoracic anatomy.
Ventricular long-axis (RVLA, LVLA)	Breath-held, ECG-gated, bSSFP cine images.	From axial stack Place perpendicular plane through long axis of ventricle, from mid-atrioventricular (AV) valve to ventricular apex.	Planning the true 4-chamber image.	Assessment of anterior and inferior myocardium, AV valves, ventricular sizes.
AV Valves	Breath-held, ECG-gated, bSSFP cine image.	From axial stack Place perpendicular plane parallel to, and on apical side of AV valve. Check orientation is parallel to the vertical axis of the AV valves on RVLA and LVLA views. The image should include base of aortic valve in systole.	Planning the 4-chamber and LV outflow tract (LVOT) images.	Subjective evaluation of AV valve morphology and function.
4-chamber view	Breath-held, ECG-gated, bSSFP cine image.	From AV valves and VLA views. Place perpendicular plane across both AV valve orifices. From LVLA cine check that this plane passes through mid-mitral valve and LV apex. From RVLA check that the plane passes through mid-tricuspid valve and RV apex.	Subjective assessment of atrial volumes, biventricular volumes and function, ventricular wall motion, AV valve regurgitation.	Planning short axis (SA) stack.
Short-axis (SA) stack	Breath-held, ECG-gated, bSSFP cine image.	From end-diastolic frame of 4-chamber cine. Place perpendicular plane at hingepoints of both AV valves, with special care to include the entire basal ventricular blood pool. From VLA views, check the first slice is perpendicular to AV valve hingepoints Contiguous slices are then placed to cover the entire ventricular mass to the apex.	Provides the images required for segmentation of ventricular volumes.	Assessment of the ventricular septum, ventricular myocardial morphology, wall motion abnormalities and outflow tracts.

MR angiogram	Breath-held, not ECG-gated.	Isotropic voxels (1.1–1.6 mm)	Angiographic views of large and small thoracic vessels. Images less subject to artifact caused by low velocity or turbulent flow.	Subjective determination of preferential blood flow.
	Gadolinium injection 0.2–0.4 mL/kg.	Planned on axial HASTE stack, for sagittally-orientated raw data.	The second pass acquisition allows assessment of systemic and pulmonary venous anatomy	Can be expanded to perform time-resolved angiography or four-dimensional angiography.
	Infants: injection rate 2 mL/s with 5 mL flush.	Include antero-posterior chest wall, lung fields		
	Older children: injection rate	Image acquisition triggered with bolus-tracking to ensure maximum signal in structure of interest.		
	3 mL/s, 10 mL flush.	Two acquisitions routinely acquired, with no interval in young children, or a 15 s interval in older children.		
3D bSSFP	Free breathing, respiratory navigated, ECG-gated.	Planned on axial HASTE stack for sagittally oriented raw data.	Provides high-resolution images of intracardiac anatomy, including coronary arteries.	Planning further imaging planes in patients with complex anatomy.
	Data acquisition optimized to occur during cardiac standstill.	Include entire heart, pulmonary arteries and veins, aortic arch.	Allows multiplanar reformatting.	
	Signal improved following gadolinium injection.	Isotropic voxels (1.1–1.6 mm).		
	Signal improved in tachycardic patients by triggering acquisition with every second heartbeat.	Respiratory navigator placed mid-right dome of diaphragm, avoiding cardiac region of interest.		
	Acquisition time 8–15 min.			
Delayed Enhancement	Free breathing, single shot true-FISP inversion recovery images.	Copy image position and parameters of the SA stack.	Screen for myocardial fibrosis or scar.	Determine if segmented, breath-held delayed enhancement should be performed.
		Adjust inversion time (TI) to null normal myocardium.		
LV outflow tract	Breath-held, ECG-gated, bSSFP cine image.	From the AV valves cine.	Outflow tract morphology, subjective assessment of semilunar valve function.	Planning phase contrast velocity mapping.
		Place a perpendicular plane through both basal aortic valve and mid-mitral valve orifice.		Planning "en-face" view of semilunar valve.
		Check orientation passes through LV apex using LVLA cine.		
		Cross-cut this view to obtain two orthogonal cine views of LVOT.		

(continued)

Table 6.1 (continued)

	Sequence	Planning	1° purpose	2° purpose
RV outflow tract	Breath-held, ECG-gated, bSSFP cine image.	From axial stack. Place perpendicular plane through the pulmonary trunk. Cross-cut this view to obtain two orthogonal cine views of RVOT.	Outflow tract morphology. Subjective assessment of semilunar valve function.	Planning phase contrast velocity mapping. Planning "en-face" view of semilunar valve.
*RV in/out	Breath-held, ECG-gated, bSSFP cine image.	From 4-chamber cine and RVOT sagittal cine. Place a perpendicular plane across the TV in 4-chamber cine. Ensure the plane crosses the RVOT in the RVOT sagittal cine.	Assess RV free wall motion. Additional profile of infundibulum.	
*Branch PA	Breath-held, ECG-gated, bSSFP cine images.	Images 1 and 2: From MRA, create MPR of the sagittal and coronal view of the RPA and of the LPA. Image 3: from images 1 and 2, plan the axial image of the confluence of the branches.	Assess the dynamic nature of the branch PAs Assess the PA confluence.	
Great artery flow	Non-breath held, ECG-gated, through-Plane Phase contrast flow velocity mapping.	From the orthogonal outflow tract images. Place a perpendicular plane across the vessel of interest. Place plane just distal to valve leaflets in systole, to avoid turbulent areas of flow. Optimise velocity encoding to maximize accuracy and prevent aliasing.	Vessel flow volume. Calculate regurgitant fractions (RF%). Validate ventricular stroke volume measurements.	Calculate pulmonary blood flow to systemic blood flow ratio (Qp:Qs), Evaluate presence and location of shunts. Calculate flow velocity.
*Branch PA flow	Non-breath held, ECG-gated, through-plane phase contrast flow velocity mapping.	From orthogonal views of the branch PA. Place perpendicular plane across the RPA and the LPA.	Assess the ratio of net forward branch PA flow. Assess regurgitant fraction of each PA.	Calculate flow velocity. Validate MPA flow.

in a plane parallel to the right-sided atrioventricular valve (AVV) and perpendicular to the ventricular septum in order to minimize partial-volume effects caused by the myocardial-blood pool interface. In cases of dilated right ventricles, one must take care to acquire sufficient slices into the right atrium to obtain the entire basal ventricular volume, particularly in diastole. Inaccurate interpretation of ventricular volumes at the basal slices is frequently responsible for observer variation in short axis stack volumetric analysis [1] and must not be overlooked at the time of image acquisition.

Post-processing of cine images to calculate ventricular volumes and systolic function is usually performed off-line, using commercially available software. The segmentation of the blood pool and myocardial border can be performed manually, or by using a variety of automated signal thresholding techniques. A fundamental issue, particularly for the RV in patients with congenital disease, is that of inclusion or non-inclusion of the trabeculae in the blood pool. This is illustrated in Fig. 6.1. If a simple endocardial contour is drawn ignoring the trabeculae and therefore including them in the blood pool, the manual segmentation process is more efficient and more reproducible [2]. However, this leads to erroneously large volume estimates for the ventricles, and prohibits internal validation of stroke volumes using great

arterial flow volumes [3]. Calculation of the difference between stroke volumes and great arterial flow to quantify tricuspid regurgitation and the presence or absence of intra-cardiac shunts will therefore also be inaccurate when major trabeculae are included in the blood pool volume rather than myocardial volume.

Although the plane of image acquisition for volumetric analysis has conventionally been the short axis stack [4, 5], there may be limitations when using this imaging plane. In complex congenital heart disease, conventional anatomic landmarks used for planning of the short axis stack may be lost, making axial stacks much simpler to acquire. Another limitation arises in right ventricles impaired by excessive afterload (e.g. pulmonary arterial hypertension) (see Sec. 6.6.2) when the loss of systolic contraction in the radial plane often exceeds that in the longitudinal plane [6]. In these severely depressed ventricles, the small changes between end-systolic and end-diastolic volumes may be more readily detected in the longitudinal plane than in the short axis plane. Finally, in the short axis plane, suboptimal visualization of the valvular attachments in the RV inflow and outflow tracts may make it difficult to distinguish atrial from ventricular volumes. These issues could all impair the accuracy and reproducibility of volumetric analysis using short axis images [7, 8].

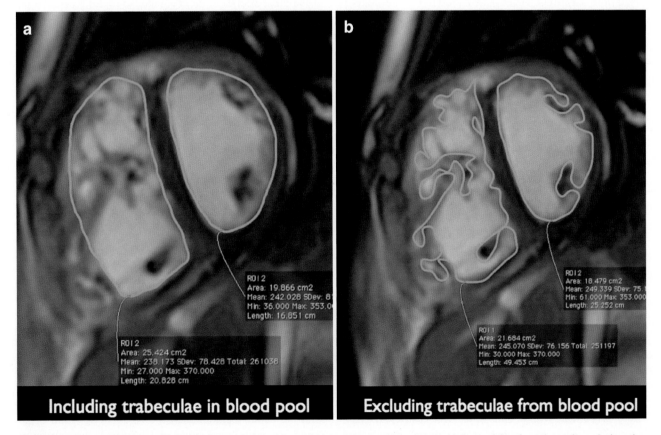

Fig. 6.1 A diagrammatic illustration of the varying modes of manual segmentation of the right and left ventricles, for volumetric analysis, using a representative mid-short axis cine view

Conversely, in the axial image plane, through-plane motion of the myocardium, with loss of clarity of the myocardial–blood pool interface can render the inferior border of the right ventricle difficult to accurately identify [7]. Moreover, any inconsistency in the patient's breath-holding position during acquisition of an axial stack will alter diaphragmatic position and therefore increase the likelihood that slices are not contiguous, significantly impairing accuracy. Although the reproducibility of volumetric analysis from axial stacks of images has been portrayed in groups of normal patients, and in a group of patients with repaired tetralogy of Fallot, it has not been evaluated in more complex congenital heart disease nor has it been directly compared to measurement reproducibility from meticulously planned and segmented short axis images.

The post-processing software used greatly influences the accuracy and reproducibility of ventricular volumetric assessment, particularly for the right ventricle. This applies to the issue of manual segmentation versus thresh-holding techniques [9]. It also applies to the means of image display. Our unit uses software [10], which permits multiple cine series to be displayed on a single screen simultaneously and allows the relative position of each cine view (or slice) to be marked in relation to other cine views at any phase of the cardiac cycle. This slice-positioning tool enables the exact position of any short or long-axis slice to be visualized in relation to the inflow and outflow tract in systole and diastole, so that the ventricular margins of the slice can be accurately segmented. While this technique greatly improves accuracy, there remains individual subjectivity with manual segmentation techniques. One method to minimize inter-observer variability is to actively archive images that include the manually drawn regions of interest, to allow comparison with future manual segmentation in serial studies.

At the present time, our lab conforms to the published standard protocols [4, 5] and performs a short axis stack for ventricular volumetric analysis, excluding papillary muscles and trabeculae from the blood pool and using the slice-position tool (available with Osirix) for general volumetric assessment. However, for isolated clinical scenarios such as pulmonary arterial hypertension (Sect. 6.6.2), an axial stack is used for volumetric analysis.

6.3 The RV with Abnormal Great Artery Position: Double Outlet Right Ventricle (DORV)

6.3.1 Definition of DORV

Although patients with double outlet right ventricle (DORV) can exist in the setting of heterotaxy, single ventricles and atrioventricular septal defects, the following discussion will be limited to those patients with situs solitus and balanced ventricles and atrioventricular valves.

The term DORV describes congenital malformations in which greater than 50 % of the circumference of both of the great arteries arises from the RV in the presence of a ventricular septal defect (VSD). It accounts for 1–1.5 % of all congenital heart disease. Echocardiography establishes the commitment of the great arteries to the right ventricle in the more extreme forms of DORV. In more subtle cases, with only a slight deviation from the traditional imaging planes, the two-dimensional images of echocardiography can be misleading and give the appearance of DORV when in fact only one great artery arises from the RV [11]. Clinicians have therefore used other morphologic criteria such as the absence of atrioventricular to semilunar valve continuity and/or the presence of bilateral infundibulum to solidify the diagnosis of DORV. Unfortunately, these criteria do not equivocally establish the diagnosis: DORV with subpulmonary VSD may exist with mitral-pulmonary continuity and thus without bilateral infundibulum [12]. In the past, the diagnosis of the more difficult cases of DORV could only be confirmed by surgical inspection.

Multiplanar reconstructions (MPRs) of intracardiac anatomy provided by CMR imaging have provided clinicians with a tool to accurately determine not only the relationship of the great arteries to the RV, but also to describe the location of the ventricular septal defect. It is this relationship of the ventricular septal defect to the great arteries that defines the physiology of patients with DORV and is the basis for the most commonly used classification of DORV, first described by Lev et al. [13]. It is important to note that in spite of the Lev classification, DORV is a continuum of anomalies with physiology of tetralogy of Fallot on one end and physiology of transposition of the great arteries on the other end. Lesions in the middle of the spectrum may not easily be described by the Lev classification, complicating the surgical decision making [14]. The major variations of DORV are discussed below.

6.3.2 DORV with Subaortic Ventricular Septal Defect (VSD) and Pulmonary Stenosis(PS)

6.3.2.1 Anatomy

DORV with a subaortic VSD accounts for two thirds of cases of DORV and is part of the continuum of tetralogy of Fallot (TOF). The great arteries lie side-by-side with the aorta rightward of the pulmonary artery (PA) and slightly posterior, thus similar to a normal heart. The rarely restrictive VSD sits between the limbs of the septomarginal trabeculations with the outlet septum attached to the anterior limb of the septomarginal trabeculations, which isolates the pulmonary artery from the left ventricle (LV) [12]. As in patients with

TOF, the severity of pulmonary stenosis will determine the degree of hypoxemia and therefore both the type and timing of surgical repair. Associated lesions, easily identified in the neonate by echocardiography, include arch anomalies, additional ventricular septal defects, branch pulmonary artery hypoplasia and anomalous coronary arteries.

6.3.2.2 Surgery

Surgical intervention consists of closing the VSD with a patch incorporating the aorta into the left ventricle. If the aorta is significantly rightward and/or anterior, the distance between the tricuspid and pulmonary valve may be less than the aortic root diameter. In this case, a baffle from the LV to the aorta passing between the tricuspid valve and pulmonary valve will be compromised [14]. Depending on the degree and location of the pulmonary stenosis, repair will also comprise of a combination of infundibular resection, right ventricular outflow tract (RVOT) patch augmentation, pulmonary valvotomy, transannular patch and branch pulmonary artery augmentation.

6.3.2.3 Imaging

Most infants with DORV/subaortic VSD/PS will not require pre-operative CMR imaging in addition to echocardiography. Rarely, a patient with an unexpected or complex pre-operative course will prompt CMR imaging. This may be a focused exam guided by the pre-operative course and query. In the event of questioning the feasibility of an intracardiac repair, the essential sequence is the three-dimensional balanced steady state free precession (3D bSSFP) whole heart sequence. By acquiring data with isotropic voxels and using MPRs, the distance between the tricuspid and pulmonary valves can be measured, thereby allowing an assessment of the likelihood of successful intracardiac baffling. During imaging, MPRs are created to prescribe complex non-traditional imaging planes to be acquired as bSSFP cine images, to demonstrate the dynamic relationship of the VSD, the aorta and the pulmonary and tricuspid valves. In patients who have mild pulmonary stenosis, in whom deferring surgical repair is favored, documenting the pulmonary blood flow, and therefore risk of developing pulmonary hypertension, may be desirable. In these patients, the exam should focus on obtaining an accurate measure of the ratio of pulmonary to aortic blood flow (Qp:Qs) and of ventricular volumes. Branch pulmonary artery flow should be obtained as validation of values obtained from the main pulmonary artery flow. In the event that the branch pulmonary artery anatomy is questioned, if only one 3D sequence may be obtained due to time constraints, magnetic resonance angiography (MRA) is the preferred sequence over the 3D bSSFP whole heart sequence. In the setting of significant pulmonary stenosis, the 3D bSSFP whole heart is at risk of dephasing artifact from turbulent flow in the pulmonary trunk. When performing MRA in patients with DORV, a prior understanding of the physiology and shunting across the VSD is necessary to anticipate the path of contrast and allow appropriately timed triggering of image acquisition. For example, in patients with near-critical pulmonary stenosis, contrast in the RV will fill the ascending aorta prior to the pulmonary arteries and branch PA imaging may be best obtained on the second pass of the MRA sequence or, should a patent ductus arteriosus (PDA) be present, with a delayed triggering of image acquisition in the ascending aorta.

Although coronary artery anatomy may be shown by the 3D bSSFP whole heart sequence, CMR imaging cannot reliably define coronary arteries in neonates. Neonatal coronary imaging is best attained with cardiac catheterization or CT angiography.

In the older child or adult, CMR plays an important role in the long-term assessment of patients with DORV/subaortic VSD/PS. There is the potential for residual pulmonary stenosis, pulmonary regurgitation and branch pulmonary artery stenosis. Serial, systematic evaluation of residual lesions and their hemodynamic consequence should utilize a 'RV assessment' protocol obtained by addition of certain relevant images to a basic protocol (Table 6.1). The RV inflow/outflow cine profiles the tricuspid valve, the RV free wall and provides an additional dynamic view of the RVOT. This view often portrays aneurismal motion of the RVOT, as defined by systolic expansion of the outflow tract. Cine imaging of the branch pulmonary arteries in orthogonal planes define the cyclic pulsatility of the vessels and areas of focal narrowing. Through-plane phase-encoded flow velocity mapping of each of the branch pulmonary arteries allows evaluation of the net ratio of forward flow to each lung. In the presence of turbulent flow in a pulmonary artery due to stenosis, phase-encoded velocity mapping will be unreliable. In this situation flow volume quantification is more accurately ascertained by summing through-plane flow volumes in the four pulmonary veins.

The remainder of a basic congenital heart disease protocol should be followed, assessing the findings in the context of past surgical intervention and the current pathology. Ventricular compliance can be assessed by the flow pattern across the pulmonary valve. A non-compliant right ventricle becomes a conduit for blood flow during atrial systole and through-plane phase-encoded velocity mapping of the pulmonary artery may demonstrate antegrade flow in late diastole. As ventricular compliance decreases, the pulmonary regurgitant fraction may decrease.

With abnormal RV loading, the hemodynamic effect on the LV must be considered. Patients with severe pulmonary regurgitation exhibit smaller left ventricular volumes as a result of decreased right ventricular output [15]. LV filling has been shown to improve after percutaneous pulmonary valve implantation [16]. Thus one should not ignore the clinical implication of RV abnormalities on left sided hemo-dynamics which must be followed just as meticulously.

6.3.3 DORV with Subaortic VSD Without Pulmonary Stenosis

6.3.3.1 Imaging

Infants with DORV and a subaortic VSD without pulmonary stenosis rarely have indications for preoperative CMR imaging. The anatomy is straightforward and can be delineated by echocardiography. The physiology is that of a large VSD. Uncomplicated surgical closure of the defect is expected to result in normal physiology and anatomy without significant residua.

Post-operative assessments using CMR would be indicated if clinical and echocardiographic screening suggested hemodynamic compromise. The protocol suggested above would apply.

6.3.4 DORV with Subpulmonary VSD

6.3.4.1 Anatomy

DORV with subpulmonary VSD accounts for one quarter of cases of DORV. It is frequently referred to as the "Taussig-Bing" variety of DORV although this term has also been used to describe complete transposition of the great arteries with subpulmonary VSD [12]. The aorta and pulmonary artery lie side-by-side with the aorta rightward of the pulmonary artery or may lie in anterior-posterior orientation with the aorta anterior and slightly rightward [17]. The VSD sits between the limbs of the septomarginal trabeculations, but in contrast with the subaortic VSD, the outlet septum attaches to the ventriculo-infundibular fold or to the posterior limb of the septomar-ginal trabeculations therefore isolating the aorta from the left ventricle. Associated findings include a constellation of left heart anomalies: coarctation of the aorta, straddling of the mitral valve and subaortic stenosis. Pulmonary stenosis is rare. As many as 27 % of patients with DORV and subpulmonary VSD have coronary artery anomalies [17]. The streaming effect of oxygenated blood from the left ventricle into the pulmonary artery results in physiology resembling that of transposition of the great arteries. Depending on the size of the VSD and associated mixing lesions (atrial septal defect, PDA), patients will present with varying degrees of cyanosis.

Echocardiography is expected to provide sufficient information for operative planning during early infancy. Rarely, a patient will require pre-operative CMR imaging to further delineate the degree of aortic arch anomalies and subaortic stenosis. The relevant images will be obtained by following the basic protocol with additional images as necessary (Table 6.2). MR angiography will demonstrate focal or tubular narrowing of the aortic arch. Additional long axis cine images of the aortic arch may be useful to demonstrate areas of flow acceleration. These may be planned from MPRs using the 3D data set or by prescribing a perpendicular plane through the ascending and descending aorta from axial images.

6.3.4.2 Surgery

The preferred surgical repair in some centers now consists of an arterial switch operation (ASO) with closure of the VSD by baffling the native pulmonary trunk, now neo-aorta, into the LV [18]. Alternatively, patients may undergo oversewing of the pulmonary trunk, baffling of the LV to the aorta incorporating the pulmonary trunk in the LV, with an RV to PA conduit completing the repair (Rastelli procedure) [19]. Patients with great arteries in the antero-posterior relationship have greater mortality when undergoing ASO than those with side-by-side great arteries. It is postulated to be due to a higher prevalence

Table 6.2 Pre-operative images often obtained in addition to the 'RV assessment' protocol given in Table 6.1, for patients with DORV/subpulmonary VSD

	Sequence	Planning	Purpose
Aortic outflow tract	Breath-held, ECG-gated, bSSFP cine images.	Image 1: From axial stack, place perpendicular plane through the aorta and angle this toward apex of the RV.	Replaces the LV outflow tract view.
		Image 2: Cross-cut image 1 with a perpendicular plane.	Assessment of subaortic stenosis if present.
			Allows planning of aortic flow.
Aortic arch	Breath-held, ECG-gated, bSSFP cine image.	From HASTE axial stack.	Subjective assessment of degree of obstruction.
		Place a perpendicular plane across the ascending aorta and ensure it passes through the descending aorta.	Assessment of area of flow acceleration.
Atrial septal defect flow	Non-breath held, ECG-gated, through-plane phase contrast flow velocity mapping.	From 4-chamber and short-axis stack.	Profiles the size of the atrial septal defect.
		Place a perpendicular plane on the right atrial side of the atrial septum, parallel to the septum.	
		Ensure the plane is parallel to the septum in the short-axis plane.	
		Venc = 180 cm/s	

of coronary artery anomalies in patients with antero-posterior great arteries and for some centers, results in a greater number of patients undergoing the Rastelli procedure [18].

6.3.4.3 Imaging

The long-term assessment of patients with DORV/subpulmonary VSD is guided by the past surgical intervention and associated residual lesions. Patients with a history of ASO and Rastelli procedure should be assessed routinely for the development or progression of branch pulmonary artery or RV-PA conduit stenosis respectively (See Fig. 6.2a, b, and Movies 6.1 and 6.2). An RV assessment protocol as described above should be followed. Reimplantation of the coronary arteries carries a risk of coronary dysfunction as demonstrated by abnormal coronary flow reserve in patients after ASO [20, 21]. Short and long axis cine images of the LV

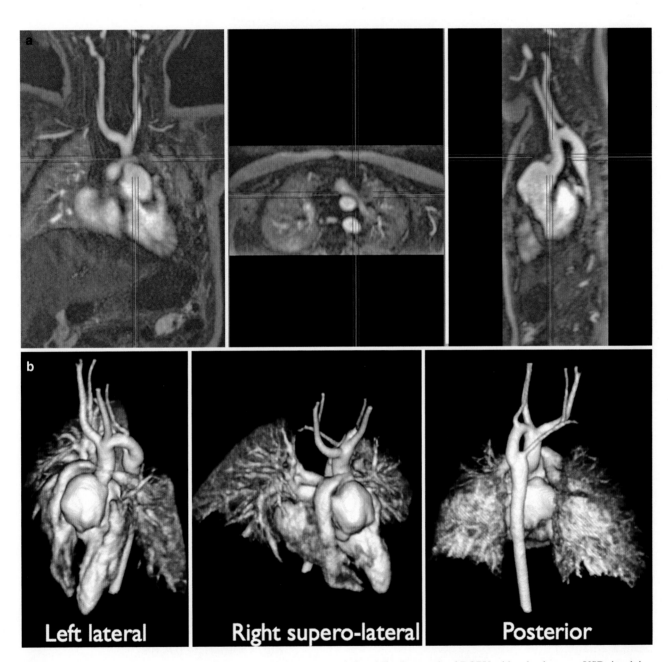

Fig. 6.2 (**a**) From the raw data described in Movie 6.1, this is a representative view using 3D image viewing software. The three planes focus on the severely stenotic left pulmonary artery, and the image demonstrates the value of isotropic data for assessing complex anatomy. (**b**) Three views from different aspects of a 3D volume-rendered model, using data derived from the MR angiogram of the above patient; an infant following repair of DORV with subpulmonary VSD, involving arterial switch operation with Le Compte maneuver and VSD closure. This image demonstrates the pertinence of 3D data, allowing visualization of the RV outflow tract, the narrowed branch pulmonary arteries and the aortic arch

should be closely evaluated for wall motion abnormalities. If found, segmented, breath-held delayed enhancement imaging, to optimize spatial resolution and sensitivity for detection of myocardial fibrosis or scar, should be performed.

6.3.5 DORV/Noncommitted VSD (ncVSD)

6.3.5.1 Anatomy

A non-committed VSD is a more unusual location for a VSD in DORV, and accounts for approximately 10 % of patients with DORV [12]. The non-committed VSD may be restrictive and does not sit between the limbs of the septomarginal trabeculations as in other types of DORV. Instead, the VSD may be perimembranous, with inlet extension, or may be muscular [11, 22]. The great arteries generally lie side-by-side with the aorta slightly posterior. Associated anomalies include pulmonary stenosis, straddling atrioventricular valves, subaortic stenosis, LV hypoplasia and coarctation of the aorta [22, 23]. Depending on the size of the VSD and degree of great artery obstruction, patients can present with cyanosis or pulmonary overcirculation.

6.3.5.2 Surgery

The remoteness of the VSD from both of the great arteries complicates the surgical repair. The aorta is located not only rightward of the pulmonary artery but high in the right ventricle and in the past, these patients were committed to a single ventricle palliation [22]. More recently, patients have successfully undergone biventricular repair by enlargement of the VSD and tunneling the left ventricle to the aorta or ASO with tunneling the left ventricle to the native pulmonary artery [22–24]. In centers which prefer the intracardiac repair to the ASO, as many as 50–100 % of patients will require VSD enlargement [23, 24]. Straddling atrioventricular valves and the location of chordal attachments play an important role in the surgical management of these patients. Attachments to the crest of the ventricular septum complicate VSD enlargement, but do not always preclude it. In contrast, attachments of the tricuspid valve crossing the subaortic pathway are more likely to prevent biventricular repair [23]. The complexity of either surgical option frequently results in patients undergoing repair at an older age predisposing patients to the need for palliative procedures such as pulmonary artery band for overcirculation and aorto-pulmonary shunts for hypoxemia as neonates [11, 23, 24].

6.3.5.3 Imaging

Pre-operative CMR imaging in patients with DORV/ncVSD will focus on the feasibility of intracardiac repair which can be determined by following the 'RV assessment' protocol. The distance between the tricuspid and pulmonary valves may be measured from the 3D bSSFP whole heart sequence. The VSD will be seen in the same sequence and will addi-tionally be profiled by the short axis cine images. The atrio-ventricular valve apparatus should carefully be evaluated for chordal attachments to the crest of the septum, using long and short axis bSSFP cine views. Critical attention must be focused on the technical quality of the images, to achieve optimal spatial resolution in order to sensitively visualize the fine fibrous structures of the chordae tendinae. The degree and location of aortic and pulmonary stenosis will be seen in both 3D datasets and bSSFP cine images.

Post-operatively, patients who have undergone tunneling of the LV to the aorta will likely have an elongated, akinetic left ventricular outflow tract (LVOT). Up to 30 % of these patients are at risk of developing subaortic stenosis [23, 25]. The preferred method of imaging the LV outflow tract involves a combination of cine imaging and 3D datasets. Cine images in orthogonal planes will demonstrate the contractility of the LVOT and the 3D bSSFP sequence by allowing multiplanar reconstructions, that will profile the length and narrowing of the outflow tract. Patients who undergo repair by ASO and tunneling of the LV to the native pulmonary trunk will need to be imaged to evaluate the potential for branch pulmonary artery stenosis and for evidence of coronary artery anomalies. As above, concerns regarding coronary artery integrity and/or wall motion abnormalities should prompt segmented, breath-held delayed-enhancement imaging.

6.3.6 DORV/Doubly Committed VSD

A doubly committed VSD in DORV occurs in approximately 10 % of patients with DORV [12]. A thin, fibrous raphe separates the rightward aorta from the pulmonary trunk. Patients present with early signs of congestive heart failure due to unrestricted pulmonary blood flow. Surgical repair consists of closing the VSD to the aorta. Pre-operatively, there are rarely indications for CMR.

Uncomplicated surgical closure of the defect is expected to result in normal physiology and anatomy without significant residua. Post-operative assessments using CMR would be indicated if clinical and echocardiographic screening suggested hemodynamic compromise. The protocols suggested above would apply.

6.4 The RV with Abnormal Division of the Trabeculations: Double-Chambered Right Ventricle (DCRV)

6.4.1 Anatomy

The double-chambered RV (DCRV) is a rare anomaly created by hypertrophied muscle bundles that divide the trabeculated apex of the RV. Various origins of the muscle bundles have been described including a hypertrophied moderator band with a high insertion site on the septal surface, and anomalous muscle bundles arising from the supraventricular crest [26]. Others describe DCRV as occurring from hypertrophied septoparietal trabeculations that create a muscular shelf, either in a high and horizontal position or in a low and oblique plane [27]. In all cases, the resultant physiology is of a high-pressure proximal chamber and a low-pressure distal chamber, both containing apical trabeculations, thus distinguishing the obstruction of DCRV from the infundibular obstruction of tetralogy of Fallot [27]. DCRV, in 70–90 % of patients, is associated with an existing or pre-existing perimembranous VSD [26–28].

6.4.2 Imaging

In small children with pristine echocardiographic acoustic windows, the diagnosis may easily be made using modified subcostal right ventricular views. In older children and adults, limited views of the right ventricle may result in poor detection of obstructive right ventricular muscle bundles, particularly when the high velocity jet of the obstruction is mistaken for shunting across the VSD. In a recent retrospective review of 32 adult patients with DCRV, transthoracic echocardiography correctly identified a DCRV in only 5 % of patients [28]. Missed diagnoses have been reported in multiple patients, leading to inappropriate surgical and medical management [29]. Suspicion of the presence of DCRV, based on physical exam and on an unexpectedly hypertrophied RV on echocardiography, should prompt additional imaging by a modality that provides unrestricted views of the right ventricle such as CMR or transesophageal echocardiography. The degree of obstruction across the hypertrophied muscle bundles will determine timing of surgical intervention. Progression of the obstruction occurs at a highly variable rate; patients

have required surgical resection anytime between infancy and adulthood [26, 27].

CMR imaging should follow the 'RV assessment' protocol with additional images focused on the intra-cavitary anatomy (Table 6.3). Cine imaging of the right ventricular obstruction will identify the location of maximal obstruction and may need to be obtained from non-traditional oblique planes through the RV cavity (Fig. 6.3 and Movies 6.3, 6.4 and 6.5). The peak gradient across the area of greatest obstruction can be obtained by applying the Bernoulli equation to velocity data obtained from phase contrast velocity mapping of the area, potentially obviating the need for cardiac catheterization. In the presence of a VSD, the size and extension of the defect should be profiled by a short axis or axial stack through the ventricles. The 3D bSSFP dataset will allow multiplanar reconstruction of the obstruction and of the VSD. MR angiography will unlikely provide additional pre-operative information and may be removed from the protocol.

Surgical repair consists of an atrial approach, although in more complicated cases, a ventriculotomy may be necessary. Resection of the muscle bundles carries excellent mid and long-term outcomes [26, 30]. Nonetheless, the potential for post-operative residual or recurrent obstruction requires long-term follow-up [26]. CMR imaging should be performed as described above with a focus on profiling the anatomy of the resected area and quantifying the right ventricular pressure gradient.

6.5 The RV with Abnormal Pulmonary Outlet: Pulmonary Atresia with Intact Ventricular Septum (PA/IVS)

6.5.1 Anatomy

Accounting for less than 2.5 % of congenital heart disease [31] PA/IVS presents a spectrum of right ventricular anomalies from a severely hypoplastic RV to a near-normal volume RV.

Table 6.3 Images often obtained in addition to the 'RV assessment' protocol given in Table 6.1, for patients with double-chambered RV

	Sequence	Planning	Purpose
RV cavity	Breath-held, ECG-gated, 'black-blood' images (HASTE or TSE). Contiguous, high resolution slices.	From scouts.	Define location of muscle bands including attachments.
		Stacks covering the RV in sagittal, axial and coronal planes.	Help plan cine imaging of obstruction.
RV obstruction cine	Breath-held, ECG-gated, bSSFP cine images.	Image 1: From HASTE axial stack. Place perpendicular plane through the RV outlet by scrolling through axial stack.	Obtain dynamic profile of area of obstruction.
		Image 2: Orthogonal view through image 1.	Help plan phase-contrast velocity mapping of obstruction.
RV obstruction flow	Non-breath held, ECG-gated, through-plane phase contrast flow velocity mapping.	From orthogonal cine views of the RV obstruction.	Obtain peak velocity to estimate gradient across the obstruction, with Bernoulli equation.
		Place a perpendicular plane just distal to point of maximal jet acceleration.	
		Venc at least 4 m/s, or greater based on estimate of gradient.	

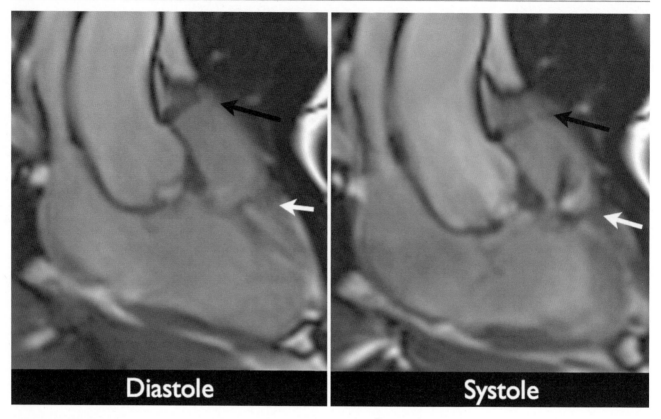

Fig. 6.3 A segmented, bSSFP cine, showing a skewed sagittal view of the right ventricle that includes both inflow and outflow tracts. This adult patient has unoperated, double-chambered right ventricle, associated with a perimembranous ventricular septal defect. Persistent, native, septo-parietal fibromuscular bands occupy a high horizontal position, proximal to the infundibular region, and give rise to dynamic obstruction. The level of the obstruction is shown with a *white arrow*, the level of the pulmonary valve is shown with a *black arrow*. The unobstructed infundibular region lies between these levels

Bull et al. classified patients with PA/IVS based on the tripartite nature of the RV that consists of an inlet, a trabecular apex and an infundibulum [32]. It is myocardial overgrowth of one or more of these components that results in the characteristic hypoplastic and thick-walled RV. Muscular overgrowth of the infundibulum only occurs in the setting of apical overgrowth, thus patients with muscular pulmonary atresia will likely have unipartite ventricles. Valvar atresia, which occurs in 75 % of patients with PA/IVS [33], is associated 50 % of the time with a well-developed infundibulum. The remainder of patients will have some degree of stenosis [34]. It has been postulated that the embryological insult in PA/IVS occurs later in development than in tetralogy of Fallot with pulmonary atresia (TOF/PA). As a result, and in contrast to patients with TOF/PA, the pulmonary valve, branch pulmonary arteries and ductus arteriosus in patients with PA/IVS will frequently be of near normal size and morphology [35]. Occasionally, one may find discontinuous pulmonary arteries supplied by bilateral ducti and more infrequently, multiple aorto-pulmonary collateral vessels. Other associated findings include an obligatory right to left shunt at the atrial septum, which if absent results in fetal death. The tricuspid valve is frequently both hypoplastic and dysplastic but only the degree of hypoplasia correlates with right ventricular size. In fact, patients may have a severely dysplastic valve in the setting of a normal sized RV [31]. In addition to nonspecific tricuspid valve dysplasia, up to 10 % of patients will have true Ebstein's anomaly [33].

There is a high prevalence of important coronary artery abnormalities in patients with PA/IVS. From two large population-based studies, between 8 and 23 % of patients with PA/IVS have right ventricular dependent coronary circulation (RVDCC) at presentation [34, 36]. RVDCC is defined as atresia or severe stenosis of a coronary artery at its orifice or along its course, with coronary perfusion maintained by communication of the distal coronary to the RV cavity. Coronary perfusion pressure is therefore dependent on elevated right ventricular pressure. In these patients, any procedure that results in a decrease in right ventricular pressure, such as relief of the right ventricular outflow tract obstruction, results in reduced coronary perfusion. In addition to RVDCC, as many as 45–55 % of patients with PA/IVS have RV to coronary artery fistulae, defined as communications between the epicardial coronary arteries and the right ventricular cavity but without stenosis. In 80 % of the time, both coronary arteries are involved [34, 36]. Over time, the elevated right ventricular systolic pressure promotes myointimal thickening of the fistulous connections and can progress to clinically significant stenosis or interruption of the coronary artery from the aortic origin, therefore developing RVDCC [37]. For this reason, patients with coronary artery fistulae should undergo relief of the elevated RV pressure in a timely fashion in order to prevent the development of RVDCC.

6.5.2   Surgery

The options and timing of interventions are varied and may be staged, depending on the functionality of the RV and its potential for growth. Patients with valvar atresia and mild infundibular hypoplasia will likely undergo an RV decompression procedure such as percutaneous catheter-based pulmonary valvotomy or a combination of surgical procedures such as RVOT patch augmentation, transannular patch placement and/or infundibular resection. In the event that the RV remains unable to sustain adequate forward pulmonary blood flow, an aorto-pulmonary shunt may be placed. The goal is to promote right ventricular growth and eventually complete a biventricular repair. Patients in this pathway that fail to develop adequate RV stroke volume will undergo a bidirectional cavo-pulmonary connection and remain with 'one and a half ventricle' physiology (Fig. 6.4 and Movie 6.6). The principle of the one and a half ventricle is to unload an RV inadequate to maintain full cardiac output while at the same time avoiding the dreaded complications of the Fontan physiology. Patients with a tripartite ventricle, without significant tricuspid valve dysplasia, may successfully undergo biventricular repair in the neonatal period. Patients with unipartite ventricles and those with RVDCC, regardless of RV size, will begin single ventricle palliation. It is important to realize that patients with RVDCC, until completion of the Fontan, will have coronary blood flow supplied by deoxygenated blood from the RV. These patients therefore have an additional risk of developing myocardial dysfunction and Fontan completion will be performed as early as technically possible.

Overall 5-year survival in the modern era is 80 %, with only 55–72 % of patients having reached a definitive surgical endpoint by that time [38]. In a prospective study of 408 patients with PA/IVS from 33 institutions between 1987 and 1997, 60 % were predicted to undergo biventricular repair based on pre-operative imaging but only 30 % were able to do so. The authors found a statistically significant increased mortality of 54 versus 31 % in those neonates who did not follow their predicted clinical course, thus emphasizing the need for accurate pre-operative imaging and planning [38].

6.5.3   Imaging

6.5.3.1   Neonatal Period

Echocardiography establishes the diagnosis of PA/IVS in infancy. In the extremely severe cases of RV hypoplasia, and in patients with a very mildly hypoplastic RV with normal tricuspid valve, choosing the appropriate surgical intervention may be straightforward. In contrast, in borderline cases, determining the ability of a RV to eventually sustain systemic venous return can be extremely difficult. Complicated formulas utilizing the variables of right-sided structures, such as tricuspid valve area, RV end diastolic volume (EDV), RV length, and RV outflow diameter have been created in attempts to predict the optimal surgical management [39]. Others have relied on tricuspid valve annulus Z-score to estimate the

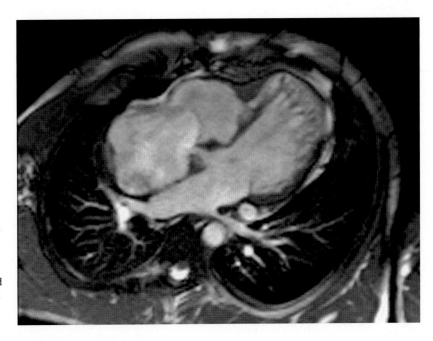

Fig. 6.4 A segmented, bSSFP cine, showing a 4-chamber view from an adult patient following "one and a half ventricle" repair of PA/IVS. This patient has a pulmonary valve homograft and a bidirectional cavopulmonary anastomosis. The right ventricle is hypoplastic with impaired systolic function (RV ejection fraction 47 %) and severe diastolic dysfunction. Note the sharp shift of the interventricular septum towards the left during diastole

potential for RV growth and successfully assign patients to a univentricular or biventricular repair. Unfortunately, there traditionally has been significant overlap between patient groups classified by tricuspid valve Z-scores and type of successful surgical intervention. To date, there is no unifying Z-score that can be utilized to predict the appropriate surgical course [38, 40, 41].

One of the difficulties in isolating a tricuspid valve Z-score as a predictor of outcome has been the significant inter-observer and intra-observer variability in the method of obtaining tricuspid valve measurements by echocardiography [41]. CMR imaging has the potential to overcome the limitations of echocardiography that have negatively impacted studies of predictors of outcome but has not been studied in this setting. It is conceivable that by providing CMR-derived, reproducible measurements of tricuspid valve area, RV volumes, ejection fraction and atrial shunting, multi-center trials could arrive at a more robust management algorithm.

In the current era, CMR would therefore unlikely alter planning in the neonatal period and is usually not performed. Patients suspected of having coronary anomalies will undergo cardiac catheterization to identify coronary artery blood supply and obtain a risk assessment of right ventricular decompression prior to intervention.

6.5.3.2 CMR After RV Decompression

CMR will provide more useful information in patients who have undergone RV decompression followed by a period of RV growth. In these patients, measurements of tricuspid valve area, RV volumes and forward pulmonary blood flow may be useful to document progression of RV output and function (Fig. 6.4). The 'RV assessment' protocol should be followed, with RV volume assessment using a short axis or axial long axis stack (for centers not using slice positioning tools during post-processing), of 2D cine images. Ventricular segmentation with exclusion of trabeculations from the ventricular volumes should be performed consistently and meticulously and indexed to body surface area to provide accurate comparisons of volumes over time. The tricuspid valve should be adequately profiled both in the long axis and short axis. Valve orifice area can be planimetered at the tips of leaflets from an 'en-face' view. The volume of pulmonary blood flow can be quantified and the contribution from multiple sources (e.g. both forward flow across the RVOT and via a cavo-pulmonary connection) defined, using through-plane phase-contrast flow volumetry. Pulmonary venous flow volumes can be ascertained to estimate total pulmonary flow and to quantify any collateral flow. Should the atrial septal communication need to be imaged, the 3D bSSFP whole heart sequence may provide adequate delineation of the septal defect, but because the atrial septum is thin, the image resolution is not always sufficient. Instead, an 'en-face' view

of the atrial septum imaged by through-plane phase-encoded velocity mapping will demonstrate the defect size, the direction of shunt through the cardiac cycle and the estimated net shunt through the defect (Fig. 6.5). The image plane can be planned from the four-chamber cine view and atrial short axis cine views by prescribing a perpendicular image plane, parallel to the atrial septum. The image plane is best prescribed on the left atrial side of the defect when net shunting is right to left and on the right atrial side when net shunting is left to right.

6.5.3.3 CMR After Biventricular Repair

It is expected that 50 % of patients with PA/IVS will successfully undergo biventricular repair [38], although most series to date have reported at most, one third of patients with PA/IVS completing a biventricular pathway [25, 36, 39]. CMR is a valuable tool for routine, serial RV assessment. It has been shown that restrictive RV physiology persists in patients with PA/IVS after biventricular repair [42], which can be demonstrated by the presence of antegrade diastolic pulmonary flow on phase contrast flow mapping (Fig. 6.6). Additional support for restrictive physiology can be demonstrated with abnormal tricuspid valve inflow pattern, a dilated right atrium and vena cavae, and RV fibrosis assessed by delayed-enhancement imaging. Branch PA size, particularly at the site of previous aorto-pulmonary shunts or surgical arterioplasties should be assessed.

6.5.3.4 CMR in the Single Ventricle (Table 6.4)

CMR imaging provides valuable clinical information prior to completion of a bidirectional cavopulmonary connection (BCPC) or total cavo-pulmonary connection (TCPC). Prior to BCPC, the basic imaging protocol (Table 6.1) should be followed paying particular attention to LV function, (particularly in the setting of RVDCC), the patency of the atrial communication, the size of the branch pulmonary arteries and presence of bilateral superior vena cavae. The atrial septum can be profiled by cine imaging or phase-encoded velocity mapping with an 'en-face' view as described above. Prior to completion of a TCPC, to assess pulmonary hemodynamics, a jugular venous pressure, reflective of pulmonary artery pressure, can be obtained under general anesthetic at the time of CMR.

Although 3D imaging using a bSSFP sequence may preclude the need for MRA, angiographic views can identify significant collateral vessels and further delineate the surgical anastomoses. MRA acquisition early after bolus administration in the upper extremities will likely be confounded by signal loss from a T2* effect in the superior vena cava and pulmonary arteries. In this case, the T1 shortening effects of the contrast will only be useful for imaging during the second pass acquisition. Administration of gadolinium contrast for MRA should therefore ideally be administered in a lower

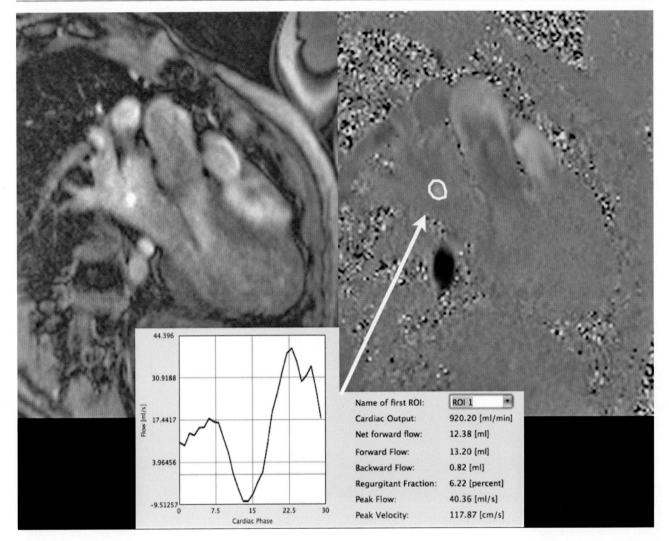

Fig. 6.5 This is the magnitude and matching phase contrast flow velocity image, planned perpendicular to the atrial septum in order to measure the through-plane flow through a small residual ASD in an adult following biventricular repair of PA/IVS. The region of interest (ASD) is *circled* (*white arrow*). The flow data is illustrated and shows phasic, but net right atrial to left atrial flow

extremity vein and triggered in the LV to opacify the inferior vena cava and the aorta during the first acquisition. The second pass acquisition of the MRA will then provide imaging of the BCPC.

Through-plane phase-encoded velocity mapping of the pulmonary arterial flow volume, compared to total pulmonary venous flow volume can be obtained to calculate the degree of systemic arterial to pulmonary collateral flow [43, 44]. An acceptable alternative method of measuring the amount of systemic arterial to pulmonary collateral flow is by measuring the discrepancy between ascending and descending aorta flow [43]. Should there be suspicion of supra-diaphragmatic systemic venous to pulmonary venous collaterals, which can develop in patients after the BCPC in patients with elevated PA pressure, both methods could be performed to quantify the contribution of each group of collaterals (Table 6.4).

Routine, serial, surveillance CMR studies are valuable in patients with single ventricle palliation of PA/IVS to ensure patency of the Fontan circuit, evaluate collateral flow, quantify atrioventricular valve regurgitation and follow ventricular systolic function.

6.6   The RV with Abnormal Afterload: Pulmonary Arterial Hypertension (PAH)

6.6.1   Classification and Diagnosis

Pulmonary hypertension is a term used to describe the presence of mean pulmonary artery pressure of 25 mmHg or higher. The term in isolation does not imply an etiology. The process by which patients develop pulmonary hypertension is highly varied and gaining an understanding of the

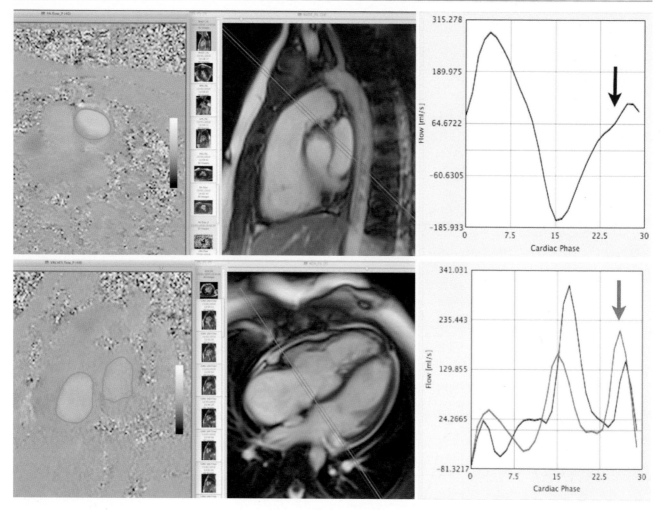

Fig. 6.6 Phase contrast flow velocity maps, measuring through-plane flow in both the pulmonary and tricuspid valves, with image planes marked in the neighboring cine image. This data is from an adult patient, with restrictive RV physiology, following biventricular repair of PA/IVS. There is forward flow in the pulmonary artery in late diastole, limiting the regurgitant fraction from the RV-PA homograft valve, marked with a *black arrow*. There is reversal of the usual E/A ratio, seen in the transtricuspid valve flow map, (*red graph*, superimposed on the *black*, transmitral flow map), marked with a *red arrow*

various pathophysiologic processes has resulted in a constantly changing nomenclature and classification scheme. As of 2008, the classification system defined by the *4th World Symposium on Pulmonary Hypertension* comprises of five groups, based on similar clinical presentations and historical response to treatment. Group 1 clusters patients with pulmonary arterial hypertension including patients with idiopathic pulmonary hypertension (IPAH) once known as primary pulmonary hypertension and patients with irreversible pulmonary arterial hypertension due to a chronic aorto-pulmonary shunt or Eisenmenger syndrome. Patients with pulmonary hypertension owing to long standing left heart disease fall under Group 2. Group 3 encompasses pulmonary hypertension secondary to primary lung disease. Pulmonary hypertension in Group 4 is caused by thrombotic disease and Group 5 combines all miscellaneous causes [45].

The diagnosis is suspected by echocardiography based on tricuspid valve regurgitation velocity, a flattened ventricular septum in systole and right ventricular hypertrophy when long-standing. The diagnosis of PAH is confirmed by cardiac catheterization with a mean pulmonary artery pressure greater than or equal to 25 mmHg. The previous criteria of a mean pulmonary artery pressure of 30 mmHg with exercise and pulmonary vascular resistance (PVR) of 3 Wood units were eliminated at the *4th World Symposium on Pulmonary Hypertension.*

Committing a patient to the diagnosis of PAH is ominous with the natural history predicting a 3-year survival of 35–45 % in IPAH and 77 % in Eisenmenger syndrome [46]. Over the past 20-years, the routine use of anticoagulants and targeted therapies such as prostanoids, phosphodiesterase inhibitors and endothelin-receptor antagonists, has resulted in an overall 40 % decrease in mortality [47]. Although diagnostic

Table 6.4 Images often obtained in addition to the 'RV assessment' protocol given in Table 6.1, for patients with PA/IVS undergoing single ventricle palliation

	Sequence	Planning	Purpose
Tricuspid valve	Breath-held, ECG-gated, bSSFP cine images.	Perpendicular plane from 4-chamber and RVLA, parallel to TV	En face view.
		5 mm contiguous slices from right atrium into ventricle	Identify dysplastic leaflets. Measure inflow and regurgitant orifices.
SVC flow	Non-breath held, ECG-gated, through-plane phase contrast flow velocity mapping.	From 3D whole heart. Ensure orthogonal planes. Close to the SVC-RA junction to avoid exclusion of azygos flow. Venc = 150 cm/s.	Assessment of proportion of Qp supplied by BCPC.
Pulmonary venous flow	Non-breath held, ECG-gated, through-plane phase contrast flow velocity mapping.	From 3D whole heart. Ensure orthogonal planes of each of the pulmonary veins. Venc = 80 cm/s.	Assessment of collateral flow.
Descending aorta flow	Non-breath held, ECG-gated, through-plane phase contrast flow velocity mapping.	From 3D whole heart. Ensure orthogonal planes of aorta at the diaphragm. Venc = 180 cm/s	Assessment of collateral flow.
Atrial septal communication	Non-breath held, ECG-gated, through-plane phase contrast flow velocity mapping.	From 4-chamber and short axis stack. Place a perpendicular plane on the left atrial side of the atrium septum, parallel to the septum. Ensure the plane is parallel to the septum in the short-axis plane. Venc = 180 cm/s	Profiles the size of the atrial septal communication.

and goal-oriented treatment algorithms have been refined to optimize the care of patients with PAH, follow-up has not been standardized. In most centers, various combinations of the 6 minute walk distance test, echocardiography and cardiac catheterization are used every 3–6 months to escalate treatment when specific goals are not met, prior to irreversible clinical deterioration.

6.6.2 Imaging

The frequency of evaluations has prompted the need for non-invasive modalities that can provide reproducible diagnostic markers. CMR imaging has been studied in the hopes of obviating the need for frequent catheterizations, by identifying markers that reliably predict PA pressure and/or PVR. Saba et al. found RV mass index to be proportional to the mean PA pressure in patients with pulmonary hypertension, but the findings were not supported in a study by Hoeper et al. [48, 49]. In a study of ten patients, Kondo et al. describe retrograde flow in the MPA to be proportional to pulmonary vascular resistance and the cross sectional area of the vessel [50]. The findings have not yet been reproduced. Alunni et al. [51] attempted to ascribe a range of mean PA pressure based on the degree of septal flattening but significant pressure measurement overlap occurred between the grades of septal abnormalities (Fig. 6.7 and Movie 6.7). Roeleveld et al. [52] sought to reproduce findings of others using the

ratio of acceleration time to ejection time in the PA, acceleration time by itself, calculations of pulse wave velocity and cross sectional vessel area to estimate mean PA pressure, and found all measurements unreliable.

In summary, CMR by itself is unable to replace direct measurements of pulmonary artery pressure by cardiac catheterization, but there is a role for CMR and cardiac catheterization in concert, to provide more reliable measurements of pulmonary vascular resistance. Cardiac catheterization relies on the Fick equation or thermodilution to estimate pulmonary blood flow which, with mean PA pressure, is then utilized to calculate pulmonary vascular resistance and cardiac output. Studies have shown that both methods of calculating pulmonary blood flow become less reliable in the setting of critically ill patients [53, 54]. In contrast, phase-encoded velocity mapping in CMR provides a direct measurement of vessel blood volume. When combined with near simultaneous measurements of pulmonary artery pressure obtained by catheterization, the two allow a very precise measure of pulmonary vascular resistance. Centers with the ability to perform hybrid procedures using simultaneous catheterization and CMR can use both modalities to evaluate pulmonary vasoreactivity and guide treatment management [55].

Efforts have also been made to identify CMR findings that can be used as prognostic markers in PAH. Few have found reliable predictors and others have refuted previous observations. Wolferen et al. determined that progressive RV

Fig. 6.7 This is a segmented, breath-hold bSSFP cine view in the mid-ventricular short axis plane, from an 11-year-old patient with idiopathic pulmonary hypertension. There is severe hypertrophy and dilatation of the right ventricle. The right ventricular systolic function is globally, severely reduced. There is bowing of the septum towards the left ventricle throughout the cardiac cycle and interventricular dyssynchrony

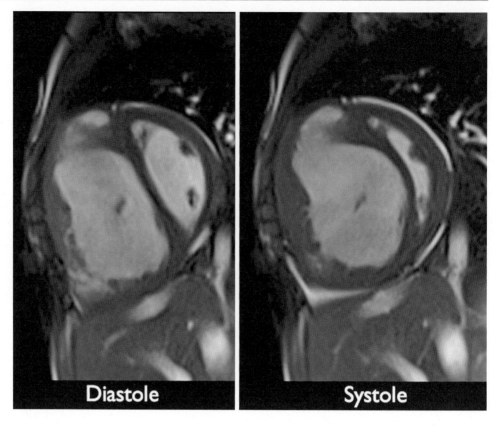

dilation, a decrease in LV end diastolic volume and a decrease in RV stroke volume predicted a worse outcome in 64 patients with PAH followed for a mean of 32 months [56]. Conversely, the degree of pulmonary artery dilatation, once thought to be proportional to the degree of pulmonary hypertension [57], has been shown to be an unreliable predictor of PAH severity. Boerritger et al. [58] have shown that pulmonary arteries continue to dilate in PAH, even in the setting of resolving hypertension by cardiac catheterization measurements (Fig. 6.8 and Movie 6.8). Overall, the most consistent marker predictive of survival is cardiac index which to date has been more extensively studied by cardiac catheterization than by CMR [56, 59].

An important observation made by CMR is that RV systemic failure in PAH occurs primarily from a decrease in transverse shortening of the RV free wall towards the septum, and is more pronounced at the apex than the base of the heart [6]. These findings are consistent with strain rate imaging by echocardiography that has demonstrated decreased apical deformation in comparison to basal deformation in PAH and is related to the degree of RV afterload [60]. The complex alteration in RV mechanics diminishes the value of estimates of RV function made by echo such as the tricuspid annular plane systolic excursion (TAPSE), which focuses on longitudinal movement at the base of the heart and will therefore overestimate RV function. The role of CMR in providing an accurate measurement of RV systolic function is amplified in the setting of PAH where traditional estimates by echocardiography will be less reliable.

In all serial CMR assessments of patients with PAH, both for monitoring disease progression and response to therapy, optimal standards of image quality and reproducibility must be maintained. Great attention must be given to ensuring technically sound and systematic methodology, in both scanning and post-processing techniques. In patients able to tolerate a slightly longer scan time, both short axis and axial stacks should be obtained to internally validate RV volumetric analysis and to measure LV volumes in the current standard of short axis images. Manual segmentation and post-processing of these hypertrophied and heavily trabeculated right ventricles may give better reproducibility than semi-automated techniques [9]. It is important to realize that abnormal flow vortices in the main pulmonary artery of patients with PAH are known to exist [61] and can limit the accuracy of phase-encoded velocity mapping of main pulmonary artery flow. Flow mapping should be performed in the proximal branch pulmonary arteries, to obtain precise measurements of blood flow for the purpose of accurate PVR calculations.

The CMR study of a patient with severe PAH can be technically challenging since dyspneic patients will frequently be unable to remain supine for extended periods, and may be unable to breath-hold comfortably and reliably. The essence of the CMR evaluation of these patients is rapid acquisition

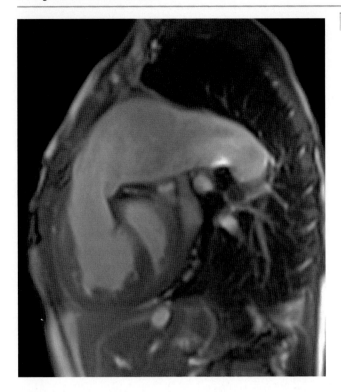

Fig. 6.8 This is a segmented, breath-hold bSSFP cine, showing a sagittal view of the RV outflow tract, dilated MPA and proximal LPA from 16-year-old patient with Eisenmenger physiology, following chronic pulmonary overcirculation due to an ASD and a large muscular VSD. The spatial and temporal resolution of the image has been lowered to give a shorter breath-hold duration, because of the poor breath-holding capacity of the patient

of critically relevant data. Real-time radial k-t SENSE imaging has been shown to provide accurate volumetric data in abnormal right ventricles and can be extremely useful in this patient population [62]. As sequence development continues to steadily progress, approaches such as higher resolution real-time imaging will allow CMR imaging of sicker and younger patients. A typical protocol in a lab performing hybrid procedures is detailed in Table 6.5 and when performed routinely, can be completed in 15–20 minute. Because a detailed anatomical evaluation is unnecessary, the examination can focus on real-time imaging of biventricular function and on non-breath-held, phase-encoded velocity mapping to quantify pulmonary blood flow. As mentioned above, because longitudinal shortening is affected later than transverse shortening [6], axial stacks may potentially provide more accurate volumetric analysis and should be considered.

The role of CMR in patients with PAH is therefore developing. It enables accurate measurements of PVR in centers with the ability to perform hybrid procedures by providing direct measurements of pulmonary artery blood flow. CMR also offers reliable, objective markers of the progression of disease, by allowing direct quantification of biventricular cardiac output, biventricular volumes and RV mass over time.

Conclusion

The abnormal right ventricle is a highly variable entity, potentially posing diagnostic and management challenges to the clinician. Prior to the advent of CMR in the clinical arena, the anatomy and physiology of abnormal right ventricles were difficult to define and the pathophysiology was frequently underestimated.

However, clinicians with access to CMR now possess a powerful resource for decision support, which is adaptable to various RV abnormalities. The use of 3D balanced SSFP imaging is ideal to understand the complex anatomy and resultant physiology of abnormal RV, particularly DORV. The ability to quantify intracardiac shunts can help to stratify risk and optimize the timing of surgical interventions. The chronic post-operative management of patients with PA/IVS, DCRV and DORV is guided by objective analysis of regurgitant valves, stenoses, RV size and function. Patients with PAH may be evaluated non-invasively for disease progression and treatment response.

In nearly all cases, attaining the full clinical potential of a CMR examination requires the presence of a cardiologist experienced in congenital and acquired heart disease in order to assimilate knowledge of the natural history of disease and the details of interventions. During the scan, continuous assessment of images as they are acquired is necessary to guide a scan beyond a basic RV assessment protocol, based on the unique hemodynamic issues of the patient. The final key to a successful scan is systematic, consistent and meticulous post-processing to give accurate and reproducible assessment of RV volumes, vessel measurements and flow analysis.

As CMR techniques evolve and a reliable body of RV data continues to develop, a greater understanding of the complex RV will ensue, allowing refinement of clinical and surgical management protocols.

6.7   Practical Pearls

1. Prepare carefully for the scan by reviewing and thoroughly understanding the patient's entire past medical history and presenting query. This will minimize the risk of overlooking relevant findings, and help explain unexpected findings that may require additional image acquisition.

2. Pay close attention to patient comfort in the scanner and to communication, so that cooperation and breath-holding capability is maximized. There are no shortcuts to a comprehensive congenital scan.

3. Patient comfort and behavior permitting, always perform a comprehensive assessment protocol for the scan, aiming

Table 6.5 Example of the standard sequences and views of a routine cardiac scan for assessment of PAH, in the order of workflow.

	Sequence	Planning	Purpose
Scout	Single shot b-SSFP images.	Contiguous axial, sagittal, coronal slices. Coverage from liver to neck in all 3 radiological planes.	Ensures isocentering of the heart in the scanner.
RVLA, LVLA	Single shot b-SSFP images. Non-breath held.	From scout images. Place a perpendicular image plane through the long axis of the ventricle from mid-AV valve to the ventricular apex.	Planning the true 4-chamber image.
4-chamber view	Breath-held, ECG-gated, bSSFP cine image.	From RVLA, LVLA. Place perpendicular plane through both AV valve orifices in each image. From LVLA cine, check that the plane passes through mid-mitral valve and LV apex. From RVLA, check that the plane passes through the-mid tricuspid valve and RV apex.	Subjective assessment of atrial volumes, biventricular volumes and function, ventricular wall motion, AV valve regurgitation.
Axial cine stack	Radial k-t SENSE. Non-breath held.	From the sagittal and coronal scout images. Plan contiguous 7–10 mm thick slices in the axial plane, covering the entire ventricular mass from diaphragm to outflow tracts.	Alternative to short axis cine stack. Provides the images required for segmentation of RV volumes.
Short axis cine stack	Radial k-t SENSE. Non-breath held.	From end-diastolic frame of 4-chamber cine. Place perpendicular plane at hinge points of both AV valves, with special care to include the entire basal ventricular blood pool. Contiguous slices are placed to cover entire ventricular mass from base to apex.	Alternative to axial cine stack. Provides the images required for segmentation of biventricular volumes.
LV outflow tract	Radial k-t SENSE. Non-breath held.	Image 1: From sagittal scout. Place a perpendicular plane through both basal aortic valve and mid-mitral valve orifice. Check orientation passes through LV apex on LVLA. Image 2: Cross-cut image 1 to obtain two orthogonal cine views of the LVOT.	Outflow tract morphology, subjective assessment of semilunar valve function. Plan AO flow.
RV outflow tract	Radial k-t SENSE. Non-breath held.	Image 1: From axial scout. Place a perpendicular plane through the pulmonary trunk and angle toward apex on RVLA. Image 2: Cross-cut image 1 to obtain two orthogonal views of the RVOT.	Outflow tract morphology, subjective assessment of semilunar valve function. Plan MPA flow.
MPA flow	Non-breath held, ECG-gated, through-plane phase contrast velocity mapping.	From the two orthogonal RVOT images. Place a perpendicular plane across the MPA. The plane should be just distal to the valve leaflets in systole, and avoid turbulent areas of flow. Optimize velocity encoding to maximize accuracy and prevent aliasing.	Calculate regurgitant fractions (RF%). Validate ventricular stroke volume measurements. Calculate PVR with simultaneous catheter-obtained pressure.

Aorta flow	Non-breath held, ECG-gated, through-plane phase contrast velocity mapping.	From the two orthogonal LVOT images. Place a perpendicular plane across the proximal ascending aorta. The plane should be just distal to the valve leaflets in systole. Optimize velocity encoding to maximize accuracy and prevent aliasing.	Validate ventricular stroke volume measurements.
Branch PA cine	Radial k-t SENSE. Non-breath held.	From axial, sagittal and coronal scout, optimize image plane to obtain 2 orthogonal planes of each branch pulmonary artery.	Plan branch PA flow.
Branch PA flow	Non-breath held, ECG-gated, through-plane phase contrast velocity mapping.	Place perpendicular image plane on two orthogonal views of each of the branch pulmonary arteries.	Validate ventricular stroke volume measurements. Calculate PVR with simultaneous catheter-obtained pressure. Validate MPA flow.

to acquire morphologic data in 3D, ventricular functional data and arterial flow data for every scan. Unexpected findings occur frequently with congenital disease, and presumed "redundant" data may be necessary at the reporting stage to resolve these.

4. Take care to optimize the sequences used, by maximizing the temporal and spatial resolution of the images, particularly in images obtained for volumetric and flow analysis. Modify these resolutions for patient body size and heart rate.

5. Carefully plan acquisition of cine image stacks for volumetric analysis. Include the whole ventricle in the stack in systole and diastole, and modify slice position to minimize partial voluming of ventricular septum and free walls.

6. Establish a consistent and systematic approach to postprocessing to minimize inter-observer variability in serial studies.

7. Use slice-positioning tools to accurately analyze basal slices for segmentation.

8. Utilize arterial and venous flow volumes as well as left ventricular volumes for quality assurance and to improve the accuracy of right ventricular volumetric analysis. Ensure that all volumetric and flow data make hemodynamic sense in the context of the patient's history.

9. Always look for non-RV causes of RV abnormality, such as anomalous pulmonary venous drainage, intracardiac shunts and valvar regurgitation.

References

1. Luijnenburg SE, Robbers-Visser D, Moelker A, Vliegen HW, Mulder BJM, Helbing WA. Intra-observer and inter-observer variability of biventricular function, volumes and mass in patients with congenital heart disease measured by CMR imaging. Int J Cardiovasc Imaging. 2010;26:57–64.

2. Winter MM, Bernink FJP, Groenink M, Bouma BJ, van Dijk AP, Helbing WA, Tijssen JG, Mulder BJ. Evaluating the systemic right ventricle by CMR: the importance of consistent and reproducible delineation of the cavity. J Cardiovasc Magn Reson. 2008;10:40–8.

3. Devos D, Kilner P. Calculations of cardiovascular shunts and regurgitation using magnetic resonance ventricular volume and aortic and pulmonary flow measurements. Eur Radiol. 2010;20:410–21.

4. Kramer C, Barkhausen J, Flamm S, Kim R, Nagel E. Standardized cardiovascular magnetic resonance imaging protocols, society for cardiovascular magnetic resonance: board of trustees task force on standardized protocols. J Cardiovasc Magn Reson. 2008;10:35–44.

5. Pennell DJ, Sechtem UP, Higgins CB, Manning WJ, Pohost GM, Rademakers FE, van Rossum AC, Shaw LJ, Yucel EK. Clinical indications of cardiovascular magnetic resonance: consensus panel report. Eur Heart J. 2004;25:1940–65.

6. Kind T, Mauritz GJ, Marcus JT, van de Veerdonk M, Westerhof N, Vonk-Noordegraaf A. Right ventricular ejection fraction is better reflected by transverse rather than longitudinal wall motion in pulmonary hypertension. J Cardiovasc Magn Reson. 2010;12:35–46.

7. Alfakih K, Plein S, Bloomer T, Jones T, Ridgway J, Sivananthan M. Comparison of right ventricular volume measurements between axial and short axis orientation using steady-state free precession magnetic resonance imaging. J Magn Reson Imaging. 2003;18:25–32.

8. Fratz S, Schuhbaeck A, Buchner C, Busch R, Meierhofer C, Martinoff S, Hess J, Stern H. Comparison of accuracy of axial slices versus short axis slices for measuring ventricular volumes by cardiac magnetic resonance in patient with corrected tetralogy of Fallot. Am J Cardiol. 2009;103:1764–9.

9. Bradlow WM, Hughes ML, Keenan NG, Bucciarelli-Ducci C, Assomull R, Gibbs JS, Mohiaddin RH. Measuring the heart in pulmonary arterial hypertension (PAH): implications for trial study size. J Magn Reson Imaging. 2010;31:117–24.

10. Rosset A, Spadola L, Ratib O. OsiriX: an open-source software for navigating in multidimensional DICOM images. J Digit Imaging. 2004;17(3):205–16.

11. Mahle WT, Martinez R, Silverman N, Cohen M, Anderson R. Anatomy, echocardiography, and surgical approach to double outlet right ventricle. Cardiol Young. 2004;18 Suppl 3:39–51.

12. Wilkinson JL. Double outlet ventricle. In: Anderson RH, Baker EJ, Macartney FJ, Rigby ML, Shinebourne EA, Tynan M, editors. Paediatric cardiology. 2nd ed. London: Churchill Livingstone; 2002. p. 1353–81.

13. Lev M, Bharati S, Meng CC, Liberthson RR, Paul MH, Idriss F. A concept of double-outlet right ventricle. J Thorac Cardiovasc Surg. 1972;64:271–81.

14. Jonas R. Double outlet right ventricle. In: Jonas RA, Dinardo J, Laussen PC, Howe R, LaPierre R, Matte G, editors. Comprehensive surgical management of congenital heart disease. London: Arnold Publishers; 2004. p. 413–28.

15. Coats L, Khambadkone S, Derrick G, Hughes M, Jones R, Mist B, Pellerin D, Marek J, Deanfield JE, Bonhoeffer P, Taylor AM. Physiologic consequences of percutaneous pulmonary valve implantation: the different behaviour of volume and pressure overloaded ventricles. Circulation. 2007;28:1886–93.

16. Lurz P, Puranik R, Nordmeyer J, Muthurangu V, Hansen MS, Schievano S, Marek J, Bonhoeffer P, Taylor AM. Improvement in left ventricular filling properties after relief of right ventricle to pulmonary artery conduit obstruction: contribution of septal motion and interventricular mechanical delay. Eur Heart J. 2009;30:2266–74.

17. Uemura H, Yagihar T, Kawashima Y, Nishigaki K, Kamiya T, Ho SY, Anderson RH. Coronary arterial anatomy in double-outlet right ventricle with subpulmonary VSD. Ann Thorac Surg. 1995;59: 591–7.

18. Takeuchi K, McGowan F, Moran AM, Zurakowski D, Mayer JE, Jonas RA, del Nido PJ. Surgical outcome of double-outlet right ventricle with subpulmonary VSD. Ann Thorac Surg. 2001;71: 49–53.

19. Brown JW, Ruzmetov M, Okada Y, Jiay P, Turrentine MW. Surgical results in patients with double outlet right ventricle: a 20-year experience. Ann Thorac Surg. 2001;72:1630–5.

20. Bengel FM, Hauser M, Duvernoy CS, Kuehn A, Ziegler SI, Stollfuss JC, Beckmann M, Sauer U, Muzik O, Schwaiger M, Hess J. Myocardial blood flow and coronary flow reserve late after anatomical correction of transposition of the great arteries. J Am Coll Cardiol. 1998;32(7):1955–61.

21. Gagliardi MG, Adorisio R, Crea F, Versacci P, Di Donato R, Sanders SP. Abnormal vasomotor function of the epicardial coronary arteries in children five to eight years after arterial switch operation. J Am Coll Cardiol. 2005;46(8):1565–72.

22. Lacour-Gayet F, Haun C, Ntalakoura K, Belli E, Houyet L, Marcsek P, Wagner F, Weil J. Biventricular repair of double outlet right ventricle with non-committed ventricular septal defect (VSD) by VSD rerouting to the pulmonary artery and arterial switch. Eur J Cardiothorac Surg. 2002;21:1042–8.

23. Belli E, Serraf A, Lacour-Gayet F, Hubler F, Zoghby J, Houyel L, Planche C. Double-outlet right ventricle with non-committed ventricular septal defect. Eur J Cardiothorac Surg. 1999;15:747–52.

24. Artrip JH, Sauer H, Campbell DN, Mitchell MB, Haun C, Almodovar MC, Hraska V, Lacour-Gayet F. Biventricular repair in double outlet right ventricle: surgical results based on the STS-EACTS International Nomenclature classification. Eur J Cardiothorac Surg. 2006;29:545–50.

25. Rychik J, Jacobs ML, Norwood WI. Early changes in ventricular geometry and ventricular septal defect size following Rastelli operation or intraventricular baffle repair for conotruncal anomaly. A cause for development of subaortic stenosis. Circulation. 1994;90(5 Pt 2):II13–9.

26. Telagh R, Alex-Mekishvili V, Hetzer R, Lange PE, Berger F, Abdul-Khaliq H. Initial clinical manifestations and mid-long-term results after surgical repair of double-chambered right ventricle in children and adults. Cardiol Young. 2008;18:268–74.

27. Alva C, Ho SY, Lincoln CR, Rigby ML, Wright A, Anderson RH. The nature of the obstructive muscular bundles in double-chambered right ventricle. J Thorac Cardiovasc Surg. 1999;117:1180–9.

28. Hoffman P, Wojcik AW, Rozanski J, Siudalska H, Jakubowska E, Wlodarska EK, Kowalski M. The role of echocardiography in diagnosing double chambered right ventricle in adults. Heart. 2004;90:789–93.

29. Kilner PJ, Sievers B, Meyer GP, Ho SY. Double-chambered right ventricle or sub-indundibular stenosis assessed by cardiovascular magnetic resonance. J Cardiovasc Magn Reson. 2002;4:373–9.

30. Hachiro Y, Takagi N, Koyanagi T, Morikawa M, Abe T. Repair of double-chambered right ventricle: surgical results and long-term follow-up. Ann Thorac Surg. 2001;72:1520–2.

31. Fricker FJ, Zuberbuhler JR. Pulmonary atresia with intact ventricular septum. In: Anderson RH, Baker EJ, Macartney FJ, Rigby ML, Shinebourne EA, Tynan M, editors. Paediatric cardiology. 2nd ed. London: Churchill Livingstone; 2002. p. 1177–89.

32. Bull C, de Leval MR, Mercanti C, Macartney FJ, Anderson RH. Pulmonary atresia and intact ventricular septum: a revised classification. Circulation. 1982;66(2):266–72.

33. Shinebourne EA, Rigby ML, Carvalho JS. Pulmonary atresia with intact ventricular septum: from fetus to adult. Heart. 2008;84:1350–7.

34. Dyamenahalli U, McCrindle BW, McDonald C, Trivedi KR, Smallhorn JF, Benson LN, Coles J, Williams WC, Freedom RM. Pulmonary atresia with intact ventricular septum: management of, and outcomes for, a cohort of 210 consecutive patients. Cardiol Young. 2004;14:299–308.

35. Kutsche LM, Van Mierop LHS. Pulmonary atresia with and without ventricular septal defect: a different etiology and pathogenesis for the atresia in the 2 types? Am J Cardiol. 1983;51:932–5.

36. Daubeney P, Delany DJ, Anderson RH, Sandor GG, Slavik Z, Keeton BR, Webber SA. Pulmonary atresia with intact ventricular septum: range of morphology in a population based study. J Am Coll Cardiol. 2002;39:1670–9.

37. Freedom RM, Nykanen DG. Pulmonary atresia and intact ventricular septum. In: Adams F, Allen M, Moss A, editors. Moss and Adams' heart disease in infants, children, and adolescents: including the fetus and young adult. 6th ed. Philadelphia: Lippincott Williams and Wilkins; 2001. p. 845–79.

38. Ashburn DA, Blackstone EH, Wells WJ, Jonas RA, Pigula FA, Manning PB, Lofland GK, Williams WG, McCrindle BW. Determinants of mortality and type of repair in neonates with pulmonary atresia and intact ventricular septum. J Thorac Cardiovasc Surg. 2004;127(4):1000–8.

39. Yoshimura N, Yamaguchi M, Ohashi H, Oshima Y, Oka S, Yoshida M, Murakami H, Tei T. Pulmonary atresia with intact ventricular septum: strategy based on right ventricular morphology. J Thorac Cardiovasc Surg. 2003;126(5):1417–26.

40. Hannan RL, Zabinsky JA, Eng M, Stanfill RM, Ventura RA, Rossi AF, Nykanen DG, Zahn EM, Burker RP. Midterm results for collaborative treatment of pulmonary atresia with intact ventricular septum. Ann Thorac Surg. 2009;87:1227–33.

41. Bull C, Kostelka M, Sorensen K, de Leval M. Outcome measures for the neonatal management of pulmonary atresia with intact ventricular septum. J Thorac Cardiovasc Surg. 1994;107:359–66.

42. Liang XC, Lam WWM, Cheung EWY, Wong SJ, Cheung YF. Restrictive right ventricular physiology and right ventricular fibrosis as assessed by cardiac magnetic resonance and exercise capacity after biventricular repair of pulmonary atresia and intact ventricular septum. Clin Cardiol. 2010;33(2):104–10.

43. Grosse-Wortmann L, Al-Otay A, Yoo SJ. Aortopulmonary collaterals after bidirectional cavopulmonary connection or Fontan completion: quantification with MRI. Circ Cardiovasc Imaging. 2009;2:219–25.

44. Whitehead K, Gillespie MJ, Harris MA, Fogel MA, Rome JJ. Non-invasive quantification of systemic-to-pulmonary collateral flow: a major source of inefficiency in patients with superior cavopulmonary connections. Circ Cardiovasc Imaging. 2009;2:405–11.

45. Simonneau G, Robbins IM, Beghetti M, Channick RN, Delcroix M, Denton CP, Elliott G, Gaine SP, Gladwin MT, Jing ZC, Korwka MJ, Langlenben D, Nakanishi N, Souza R. Updated clinical classification of pulmonary hypertension. J Am Coll Cardiol. 2009;54:s43–54.

46. Hopkins WE, Ochoa LL, Richardson GW, Trulock EP. Comparison of the hemodynamics and survival of adults with severe primary pulmonary hypertension or Eisenmenger syndrome. J Heart Lung Transplant. 1996;15:100–5.

47. Galie N, Manes A, Negro L, Palazzini M, Bacchi-Reggiani ML, Branzi A. A meta-analysis of randomized controlled trials in pulmonary arterial hypertension. Eur Heart J. 2009;30:394–403.

48. Saba TS, Foster J, Cockburn M, Cowan M, Peacock AJ. Ventricular mass index using magnetic resonance imaging accurately estimates pulmonary artery pressure. Eur Respir J. 2002;20:1519–24.

49. Hoeper MM, TOngers J, Leppert A, Baus S, Maier R, Lotz J. Evaluation of right ventricular performance with a right ventricular ejection fraction thermodilution catheter and MRI in patients with pulmonary hypertension. Chest. 2001;120:502–7.

50. Kondo C, Caputo GR, Maui T, Foster E, O'Sullivan M, Stulbar MS, Golden J, Caterjee K, Higgins CB. Pulmonary hypertension: pulmonary flow quantification and flow profile analysis with velocity-encoded cine MR imaging. Radiology. 1992;183:751–8.

51. Alunni JP, Degano B, Arnaud C, Tetu L, Blot-Souletie N, Didier A, Otal P, Rousseau H, Chabbert V. Cardiac MRI in pulmonary artery hypertension: correlations between morphological and functional parameters and invasive measurements. Eur Radiol. 2010;20:1149–59.

52. Roeleveld RJ, Marcus JT, Boonstra A, Postmus PE, Marques KM, Bronzwaer JG, Vonk-Noordegraaf A. A comparison of non-invasive MRI-based methods of estimating pulmonary artery pressure in pulmonary hypertension. J Magn Reson Imaging. 2005;22:67–72.

53. Dhingra VK, Fenwick JC, Walley KR, Chittock DR, Ronco JJ. Lack of agreement between thermodilution and Fick cardiac output in critically ill patients. Chest. 2002;122:990–7.

54. Van Grondelle A, Ditchey RV, Groves BM, Wagner WW, Reeves JT. Thermodiluation method overestimates low cardiac output in humans. Am J Physiol. 1983;245(4):H690–2.

55. Muthurangu V, Taylor A, Andriantsimiavona R, Hegde S, Miquel ME, Tulloh R, Baker E, Hill DLG, Razavi RS. Novel method of quantifying pulmonary vascular resistance by use of simultaneous invasive pressure monitoring and phase-contrast magnetic resonance flow. Circulation. 2004;110:826–34.

56. Van Wolferen SA, Marcus JT, Boonstra A, Marques KMJ, Bronzwaer JGF, Spreeuwenberg MD, Postmus PE, Vonk-Noordegraaf A. Prognostic value of right ventricular mass, volume and function in idiopathic pulmonary arterial hypertension. Eur Heart J. 2007;28:1250–7.

57. Ng CS, Wells AU, Padley SP. A CT sign of chronic pulmonary arterial hypertension: the ratio of main pulmonary artery to aortic diameter. J Thorac Imaging. 1999;14(4):270–8.
58. Boerritger B, Mauritz GJ, Marcus JT, Helderman F, Postmus PE, Westerhof N, Vonk-Noordegraaf A. Progressive dilatation of the main pulmonary artery is a characteristic of pulmonary arterial hypertension and is not related to changes in pressure. Chest. 2010;138:1395–401.
59. Appelbaum L, Yigla M, Bendayan D, Reichart N, Fink G, Priel I, Schwartz Y, Richman P, Picard E, Goldman S, Kramer MR. Primary pulmonary hypertension in Israel: a national survey. Chest. 2001;119:1801–6.
60. Dambrauskaite V, Delcroix M, Claus P, Herbots L, D'hooge J, Bijnens B, Rademakers F, Sutherland GR. Regional right ventricular dysfunction in chronic pulmonary hypertension. J Am Soc Echocardiogr. 2007;20(10):1172–80.
61. Reiter G, Reiter U, Kovacs G, Kainz B, Schmidt K, Maier R, Olschewsk H, Rienmueller R. Magnetic resonance derived 3-dimensional blood flow patterns in the main pulmonary artery as a marker of pulmonary hypertension and a measure of elevated mean pulmonary arterial pressure. Circ Cardiovasc Imaging. 2008;1:23–30.
62. Muthurangu V, Lurz P, Critchely JD, Deanfield JE, Taylor AM, Hansen M. Real-time assessment of right and left ventricular volumes and function in patients with congenital heart disease by using high spatiotemporal resolution radial k-t SENSE. Radiology. 2008;248(3):782–91.

Tetralogy of Fallot

7

Michael A. Quail, Vivek Muthurangu,
and Andrew M. Taylor

7.1 Introduction

Tetralogy of Fallot (TOF) is the most common form of cyanotic congenital heart disease, occurring in 1 in 3,600 live births [1]. Complete repair of TOF was devised over 50 years ago (first reported by Lillehei in 1954) and can result in complete intra-cardiac repair in early infancy [2]. However, despite excellent short- and medium-term survival rates, the 30 year actuarial survival for patients repaired before their 5th birthday is 90% of the expected survival rate and the annualized risk of death triples in the third postoperative decade [2, 3]. Late morbidity and mortality, in particular related to pulmonary incompetence, has been observed in many patients long after total repair.

Initially, pulmonary incompetence was believed to be a relatively benign condition, with few problems associated with right ventricular volume loading. However, it has become clear that chronic pulmonary incompetence and right ventricular (RV) volume loading can cause RV dysfunction, which can in turn lead to symptoms of reduced exercise tolerance, increased risk of atrial and ventricular tachyarrhythmia, and sudden death. This has lead to an increasing proportion of patients requiring operative replacement of incompetent and/or stenosed pulmonary valves and conduits.

The accurate quantification of pulmonary incompetence and stenosis and their effects on the right and left ventricles is therefore crucial: Data that can be provided by cardiovascular magnetic resonance (CMR) imaging. In this chapter, we will provide an overview of TOF, its treatment and its assessment with CMR. Ultimately, CMR may enable improvements in the management of late complications through appropriate surveillance and treatment and may extend the survival and quality of life of patients.

7.2 Morphology

Morphologically the principle defect of this condition is antero-cephalad deviation of the muscular outlet septum resulting in the tetrad of, ventricular septal defect (VSD), pulmonary outflow tract obstruction, overriding aorta and RV hypertrophy (Fig. 7.1). In TOF the malaligned outlet septum serves to narrow the sub-pulmonary outflow tract and simultaneously create an interventricular defect that is over-ridden by the aortic valve apparatus.

The VSD in TOF is usually non-restrictive and sub-aortic; however, it may occasionally extend into the sub-pulmonary region. Its inferior and anterior borders are comprised of the limbs of the septomarginal trabeculation, whilst the superior border is formed from the deviated outlet septum and poste-riorly the anteroseptal leaflet of the tricuspid valve.

Obstruction of the right ventricular outflow tract (RVOT) in TOF is most frequently in the form of infundibular stenosis (45%) with obstruction rarely isolated to the pulmonary valve alone (10%), and more usually a combination of the two (15%). In its most severe form the pulmonary valve is atretic (15%) [4]. The deviated outlet septum combined with hypertrophied septoparietal trabeculations contributes

M.A. Quail, B.Sc. (hons), MB ChB (hons), MRCPCH (✉)
Academic Clinical Fellow, Pediatric Cardiology,
Centre for Cardiovascular Imaging,
UCL Institute of Cardiovascular Sciences and Great Ormond Street
Hospital for Children, Great Ormond Street,
London WC1N 3JH, UK
e-mail: m.quail@ucl.ac.uk

V. Muthurangu, M.D., MRCPCH
UCL Centre for Cardiovascular MR,
University College London,
30 Guildford Street, London WC1N 1EH, UK
e-mail: v.muthurangu@ich.ucl.ac.uk

A.M. Taylor, M.D., FRCR, FRCP
Cardio-Respiratory Unit, UCL Institute of Child Health
and Great Ormond Street Hospital for Children,
Great Ormond Street, London, WC1N 3JH, UK
e-mail: a.taylor@ich.ucl.ac.uk

Electronic supplementary material The online version of this chapter (doi:10.1007/978-1-4471-4267-6_7) contains supplementary material, which is available to authorized users.

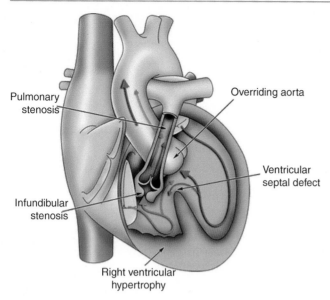

Pulmonary stenosis

Overriding aorta

Ventricular septal defect

Infundibular stenosis

Right ventricular hypertrophy

Fig. 7.1 Schematic diagram of unrepaired TOF (Copyright belongs to Gemma Price)

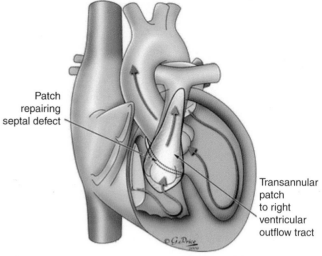

Patch repairing septal defect

Transannular patch to right ventricular outflow tract

Fig. 7.2 Schematic diagram of repaired TOF (Copyright belongs to Gemma Price)

significantly to sub-valvular obstruction and inevitably requires division at surgery. The pulmonary valve is frequently stenotic with thickened and tethered leaflets requiring valvotomy or placement of a trans-annular patch if the annulus diameter is deemed inadequate (Fig. 7.2). However, the resultant sequelae of pulmonary incompetence are now recognised to be a significant problem later in life. Stenosis of the origin of the left and/or right pulmonary arteries (PAs) is a common finding and may require resection if localised or placement of a separate patch if more diffusely hypoplastic. In a proportion of patients, there may be pulmonary atresia, particularly at an infundibular or valvular level and associated major aorto-pulmonary collateral arteries (MAPCAs). The preferred approach in this situation may be the placement of a right ventricle to pulmonary artery (RV-PA) conduit.

The individual components of the tetrad clearly show marked variability, especially the nature of pulmonary stenosis and the extent of the VSD; these variations account for the spectrum of clinical severity, and their surgical treatment can significantly influence later outcomes.

7.2.1 Associated Anomalies

Significant associated cardiac defects are uncommon. The most frequent associated lesions include: right sided aortic arch, atrial septal defect, patent ductus arteriosus, atrioventricular septal defects and additional VSDs. Less commonly, there may be a persistent left-sided superior vena cava, anomalous origin of the left anterior descending coronary artery or aortopulmonary collaterals if severe pulmonary

stenosis. Associated syndromic conditions in which TOF may occur as a major manifestation include DiGeorge syndrome (22q11.2 deletion) and Alagille syndrome (JAG1 mutation); however, the condition more often occurs as an isolated defect.

7.3 Clinical Presentation

The clinical presentation of TOF in infancy varies depending on the degree of RVOT obstruction. Typically the infant will present with cyanosis due to right-to-left shunt and diagnosis is then established by echocardiography. Surgery is usually performed around 3–6 months as cyanosis progresses, often without a prior palliative shunt procedure. In the infant with TOF and pulmonary atresia, severe cyanosis is seen immediately after birth.

The complications observed in patients beyond the immediate postoperative period relate to surgical residua and progression of the 'unnatural' history of the disease. Common problems requiring re-intervention include severe pulmonary regurgitation, residual outflow tract obstruction and conduit failure. Less commonly a residual VSD, particularly at the postero-inferior margin of the patch, and severe tricuspid regurgitation require re-operation [5]. Pulmonary regurgitation, in contrast to other residua, is remarkably well tolerated. However, over time it produces its deleterious effects through volume overload of the right ventricle. It is associated with pathological RV dilatation and dysfunction, decreased exercise tolerance, sudden cardiac death and ventricular arrhythmia associated with prolonged QRS duration. Pulmonary valve replacement (PVR) can ameliorate the volume overload imposed by pulmonary regurgitation. However, the optimal timing for this procedure remains unclear, as homograft prostheses have a limited lifespan and further reoperations may be required should these fail.

7.3.1 Primary Surgical Repair

Early primary repair is preferred because it shortens the period the patient is exposed to hypoxemia, to right ventricular (RV) pressure overload and subsequent RV hypertrophy, and is performed with a low peri-operative mortality.

The surgical approach has also shifted from a trans-ventricular approach to a trans-atrial/trans-pulmonary approach, with the aim of preserving RV structure and myocardial function and reducing the potential side effects of an RV ventriculotomy (coronary artery damage, RV contractile reduction, scar arrhythmia).

7.3.2 Late Surgical Treatment: Pulmonary Valve Replacement

Surgical PVR can be performed using a variety of valve materials including cadaveric homografts and man-made conduits. Additional procedures may also be necessary and can be performed during the same cardiopulmonary bypass including: resection of residual trabeculations, extensive enlargement of pulmonary arteries, closure of a patent foramen ovale, residual atrial and/or ventricular septal defects, tricuspid valve annuloplasty, and aortic valve replacement.

More recently, PVR has been performed with a degree of RVOT re-fashioning [6] to reduce RVOT aneurismal dilatation and optimally align the RVOT and new pulmonary trunk [7].

7.3.3 Percutaneous Pulmonary Valve Implantation

In patients who develop stenosis of their surgical PVR (homograft or conduit stenosis) percutaneous transcatheter stenting is possible. This can prolong conduit life and postpone re-operation. However bare-metal stenting can potentially convert the pressure-overloaded ventricle to one of volume-overload, through relief of obstruction and introduction of free pulmonary incompetence.

In 2000, percutaneous pulmonary valve implantation (PPVI) was described, whereby a new pulmonary valve was placed into a dysfunctional RV-PA prosthetic conduit [8]. Over the following decade, this technology has been accepted into clinical practice, with over 1,500 devices now implanted throughout the world. The Melody™ device (Medtronic Inc., Minneapolis, MN, USA) has CE marking in Europe and Canada and Food and Drug Administration (FDA) approval in the USA. Patients have been successfully treated to relieve both pulmonary stenosis and regurgitation [9, 10]. This method offers a minimally invasive alternative to open-heart surgery for RVOT/pulmonary trunk dysfunction in children and adults by restoring acceptable RV loading conditions [11].

The device is composed of a tri-leaflet bovine jugular vein sutured into a platinum-iridium, gold welded, balloon expandable stent (Fig. 7.3). When expanded, the competence of the valve is maintained at a large range of diameters: 14–22 mm. The device is implanted under general anaesthesia, usually via femoral access.

7.4 CMR Imaging

As patients with congenital heart disease in general, and TOF in particular are increasingly surviving longer, appropriate follow up and surveillance for complications is becoming more important. In this regard, echocardiography has been the mainstay of investigation – providing important information regarding intra-cardiac anatomy, assessing valvular competence, and ventricular function. However, the technique is limited by post-operative restriction of acoustic windows, inability to provide sufficient hemodynamic information and because extra-cardiac anatomy, such as branch PAs, can be difficult to assess.

CMR has become an important modality in the assessment of TOF because the technique can provide three-dimensional (3D) anatomy of the right-sided cardiac and vascular structures crucial to adequate clinical assessment. MR can provide reliable serial hemodynamic information non-invasively and unlike echocardiography, can quantify pulmonary regurgitation volume, and flow in branch PAs. MR provides a large field of view, unlimited choice of imaging planes and is much less operator dependent than echocardiography. A current limitation of MR is the inability to measure hemodynamic pressures.

7.4.1 Indications

MR is primarily used for the assessment of patients with TOF late after primary repair for the assessment of significant residual lesions that are identified at routine follow-up. Patients also undergo CMR assessment routinely before transfer from pediatric to adult congenital cardiac services to provide baseline anatomic and functional information. The exact frequency of serial scans remains to be determined; repeat scans are usually performed early if significant lesions are present, particularly where surgical or catheter intervention may be required.

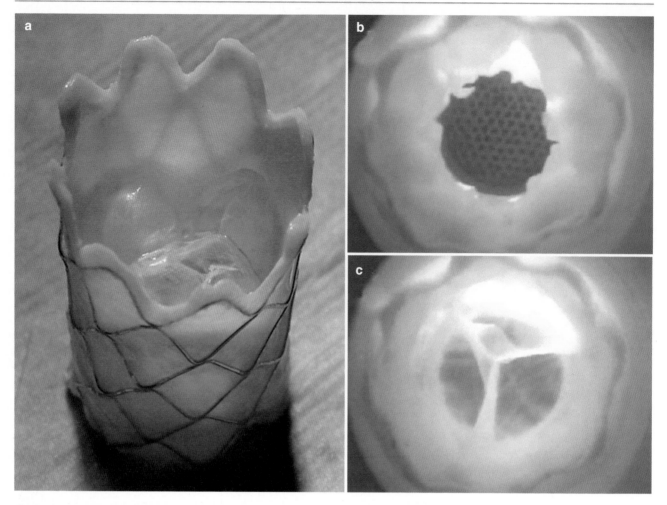

Fig. 7.3 PPVI device (**a**). Device viewed in water bath showing the valve open during forward flow (**b**) and closed during reverse flow (**c**) – note tri-leaflet morphology of the valve

7.4.2 CMR Sequences

7.4.2.1 3D Imaging

The 3D capabilities of CMR play a key role for pediatric and adult patients with congenital heart disease. There are two conventional methods of acquiring 3D data. One uses angiographic techniques with gadolinium-based contrast agents that can be injected via any peripheral vein. The other uses a 3D balanced-SSFP sequence, which is respiratory and cardiac gated, but does not require contrast [12]. Both data sets are acquired in such a way to give isotropic voxels, so that the images can be viewed with the same spatial resolution in any anatomical plane. These data can be used during the scan to plan image planes for further scanning, as well as during the reporting phase to assess 3D relationships between structures, quantify vessel size and view morphology. The high-signal, isotropic 3D images that are achieved using gadolinium-contrast angiography allow complex modelling of structures so that interventional techniques can be optimized [13].

Gadolinium-enhanced MR angiography is particularly useful in the assessment of complex pulmonary vascular anatomy associated with TOF (Movie 7.1), where the pulmonary vascular bed may be supplied with blood flow from other sources, such as surgically created shunts or aorto-pulmonary collateral vessels. Delineation of all sources of pulmonary blood supply and the size and morphology of the pulmonary arteries is essential as surgical and transcatheter procedures are often required to augment effective pulmonary blood flow or to eliminate sources of excessive pulmonary blood flow [14]. Gadolinium contrast-enhanced MR angiography relies on the T1 shortening effect of dilute gadolinium. A 3D data set is acquired at the peak of the Gadolinium bolus. Sequences are designed to ensure that tissues without Gadolinium enhancement are suppressed, resulting in prominence of contrast enhanced vessels. Images are acquired in a single breath-hold, without cardiac synchronisation. This results in two significant limitations: Image blurring due to cardiac motion reduces the ability of this technique to visualize intra-cardiac anatomy, and secondly the size of individual vessels represent an average size over the cardiac cycle which can lead to underestimation of systolic dimensions. A further disadvantage of Gadolinium-enhanced MR angiography is that fast moving turbulent blood causes signal drop out, leading to over-estimation of stenoses.

7.4.2.2 Cine Imaging

Cine imaging using balanced-SSFP, or fast gradient echo sequences, gives multiphase data that shows myocardial or valve motion over the entire cardiac cycle. These cines may have up to 40 frames per cardiac cycle, a temporal resolution adequate for accurate physiological representation. The balanced-SSFP sequences are now used as standard, as they provide improved blood-pool homogeneity throughout the cardiac cycle. Balanced-SSFP images have significantly higher contrast-to-noise ratios allowing better detection of the endocardial border than traditional gradient echo sequences [15]. The technique lends itself particularly to assessment of TOF allowing qualitative assessment of cardiac chambers, pulmonary valvular function and vascular anatomy.

Cine images are acquired in equal-width slices perpendicular to the long-axis of the heart, from base to apex, in order to assess cardiac function and measure the ventricular volumes. The post-processing of cine images to calculate ventricular volumes and function is performed off-line, using commercially available or open-source software. The segmentation of the blood pool and myocardial border can be performed manually, or by using automated signal thresholding techniques. There is currently a wide range of software available, and a wide variation in segmenting practice and procedures. A fundamental issue, particularly for pediatric patients and those with congenital disease, is that of inclusion or non-inclusion of the trabeculae in the blood pool. If a simple endocardial contour is drawn and the trabeculae ignored and included in the blood pool, the manual segmentation process is more efficient and more reproducible [16]. However, this leads to erroneously large volume estimates for the ventricles, and prohibits internal validation of stroke volumes using great arterial flow volumes.

7.4.2.3 Flow Assessment

Accurate quantification of flow volume is crucial in patients with known or suspected congenital heart disease [17]. For volume quantification we favour a free-breathing, velocity encoded phase-contrast sequence with a temporal resolution of at least 30 frames per cardiac cycle. Slice positioning and velocity encoding must be optimized [18]. If these parameters are rigorously controlled, flow can be assessed in large and small arteries, systemic and pulmonary veins [19, 20]. Aortic and pulmonary valve regurgitant volumes can be directly measured (Fig. 7.4). Phase contrast flow sequences also enable the profiling of flow acceleration jets, with

velocity estimation. More importantly, with appropriate combinations of arterial and venous flow volume assessment, the technique allows accurate assessment of inter-atrial, inter-ventricular, arterial and venous shunt volumes. In the context of atrio-ventricular valve regurgitation, knowledge of the ventricular stroke volume, combined with knowledge of the forward arterial flow volume from that ventricle allows for calculation of mitral or tricuspid valve regurgitant fraction. For every patient in whom ventricular function is quantified, the practise of our unit is to undertake great arterial flow volume assessment to guide the volumetric analysis. This greatly enhances the accuracy and reproducibility of our reporting procedure [21].

7.4.2.4 Black-Blood Imaging

Spin echo pulse sequences can still play a role in the assessment of TOF. They are good for the morphology of the blood vessels and cardiac chambers, in particular when turbulent flow at the site of stenosis reduces the accuracy of b-SSFP or MR angiography images. Black-blood imaging is also good at elucidating the relationship between airway and blood vessels. In TOF, this allows accurate assessment of branch PA abnormalities including hypoplasia, stenosis and non-confluence, which are otherwise missed by echocardiography [22].

Following treatment of PA stenoses by intravascular stenting, gradient echo sequences suffer from serious artefacts due to T2* field inhomogeneity. Though spin-echo is less susceptible to metal artefacts, this does not necessarily lead to a better assessment of stents; and may possibly lead to false re-assurance as to their patency [23]. CT imaging may be required to definitively exclude intra-stent stenosis.

7.4.2.5 Late-Gadolinium Enhancement (LGE)

Late-gadolinium enhancement (LGE) demonstrates large focal areas of fibrosis or other myocardial abnormality and is frequently observed in patients with TOF [24]. This is particularly so in areas that reflect the surgical repair – RVOT scar, site of VSD repair, ventriculotomy site; however, areas of LGE are also seen remote to sites of surgery. Importantly, LGE correlates to RV systolic function and dilatation and ultimately, may provide some prognostic information for timing PVR in repaired TOF.

7.4.2.6 Stress CMR Imaging

Stress MR imaging can be performed either with exercise (specifically designed MR bicycle) or Dobutamine administration and has been used as means of assessing global RV function in response to increased workload. An abnormal RV response to stress [25] has been demonstrated in patients with TOF and pulmonary incompetence. In normal subjects, RV ejection fraction increases during stress, whilst in patients

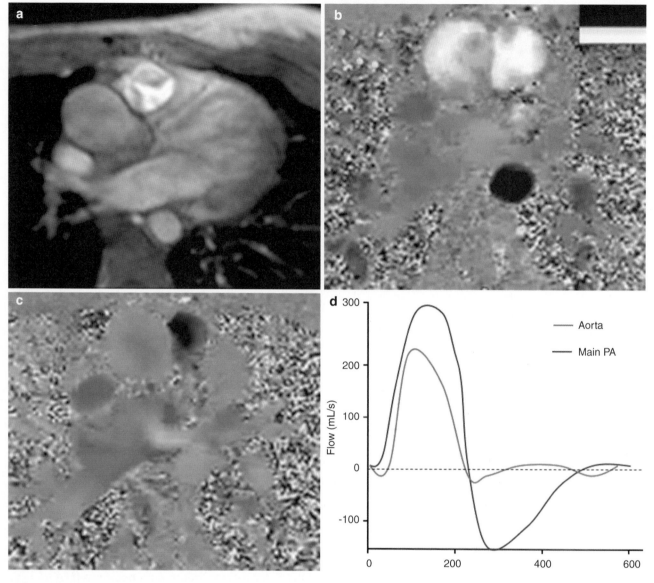

Fig. 7.4 MR phase contrast velocity mapping in pulmonary regurgitation – (**a**) diastolic, modulus image showing non-coaptation of the valve leaflets, (**b**) systolic phase contrast image with *white* forward flow (note *black* flow in the descending aorta posteriorly), (**c**) diastolic phase contrast showing pulmonary regurgitation (*black*), (**d**) flow curve over the cardiac cycle

with TOF RV function remains unchanged or reduced during stress. The responses of subjects with chronic pulmonary incompetence to stress may be able to provide important prognostic indictors to help with the timing of pulmonary valve replacement in this patient population, though further long-term studies are needed to address these issues. Importantly, the use of real-time imaging to assess flow and function [26] during exercise may mean that such studies can now be carried out, without the need for pharmacological stress or the need to breath-hold during exercise, making exercise MR more acceptable to the patient.

7.4.3 Clinical Imaging Protocol (Table 7.1)

7.5 CMR Findings in TOF

7.5.1 Pulmonary Valve and RV Assessment

The MR assessment of TOF requires comprehensive evaluation of the entire heart; however, emphasis is rightly placed on the evaluation of the right ventricle and pulmonary valve.

Table 7.1 Clinical imaging protocol

	Sequence	Planning	Purpose
Scout	Single shot bSSFP	3 images in 3 orthogonal planes	Iso-centreing
Axial stack	HASTE or TSE 'black blood' contiguous axial slices. Respiratory navigated, ECG-gated.	Coverage of heart and systemic/pulmonary vessels including proximal arch branches	Thoracic anatomy, planning
Ventricular long-axis (RV and LV)	bSSFP cine images, breath-held, ECG gated	Orthogonal plane through long axis of ventricle from AV valve to ventricular apex, planned from axial stack	AV valve function, assessment of ventricular volumes
AV Valves	bSSFP cine images, breath-held, ECG gated	Orthogonal plane parallel to AV valve, planned from axial stack	Planning 4-chamber
4-Chamber View	bSSFP cine images, breath-held, ECG gated	Orthogonal plane across AV valve orifices, planned from AV valves sequence	Atrial/ventricular size and function, AV regurgitation
Short-axis stack	bSSFP cine images, breath-held, ECG gated	Orthogonal plane at AV valve hinge-points with inclusion of basal blood pool, planned from end-diastolic frame of 4 chamber cine	Ventricular volume calculation, assessment of septum and outflow tracts
MR angiography	Gadolinium Injection. Breath held, No ECG-gating	Planned on axial HASTE stack for coronal orientation	Angiographic views of large and small vessels. Second pass allows assessment of systemic and pulmonary venous anatomy
3D bSSFP	Free breathing, respiratory navigated, ECG-gated. Data acquisition in diastole	Planned on axial HASTE stack for sagittal orientation	High resolution intra-cardiac anatomy
LV and RV outflow tracts	bSSFP cine images, breath-held, ECG gated	LV planned from AV valves cine. RV planned from axial stack.	Outflow tract morphology, subjective assessment of semilunar valve function.
Great Vessel Flow	Through-plane velocity mapping, ECG gated, Non-breath held	Planned from outflow tract images.	Vessel flow volume/velocity, calculation of regurgitant fraction and volume. Evaluate Shunts

The RV outflow tract is visualised by aligning a plane that passes through the pulmonary trunk (or conduit) and the RV inferiorly from the axial stack. An alternative RVOT plane is a sagittal or sagittal-oblique view through the pulmonary trunk and descending aorta. Pulmonary incompetence can be assessed using a plane perpendicular to the RVOT views described, just above the pulmonary valve.

7.5.1.1 Pulmonary Incompetence

Pulmonary incompetence to some degree is a predominant feature of TOF late after repair. MR can image the regurgitant jet in three dimensions and can quantify the regurgitant volume or describe it as a regurgitant fraction. This quantification is important in clinical decision-making regarding catheter or surgical valve replacement.

Turbulence of blood regurgitating through the pulmonary valve in diastole causes de-phasing and signal loss in gradient echo cine imaging (Movie 7.2). This facilitates a qualitative gradation of the regurgitant jet: Grade 1 = signal loss close to the valve; grade 2 = signal loss extending into the proximal chamber; grade 3 = signal loss filling the whole of the proximal chamber; grade 4 = signal loss in the receiving chamber throughout the relevant half of the cardiac cycle. The most accurate assessment of PR however is achieved by through-plane velocity-encoded phase-contrast

imaging. Instantaneous flow volumes in the PA are calculated by multiplying the PA contour area (drawn manually) with the spatial average flow within this contour (Fig. 7.4). Total forward and retrograde (regurgitant) flow in a cardiac cycle can be calculated by integrating the instantaneous flow volumes for all frames. This technique has been validated in TOF by comparing it to the differences in left and right stroke volume, which can also be used to quantify pulmonary regurgitation if there is no other valve regurgitation or shunt [18]. The regurgitant fraction is calculated by dividing pulmonary retrograde flow by pulmonary forward flow ×100.

7.5.1.2 Pulmonary Stenosis and RVOT Obstruction

Pulmonary stenosis and RVOT obstruction are significant and common residual lesions following TOF repair. Using MR velocity mapping and the modified Bernoulli equation, the gradient across a stenosis can be calculated. This technique is comparable to Doppler echocardiography, but is not limited by acoustic windows, allowing measurement of the velocity jet in any plane. Imaging is usually performed using a combination of through-plane (perpendicular to jet) and in-plane (parallel to jet) imaging. The latter is used to initially define the jet, with subsequent through-plane images at the site of maximum velocity.

7.5.1.3 Systolic Ventricular Function

Systolic ventricular function, in TOF is based on MR ventricular volumetric assessment. The complex geometry of the RV means that no single imaging plane is well suited to RV assessment. We recommend the use of the short axis; however, the interface between right ventricle and right atrium can be difficult to assess, and long axis imaging may help.

7.5.1.4 Diastolic Ventricular Function

Diastolic ventricular function can also be assessed using MR. Though the late forward flow of so-called 'restrictive physiology' can be seen, RV time-volume curves can be created using either cine ventricular volume data or by combining phase contrast velocity maps of flow through the tricuspid and pulmonary valve. These have not only been used to demonstrate impaired diastolic function in the RV and LV of patients with TOF, but also how early diastolic filling can improve following relief of conduit stenosis [27]. Again, further studies of diastolic properties, with both CMR and echocardiography are required to define the prognostic use of this information.

7.5.2 Unrepaired TOF

In the assessment of the patient with unrepaired TOF, the anatomical diagnosis will usually have been made previously by echocardiography. MR will therefore aim to confirm the characteristic morphology (Fig. 7.5) and assist pre-operative planning by defining any additional complex anatomy and physiology that may influence the surgical procedure. Assessment should include:

- RV outflow tract obstruction – Is narrowing of the subpulmonary infundibulum fixed or dynamic?
- Pulmonary valve morphology – Is valve sparing surgery possible?
- Quantify peak velocity across RV outflow tract
- Identify and measure any branch pulmonary stenosis/ hypoplasia
- Identify and measure any palliative shunts
- Measure differential lung perfusion
- Quantify ventricular volumes, mass and function
- Check aortic root for dilation
- Exclude additional VSDs

7.5.3 Repaired TOF

Patients who have undergone surgical repair of TOF will have had repair of VSD and relief of the RVOT obstruction. The latter may have involved surgical resection of infundibular muscle bundles and/or the insertion of a transannular patch if the annular diameter was deemed inadequate. Significant

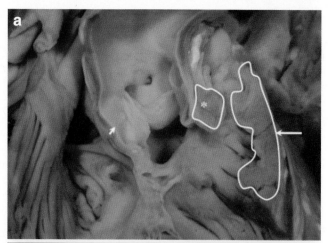
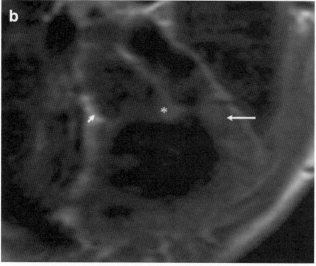

Fig. 7.5 Unrepaired TOF in neonate. (**a**) Histological specimen of showing VSD, overriding aorta (*arrowhead*), infundibular stenosis (*asterisks*) and RV hypertrophy (*arrow*). (**b**) Comparison CMR image – black-blood coronal oblique view

pulmonary regurgitation is almost always encountered following this procedure; though mild/moderate regurgitation is well tolerated. Pulmonary regurgitation may be increased by proximal or distal pulmonary artery stenosis, and chronic severe/free pulmonary regurgitation may lead to RV dilatation and dysfunction. The MR study aims to comprehensively define the hemodynamic status of the patient. Clinicians assessing patients should:

- Describe RV outflow tract and pulmonary trunk anatomy
- Identify any RV outflow tract aneurysm (Fig. 7.6)
- Quantify pulmonary valve regurgitation (Fig. 7.3)
- Assess proximal and distal pulmonary arteries for stenoses (Fig. 7.7)
- Assess bi-ventricular function, volume and mass (Movie 7.3)
- Check for the presence of MAPCAs

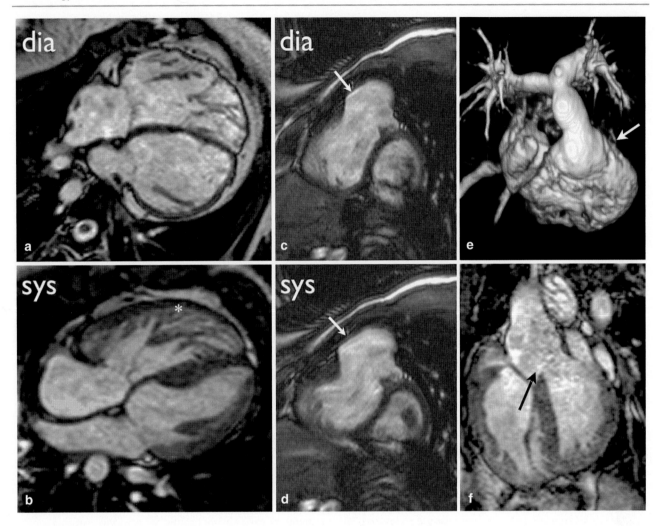

Fig. 7.6 Repaired TOF in an adolescent. (**a, b**) 4-chamber b-SSFP image showing RV dilatation in diastole (*dia*) and RV hypertrophy in systole (*sys*,*). (**c, d**) b-SSFP image showing dilated and aneurysmal RVOT (*arrow*) following transannular patch repair in oblique sagittal view (**c**) diastole and (**d**) systole – note the paradoxical increase in aneurysm size during systole. (**e**) 3D MR angiogram reconstruction of RVOT aneurysm (*arrow*). (**f**) b-SSFP image through an intact VSD patch (*arrow*)

- Measure Qp:Qs – assess for residual shunts, e.g. residual VSD, MAPCAs
- Check Aortic root for dilatation
- Assess course of coronary arteries which may be in close proximity to stent implantation sites

7.6 Clinical Use of CMR

The most commonly encountered complication of repaired TOF is severe RV dilatation and dysfunction secondary to free pulmonary incompetence. The dilemma of when to treat patients with free pulmonary incompetence, presenting late after repair of right ventricular outflow tract obstruction is one that faces all congenital heart disease clinicians. Although there is clear data to suggest that, in the long-term, pulmonary incompetence is detrimental, leading to an increased incidence of adverse events (death, sustained arrhythmias, increasing symptoms) [28], the conventional thinking has been that the benefit of treating free pulmonary incompetence is outweighed by the potential risk of surgical pulmonary valve replacement and the lack of longevity of this treatment (conduit dysfunction within 10–15 years that exposes patients to multiple operations over their life) [29, 30]. PVR has therefore often been left until patients develop symptoms; however, once symptoms develop, there is the potential that symptomatic improvement after surgery may be limited due to the fact that the right ventricle has been chronically exposed to pulmonary incompetence.

More recently, there has been a shift in this risk/benefit continuum. Operative mortality and morbidity are now small with modern operative methods and postoperative care [6, 29] and conduit life can now be extended using new non-invasive percutaneous approaches to treat conduit dysfunction.

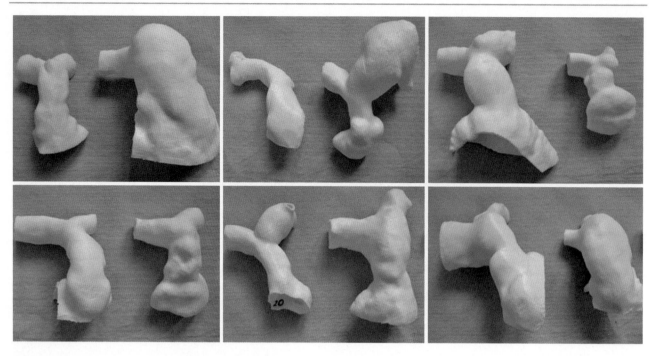

Fig. 7.7 Variations in pulmonary trunk and branch pulmonary artery anatomy. Rapid prototyping models (reconstructed from CMR contrast-enhanced angiography data) of 12 patients with TOF assessed 10–15 years after early complete repair

7.6.1 Use of CMR to Select Patients with Severe Pulmonary Incompetence for PVR

Current data from CMR assessment of patients with severe pulmonary incompetence have demonstrated elevated RV end-diastolic and end-systolic volumes and reduced RV ejection fraction compared to normal [31]. Furthermore, there is increasing evidence that RV function may be irreversibly compromised by such long-term changes [32]. This is exemplified by three findings that have been demonstrated by CMR. Firstly, RV ejection fraction has been shown to be significantly lower in patients with both RV pressure and volume overload as compared with RV pressure overload alone. Secondly, an abnormal RV response to stress has been demonstrated in patients with TOF and pulmonary incompetence. And finally, there appears to be no, or limited, improvement in RV function (ejection fraction at rest) following PVR [31, 32]. Indeed, the only study to demonstrate an improvement in RV ejection fraction following PVR was in patients with moderately dilated right ventricles [33].

Despite this lack of marked improvement in RV function by correcting pulmonary incompetence, PVR does reduce RV dimensions (Fig. 7.8), and if performed before an RV EDV index of 160 ml/m^2 or an RV ESV index of 82 ml/m^2 [34] (or RV end-diastolic volume index of 170 ml/m^2 or an RV end-systolic volume index of 85 ml/m^2) [35] RV dimensions can be normalised (defined as EDVI ≤ 108 ml/m^2 and

ESVI ≤ 47 ml/m^2). Other supportive data exists [33, 35, 36], and most centres would consider PVR if the RV EDVI is between 150 and 200 ml/m^2. However, these numbers need to be taken with caution as they represent studies done in patients of varying age groups, with varying original operations and varying PVR surgery (RVOT aneurysmal reduction or not). Furthermore, as there is no standardisation for the measurement of RV volumes, the quantitative measure of RV dimensions can vary between centres. It may be that as the RV dilates, interaction through the septum reduces LV filling [27] and reduces LV function. Importantly, there are suggestions that this may be happening at even moderate RV dilatation, because following PVR, LV EDV increases [32–35] with a subsequent increase in LV function in some studies [33, 37]. Further research is required to define CMR prognostic factors for PVR timing, and importantly other information from echocardiography, exercise testing, assessment of neurohormonal activation, ECG data and stress CMR may be useful for decision making [33].

7.6.2 Which Treatment Option?

Once a PVR has been clinically justified, there is now a choice between surgery and PPVI for approximately 15% of patients with TOF. Technical suitability for PPVI can be

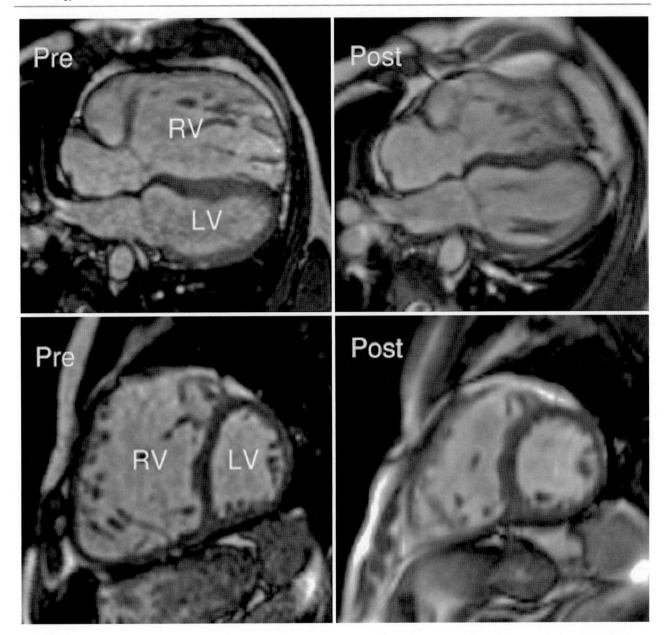

Fig. 7.8 Response to surgical PVR after 1 year. 4-chamber and short axis views showing marked RV volume reduction and increased LV volumes

defined by CMR using the protocol previously defined, but with focus on three main areas:

7.6.2.1 RVOT/Pulmonary Trunk Size and Distensibility

PPVI can be performed in RVOT/pulmonary trunks that range from 14 to 22 mm. At the lower end of the spectrum, conduits need to be of an adequate size to allow for sufficient opening without residual gradients. At the upper end, the device can only be expanded to a maximal diameter of 22 mm – any larger and valve leaflet coaptation may fail, or the device may embolise. This precludes PPVI in dilated

anatomies (Fig. 7.7). Conduit sizes can be gleaned from operative reports; however, conduits can become smaller (or larger) over time and, in order to have a full understanding of the anatomy of the outflow tract, CMR with 3D capabilities is crucial. Although the CMR-derived 3D reconstructions can be used to define size, it is important to realize that these reconstructions are performed on data acquired in diastole, or from non-ECG-gated data and, thus, maximal dimensions of very distensible anatomies may be underestimated. Cine imaging of the RVOT/ pulmonary trunk in both long and short axes overcomes this problem, enabling the measurement of the maximum diameter of the site at which PPVI may be attempted. If the results of MRI are doubtful or borderline, balloon sizing of the RVOT can be performed at the time of catheterization.

7.6.2.2 RVOT/Pulmonary Morphology

The 3D information from CMR can be used to visualize the best site for device anchorage in the RVOT/pulmonary trunk. Furthermore, certain shapes are not suitable for safe implantation of the device [13]. A morphological classification has been created according to measurements of 3D reconstructions of the RVOT [38]. Importantly, a pyramidal morphology, meaning that the RVOT funnels down toward the pulmonary bifurcation, is not suitable for PPVI because of the high risk of device dislodgement. Ideal RVOT/pulmonary trunk shapes comprise conduits with parallel borders or conduits with a narrowing in the mid-portion, since this provides a safe landing zone for the stent [38].

7.6.2.3 Proximity of the Proximal Coronary Arteries

The proximity of the proximal coronary arteries to the RVOT/ pulmonary trunk has to be assessed (Movie 7.4). On CMR 3D whole-heart b-SSFP images, the anatomical relationship of the coronary arteries and the proposed implantation site can be judged. In addition, aortic root angiography is performed at the time of catheterization. On biplane projection, the relationship between the coronaries and the pulmonary artery can be judged. In case the CMR assessment or aortic root angiography cannot fully rule out the risk for coronary compression, simultaneous high-pressure balloon inflation in the implantation site and selective coronary angiography is performed [39]. Importantly, when angiography and simultaneous balloon inflation is performed, it is crucial to expand the RVOT to a therapeutic size. This maneuver is only meaningful, when the conduit is expanded with a high-pressure balloon up to the diameter that will be reached post-PPVI.

7.6.3 Acute Hemodynamic Results and Implications for Biventricular Function Following PPVI

CMR performed before and within 1 month of the procedure, with analysis of biventricular function and calculation of great vessel blood flow, has shown an improvement in effective RV and LV stroke volume in both patients with predominantly pulmonary stenosis and those with predominantly regurgitation [9, 10, 37]. In patients with predominantly pulmonary stenosis, this is due to decreased RV ESV and improved RV ejection fraction after marked relief of afterload [10]. By contrast, RV ejection fraction remains unchanged in patients with predominantly pulmonary regurgitation, with the improvement in RV and LV effective

stroke volume due to abolishment of pulmonary regurgitation [37].

7.6.4 Development of New Percutaneous Devices

Because of the wide variation in patient morphology, size, and dynamics of the right ventricular outflow tract (RVOT)/ pulmonary trunk (Fig. 7.7), only ~15% of patients with a hemodynamic and clinical indication for PPVI can be treated with the current device. Thus, 85% of patients with pulmonary dysfunction still require open-heart surgery for treatment. The majority of these patients are those with dilated, dynamic RVOT/pulmonary trunk anatomy (patients with TOF and previous RVOT patches) in whom the current percutaneous device is too small. Over the last 3 years, we have developed a new device, which can be implanted into the dilated outflow tract (Fig. 7.9). This device has now undergone a successful 'first-in-man' implantation [40]. For this implantation, advanced cardiovascular imaging, in combination with patient-specific computer modelling is crucial to achieve procedural success. We await further human studies of this device in the near future.

7.7 Discussion

In this chapter, we have emphasised the advantages of MR imaging over other modalities to demonstrate its many strengths in the comprehensive assessment of TOF. However it is prudent to mention that there are clearly clinical situations in which other modalities are indeed superior and preferable.

Echocardiography is a very effective bedside imaging tool, and is used as the sole modality for the initial diagnosis of TOF in infancy and indeed the majority of later clinical follow-up. It could rightly be considered that MR is an adjunct to this primary imaging modality in the management of TOF.

In patients who have been treated previously with metallic stents, aneurysm clips or pacemakers, CT imaging is the preferable imaging modality. CT delineates RVOT and branch pulmonary artery morphology very well and it has a very rapid acquisition time, which is valuable for critically ill patients. As patients with TOF survive longer, the burden of acquired ischemic heart disease will increase, and it is here that CT imaging of the coronary arteries is superior to MR. However the technique cannot quantify vascular flow and of course, uses ionising radiation.

In our institution we have observed an increase in the use of cross-sectional imaging modalities with a resultant decrease in diagnostic cardiac catheterisations. Cardiac catheterisation

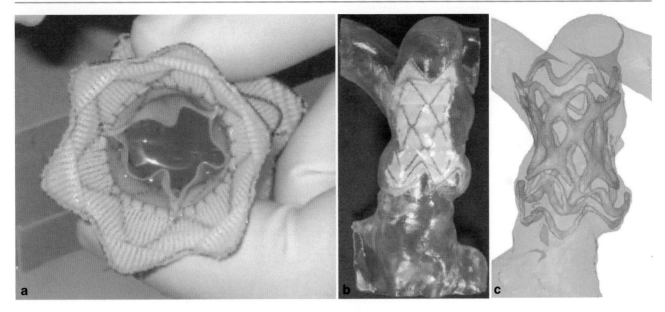

Fig. 7.9 New percutaneous device for implantation into the dilated outflow tract. (**a**) Nitinol device, (**b**) pre-implantation in rapid prototyping model, (**c**) 3D CT reconstruction post-implantation with device in-situ in 'first-in-man' case

is still necessary when therapeutic interventions are required or when intravascular pressures must be discerned. However, the fluoroscopic projections are not suitable for the characterisation of complex 3D malformations or ventricular function.

Conclusion

The tremendous advance in cross-sectional cardiovascular imaging has changed the landscape in the long-term follow-up and clinical decision-making in TOF. The wealth of reliable, reproducible hemodynamic information provided by MR studies justifies its recognition as the gold standard. The data provided by MR in TOF continues to advance our understanding of the disease and will continue to help us manage patients more effectively.

7.8 Practical Pearls

1. TOF is common and its routine assessment should be familiar to all CMR imagers.
2. Protocolised follow-up for repaired TOF is important and should include CMR as outlined in the clinical imaging protocol.
3. Debate remains about the exact timing of PVR in TOF, but an indexed RV end-diastolic volume between 150 and 200 ml/m², in the presence of severe pulmonary incompetence, seems appropriate.
4. CMR can be used to select treatment options (watchful waiting, surgical PVR or PPVI).
5. CMR provides excellent longitudinal data to track hemodynamic deterioration or responses to therapy.

References

1. Apitz C, Webb GD, Redington AN. Tetralogy of Fallot. Lancet. 2009;374(9699):1462–71.
2. Murphy JG, Gersh BJ, Mair DD, Fuster V, McGoon MD, Ilstrup DM, et al. Long-term outcome in patients undergoing surgical repair of tetralogy of Fallot. N Engl J Med. 1993;329(9):593–9.
3. Nollert G, Fischlein T, Bouterwek S, Bohmer C, Klinner W, Reichart B. Long-term survival in patients with repair of tetralogy of Fallot: 36-year follow-up of 490 survivors of the first year after surgical repair. J Am Coll Cardiol. 1997;30(5):1374–83.
4. Park MK. Pediatric cardiology for practitioners. 3rd ed. St. Louis: Mosby; 1996.
5. Oechslin EN, Harrison DA, Harris L, Downar E, Webb GD, Siu SS, et al. Reoperation in adults with repair of tetralogy of Fallot: indications and outcomes. J Thorac Cardiovasc Surg. 1999;118(2):245–51.
6. Ghez O, Tsang VT, Frigiola A, Coats L, Taylor A, Van Doorn C, et al. Right ventricular outflow tract reconstruction for pulmonary regurgitation after repair of tetralogy of Fallot. Preliminary results. Eur J Cardiothorac Surg. 2007;31(4):654–8.
7. Nordmeyer J, Tsang V, Gaudin R, Lurz P, Frigiola A, Jones A, et al. Quantitative assessment of homograft function 1 year after insertion into the pulmonary position: impact of in situ homograft geometry on valve competence. Eur Heart J. 2009;30(17):2147–54.
8. Bonhoeffer P, Boudjemline Y, Saliba Z, Merckx J, Aggoun Y, Bonnet D, et al. Percutaneous replacement of pulmonary valve in a right-ventricle to pulmonary-artery prosthetic conduit with valve dysfunction. Lancet. 2000;356(9239):1403–5.
9. Khambadkone S, Coats L, Taylor A, Boudjemline Y, Derrick G, Tsang V, et al. Percutaneous pulmonary valve implantation in humans: results in 59 consecutive patients. Circulation. 2005;112(8): 1189–97.
10. Coats L, Khambadkone S, Derrick G, Sridharan S, Schievano S, Mist B, et al. Physiological and clinical consequences of relief of right ventricular outflow tract obstruction late after repair of congenital heart defects. Circulation. 2006;113(17):2037–44.
11. Lurz P, Nordmeyer J, Muthurangu V, Khambadkone S, Derrick G, Yates R, et al. Comparison of bare metal stenting and percutaneous pulmonary valve implantation for treatment of right ventricular

outflow tract obstruction: use of an x-ray/magnetic resonance hybrid laboratory for acute physiological assessment. Circulation. 2009;119(23):2995–3001.

12. Sorensen TS, Korperich H, Greil GF, Eichhorn J, Barth P, Meyer H, et al. Operator-independent isotropic three-dimensional magnetic resonance imaging for morphology in congenital heart disease: a validation study. Circulation. 2004;110(2):163–9.

13. Schievano S, Coats L, Migliavacca F, Norman W, Frigiola A, Deanfield J, et al. Variations in right ventricular outflow tract morphology following repair of congenital heart disease: implications for percutaneous pulmonary valve implantation. J Cardiovasc Magn Reson. 2007;9(4):687–95.

14. Geva T, Greil GF, Marshall AC, Landzberg M, Powell AJ. Gadolinium- enhanced 3-dimensional magnetic resonance angiography of pulmonary blood supply in patients with complex pulmonary stenosis or atresia: comparison with x-ray angiography. Circulation. 2002;106(4):473–8.

15. Barkhausen J, Ruehm SG, Goyen M, Buck T, Laub G, Debatin JF. MR evaluation of ventricular function: true fast imaging with steady-state precession versus fast low-angle shot cine MR imaging: feasibility study. Radiology. 2001;219(1):264–9.

16. Winter MM, Bernink FJ, Groenink M, Bouma BJ, van Dijk AP, Helbing WA, et al. Evaluating the systemic right ventricle by CMR: the importance of consistent and reproducible delineation of the cavity. J Cardiovasc Magn Reson. 2008;10:40.

17. Rebergen SA, Chin JG, Ottenkamp J, van der Wall EE, de Roos A. Pulmonary regurgitation in the late postoperative follow-up of tetralogy of Fallot. Volumetric quantitation by nuclear magnetic resonance velocity mapping. Circulation. 1993;88(5 Pt 1):2257–66.

18. Taylor A, Bogaert J. Valvular heart disease. In: Bogaert J, Dymarkowski S, Taylor A, editors. Clinical cardiac MRI. Heidelberg: Springer; 2005. p. 353–79.

19. Powell AJ, Geva T. Blood flow measurement by magnetic resonance imaging in congenital heart disease. Pediatr Cardiol. 2000;21(1):47–58.

20. Grosse-Wortmann L, Al-Otay A, Goo HW, Macgowan CK, Coles JG, Benson LN, et al. Anatomical and functional evaluation of pulmonary veins in children by magnetic resonance imaging. J Am Coll Cardiol. 2007;49(9):993–1002.

21. Devos DG, Kilner PJ. Calculations of cardiovascular shunts and regurgitation using magnetic resonance ventricular volume and aortic and pulmonary flow measurements. Eur Radiol. 2010;20(2):410–21.

22. Greenberg SB, Crisci KL, Koenig P, Robinson B, Anisman P, Russo P. Magnetic resonance imaging compared with echocardiography in the evaluation of pulmonary artery abnormalities in children with tetralogy of Fallot following palliative and corrective surgery. Pediatr Radiol. 1997;27(12):932–5.

23. Nordmeyer J, Gaudin R, Tann OR, Lurz PC, Bonhoeffer P, Taylor AM, et al. MRI may be sufficient for noninvasive assessment of great vessel stents: an in vitro comparison of MRI, CT, and conventional angiography. Am J Roentgenol. 2010;195(4):865–71.

24. Babu-Narayan SV, Kilner PJ, Li W, Moon JC, Goktekin O, Davlouros PA, et al. Ventricular fibrosis suggested by cardiovascular magnetic resonance in adults with repaired tetralogy of fallot and its relationship to adverse markers of clinical outcome. Circulation. 2006;113(3):405–13.

25. Tulevski II, Hirsch A, Dodge-Khatami A, Stoker J, van der Wall EE, Mulder BJ. Effect of pulmonary valve regurgitation on right ventricular function in patients with chronic right ventricular pressure overload. Am J Cardiol. 2003;92(1):113–6.

26. Lurz P, Muthurangu V, Schievano S, Nordmeyer J, Bonhoeffer P, Taylor AM, et al. Feasibility and reproducibility of biventricular volumetric assessment of cardiac function during exercise using real- time radial k-t SENSE magnetic resonance imaging. J Magn Reson Imaging. 2009;29(5):1062–70.

27. Lurz P, Puranik R, Nordmeyer J, Muthurangu V, Hansen MS, Schievano S, et al. Improvement in left ventricular filling properties after relief of right ventricle to pulmonary artery conduit obstruction: contribution of septal motion and interventricular mechanical delay. Eur Heart J. 2009;30(18):2266–74.

28. Therrien J, Marx GR, Gatzoulis MA. Late problems in tetralogy of Fallot – recognition, management, and prevention. Cardiol Clin. 2002;20(3):395–404.

29. Oosterhof T, Meijboom FJ, Vliegen HW, Hazekamp MG, Zwinderman AH, Bouma BJ, et al. Long-term follow-up of homograft function after pulmonary valve replacement in patients with tetralogy of Fallot. Eur Heart J. 2006;27(12):1478–84.

30. Shebani SO, McGuirk S, Baghai M, Stickley J, De Giovanni JV, Bu'lock FA, et al. Right ventricular outflow tract reconstruction using Contegra valved conduit: natural history and conduit performance under pressure. Eur J Cardiothorac Surg. 2006;29(3):397–405.

31. Vliegen HW, van Straten A, de Roos A, Roest AA, Schoof PH, Zwinderman AH, et al. Magnetic resonance imaging to assess the hemodynamic effects of pulmonary valve replacement in adults late after repair of tetralogy of fallot. Circulation. 2002;106(13):1703–7.

32. Therrien J, Siu SC, McLaughlin PR, Liu PP, Williams WG, Webb GD. Pulmonary valve replacement in adults late after repair of tetralogy of Fallot: are we operating too late? J Am Coll Cardiol. 2000;36(5):1670–5.

33. Frigiola A, Tsang V, Bull C, Coats L, Khambadkone S, Derrick G, et al. Biventricular response after pulmonary valve replacement for right ventricular outflow tract dysfunction: is age a predictor of outcome? Circulation. 2008;118(14 Suppl):S182–90.

34. Oosterhof T, van Straten A, Vliegen HW, Meijboom FJ, van Dijk AP, Spijkerboer AM, et al. Preoperative thresholds for pulmonary valve replacement in patients with corrected tetralogy of Fallot using cardiovascular magnetic resonance. Circulation. 2007;116(5):545–51.

35. Therrien J, Provost Y, Merchant N, Williams W, Colman J, Webb G. Optimal timing for pulmonary valve replacement in adults after tetralogy of Fallot repair. Am J Cardiol. 2005;95(6):779–82.

36. Buechel ER, Dave HH, Kellenberger CJ, Dodge-Khatami A, Pretre R, Berger F, et al. Remodelling of the right ventricle after early pulmonary valve replacement in children with repaired tetralogy of Fallot: assessment by cardiovascular magnetic resonance. Eur Heart J. 2005;26(24):2721–7.

37. Coats L, Khambadkone S, Derrick G, Hughes M, Jones R, Mist B, et al. Physiological consequences of percutaneous pulmonary valve implantation: the different behaviour of volume- and pressure-overloaded ventricles. Eur Heart J. 2007;28(15):1886–93.

38. Schievano S, Migliavacca F, Coats L, Khambadkone S, Carminati M, Wilson N, et al. Percutaneous pulmonary valve implantation based on rapid prototyping of right ventricular outflow tract and pulmonary trunk from MR data. Radiology. 2007;242(2):490–7.

39. Sridharan S, Coats L, Khambadkone S, Taylor AM, Bonhoeffer P. Images in cardiovascular medicine. Transcatheter right ventricular outflow tract intervention: the risk to the coronary circulation. Circulation. 2006;113(25):e934–5.

40. Schievano S, Taylor AM, Capelli C, Coats L, Walker F, Lurz P, et al. First-in-man implantation of a novel percutaneous valve: a new approach to medical device development. EuroIntervention. 2010;5(6):745–50.

Ebstein's Anomaly and Other Tricuspid Valve Anomalies

8

Steve W. Leung and Mushabbar A. Syed

8.1 Introduction

Ebstein's anomaly is a rare congenital heart disease that affects approximately 1 in 200,000 live births, and <1 % of all congenital heart diseases [1]. The anomaly was originally described in 1866 by Dr. Wilhelm Ebstein in a patient with progressive tricuspid insufficiency due to a congenital malformation [2]. Until 1950s, the diagnosis of Ebstein's anomaly was mainly based on autopsy findings. It was not until 1951 when Soloff et al. first described a method of diagnosing Ebstein's anomaly while the patient is still alive by invasive angiogram [3]. In the 1970s, with the development of M-mode, two-dimensional, and Doppler echocardiography, echocardiography became the primary modality in diagnosing Ebstein's anomaly [4]. However, echocardiography is highly dependent on operator experience, the availability of good acoustic windows, and spatial resolution distal to the probe. Due to the position of the right ventricle being directly behind the sternum and its complex geometry, imaging the right ventricle with echocardiogram is often difficult (Movie 8.1).

More recently, cardiac magnetic resonance imaging (CMR) has emerged as a versatile technique for the assessment of cardiac function, morphology, vascular anatomy and flow in patients with congenital heart disease. Patients who have limited echocardiographic windows can have clearer pictures with CMR and the right ventricle can be visualized more easily. Quantification of right ventricular volume and function and identification of other associated lesions can be obtained in the management of this special population.

8.2 Definition

Ebstein's anomaly encompasses a wide spectrum of anatomic and functional abnormalities of the morphologic tricuspid valve and right ventricle. The classic description involves the apical displacement of basal attachments of the septal and posterior leaflets of tricuspid valve secondary to failed delamination of the tricuspid valve leaflets from the endocardium during fetal development leading to atrialization of the right ventricle. Apical displacement of the septal leaflet of ≥ 8 mm/m^2 indexed to body surface area relative to the mitral valve in the apical 4-chamber view is considered diagnostic [4].

8.3 Morphology

Ebstein's anomaly is characterized by the congenital malformations of the right ventricle and tricuspid valve. These malformations include adherence of the septal and posterior leaflet to the myocardium, apical displacement of the tricuspid annulus, redundancy/fenestration and tethering of the anterior leaflet, dilation of the atrialized portion of the right ventricle and dilation of the right atrioventricular junction [5]. The posterior leaflet is the most frequently affected leaflet, followed by the septal, and anterior leaflets. Depending on the severity of the tethering, patients can present as a neonate or late into adult life. Due to the developmental malformation of the tricuspid valve, patients can have tricuspid regurgitation or occasionally tricuspid stenosis.

S.W. Leung, M.D.
Department of Medicine and Radiology,
Division of Cardiovascular Disease, University of Kentucky,
900 S. Limestone St., C.T. Wethington Bldg Rm 326,
Lexington, KY, USA
e-mail: steve.leung@uky.edu

M.A. Syed, M.D., FACC (✉)
Department of Medicine and Radiology, Stritch School of Medicine,
Loyola University Chicago, IL, USA

Cardiovascular Imaging, Heart and Vascular Institute,
Loyola University Medical Center, Maywood, IL, USA
e-mail: masyed@lumc.edu

Electronic supplementary material The online version of this chapter (doi:10.1007/978-1-4471-4267-6_8) contains supplementary material, which is available to authorized users.

M.A. Syed, R.H. Mohiaddin (eds.), *Magnetic Resonance Imaging of Congenital Heart Disease*,
DOI 10.1007/978-1-4471-4267-6_8, © Springer-Verlag London 2012

The amount of tethering also determines whether the valve can be repaired or replaced by the Carpentier Classification [6].

Type A: right ventricular volume is adequate

Type B: large atrialized right ventricle with mobile anterior leaflet of the tricuspid valve

Type C: severely restricted anterior leaflet of the tricuspid valve

Type D: almost complete atrialization of the right ventricle except for a small infundibular component

Patients with Type A, B and C leaflets are likely to benefit from surgical repair. Type D patients require valve replacement.

8.4 Associated Anomalies

The most common anomaly associated with Ebstein's anomaly is interatrial connection such as atrial septal defects and perforated foramen ovale, which occurs in upwards of 80 % of patients with Ebstein's anomaly. There are numerous other abnormalities that are associated with Ebstein's anomaly asides from atrial septal defects (Table 8.1). Ebstein's anomaly, generally an isolated process, has been described in patients with Down's syndrome, Marfan syndrome, Noonan syndrome and left ventricular non-compaction.

8.5 Clinical Presentation

Due to the wide spectrum of the severity of the tricuspid malformation, clinical presentation can range from intrauterine fetal demise to incidental finding in an asymptomatic adult patient. Patients who present during their first year of life usually have more severe cardiac disease, and present with severe heart failure and cyanosis. In contrast, children and adults more often present with incidental murmurs and arrhythmias such as Wolff-Parkinson-White syndrome [7].

Symptomatic patients may present with peripheral edema, dyspnea on exertion, or other signs and symptoms of right ventricular heart failure from worsening tricuspid regurgitation. Since there is a high percentage of patients with Ebstein's anomaly that has arrhythmias, palpitations can also be a presenting symptom. Due to the high prevalence of septal defects, patients may present later in life with pulmonary hypertension, paradoxical emboli and Eisenmenger physiology.

The electrocardiogram in patients with Ebstein's anomaly often has interventricular conduction delay or right bundle branch block. The p-waves may indicate marked right atrial enlargement often described as Himalayan P-waves. Since there is a higher prevalence of pre-excitation in this popula-

Table 8.1 Anatomical anomalies associated with Ebstein's Anomaly

Septal defects
Atrial septal defect
Perforated foramen ovale
Ventricular septal defect
Aortic valve/Aorta
Bicuspid or atretic aortic valve
Aortic coarctation
Subaortic stenosis
Corrected transposition of the great arteries
Patent ductus arteriosus
Pulmonic valve/Pulmonary artery
Pulmonary stenosis
Pulmonary atresia
Hypoplastic pulmonary arteries
Hypertensive pulmonary vascular disease
Mitral valve
Parachute mitral valve
Cleft anterior leaflet of the mitral valve
Mitral valve prolapse
Other
Left ventricular outflow obstruction
Tetralogy of Fallot
Left ventricular non-compaction

tion, delta waves can be seen in some patient's ECGs. Due to the atrialization of the right ventricle, right ventricular hypertrophy is rare and if present other associated anomalies should be considered.

Most cases of Ebstein's anomaly discovered have been sporadic, but there have been some familial cases. Neonates whose mothers were exposed to lithium have been reported to develop Ebstein's anomaly.

8.6 Cardiac Magnetic Resonance Imaging

8.6.1 Indications

Echocardiography has been the main tool in the diagnosis of Ebstein's anomaly. However, in patients with poor echocardiographic windows, CMR can be an alternative method in making the diagnosis. In patients with known Ebstein's anomaly, CMR can provide valuable information in quantifying right ventricular size and function, along with severity of tricuspid regurgitation. Serial CMR can be performed to monitor right ventricular size and function, as well as severity of tricuspid regurgitation. Since patients with Ebstein's anomaly often have other associated anomalies, CMR can provide good views of the atrial and ventricular septum, aorta and pulmonary artery and quantify pulmonary and systemic flow to calculate the amount of shunt.

Table 8.2 Imaging protocol example

- Scout (localizers) scan: in three-plane (axial, sagittal, coronal), axial stack, 4-chamber, short axis plane
- SSFP cine images:
    Short axis, multislice stack from base to apex
    3-chamber, 2-Chamber, 4-Chamber views
    2-chamber of the right atrium/right ventricle
    LVOT and RVOT
    4-chamber view, stack for full volume coverage (for identification of septal defects)
    Optional: Axial plane, 10 mm stack from top to bottom of the right ventricle
- First pass contrast enhanced MRA of pulmonary arteries and aorta
- In-plane phase contrast flow imaging (ECG gated, free breathing)
    4–chamber view
    LVOT
    RVOT
    Optional: 2-chamber view of the right atrium/ventricle
- Through-plane phase contrast imaging (ECG gated, free breathing) of the main pulmonary artery (Qp) and ascending aorta (Qs)
- *Optional: Through-plane phase contrast imaging (ECG gated, free breathing) of the tricuspid valve in short axis plane using a 4-chamber cine SSFP to align the imaging plane with the valve annulus at end-systole.*
- Late gadolinium enhancement imaging in short axis stack, 2-chamber, 3-chamber, 4-chamber views (usually 10–20 min post contrast)
- *Optional: Through-plane phase contrast of static gel phantom with identical acquisition parameters as Qp and Qs*

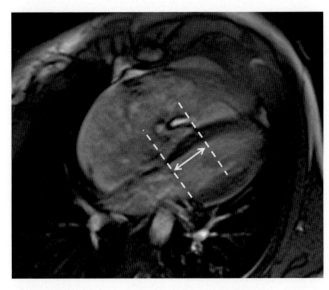

Fig. 8.1 Still frame in an SSFP 4-Chamber view shows the apical displacement (*double arrow*) of the tricuspid valve compared to the mitral valve. End-diastolic frame is used for measuring the apical displacement

8.6.2   Goals of Imaging

1. To determine the extent of apical displacement of the tricuspid valve and assess mobility of the anterior leaflet (Carpentier classification)
2. To accurately assess right ventricular size, and function
3. To identify tricuspid regurgitation, and quantify severity
4. To identify associated lesions such as perforated foramen ovale, atrial septal defect, ventricular septal defect and calculate the amount of shunt (Qp:Qs ratio)

5. To determine aortic or pulmonary artery anomalies
6. To identify right ventricular outflow tract obstructions.

8.6.3   CMR Sequences and Imaging Protocols

A sample CMR scanning protocol is listed in Table 8.2.

8.6.3.1   Scout Imaging

Scout imaging in various planes can help quickly identify any significant right ventricular enlargement, and any apparent associated lesions in the aorta or pulmonary artery such as coarctation or hypoplastic pulmonary artery. Since most patients who present have enlarged right heart, the cardiac anatomy is likely to be distorted. The scout images can then help with accurate prescription of the long and short-axis cines, and ensure adequate coverage of the ventricles for quantification of size and function.

8.6.3.2   Cine Imaging – Diagnosis, Chamber Size and Function, and Septal Defects

For the diagnosis of Ebstein's anomaly, 4-chamber steady state free precession (SSFP) cine can identify the apical displacement of the tricuspid valve compared to the mitral valve (Fig. 8.1 and Movie 8.2). The diagnosis can be made if the apical displacement of the tricuspid valve compared to the mitral valve is $\geq 8mm/m^2$ indexed to body surface area. The identification of the tricuspid leaflets and the amount of tethering can be useful in determining type of surgical treatment. However, due to the complex shape and thin tricuspid valve leaflet and relatively limited spatial resolution of CMR,

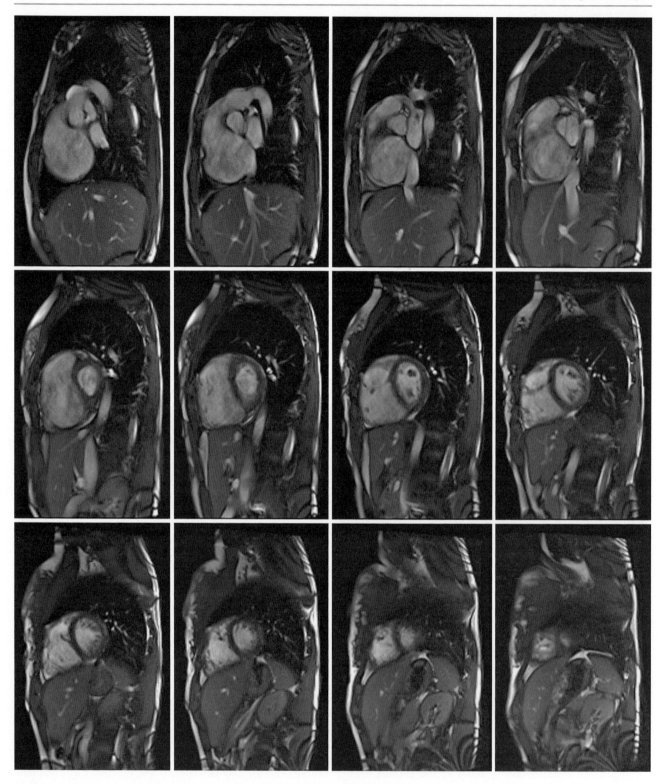

Fig. 8.2 Still frame of short axis stack for evaluation of ventricular size and function

it may be difficult to visualize leaflet adherence to the myocardium.

The short-axis cines from base to apex are routinely used for calculating LV and RV size and function (Fig. 8.2) [8]. Alternatively, axial plane cines can also be used for calculating RV size and function; however, the method of acquiring RV size and function in serial follow up studies should be consistent with the first study [9].

To identify septal defects, 4-chamber stack of cines through the atrial and ventricular septum extending from the

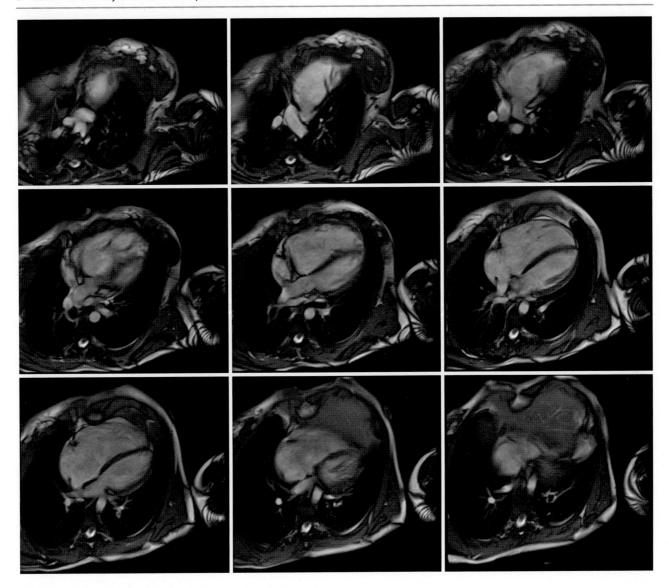

Fig. 8.3 Still frame of 4-chamber stack for evaluation of septal defects

superior vena cava to the level of AV valves should be obtained for interatrial or interventricular connections (Fig. 8.3).

8.6.3.3 In Plane Phase Contrast Imaging: Evaluation of Abnormal Flow

SSFP cine imaging can often miss valvular regurgitation or flow through septal defects as the sequence is designed to suppress flow for better delineation of endocardial borders. Therefore, ECG gated, free breathing, in-plane phase contrast imaging can be helpful in clearly identifying any tricuspid regurgitation or flow through septal defects in patients with Ebstein's anomaly. Qualitatively, tricuspid regurgitation can be evaluated by in-plane phase contrast imaging in the 4-chamber view or right atrial/ventricular 2-chamber view with the axis parallel to the predicted tricuspid regurgitant jet

(Movie 8.3). The velocity encoding (VENC) setting should be at least 150 cm/s. For septal defects, the appropriate 4-chamber view of the suspected area of the defect should be evaluated with in-plane phase contrast. Due to slow flow in the atrium, the VENC setting is usually set at 50–100 cm/s. Since patients with Ebstein's anomaly can also have left or right ventricular outflow tract (LVOT, RVOT) obstruction, LVOT and RVOT in-plane phase contrast can help identify any significant turbulent flow suggestive of obstruction across the outflow tracts (Fig. 8.4 and Movie 8.4).

Occasionally, patients with Ebstein's anomaly have tricuspid stenosis. Severe tricuspid stenosis has been identified as a right atrium to right ventricle gradient of >5 mmHg during diastole by Doppler echocardiography. In-plane phase contrast imaging in a 4 chamber or right sided 2 chamber orientation can identify increased velocity through the tricuspid

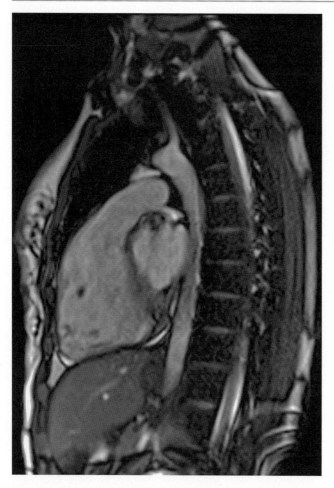

Fig. 8.4 Still frame of right ventricular outflow tract SSFP cine for evaluation of right ventricular outflow tract obstruction

valve during diastole as a sign of tricuspid stenosis. Initial VENC of 100 cm/s should be used. If the jet aliases during diastole, then the gradient across the tricuspid valve is >4 mmHg by using the simplified Bernoulli's equation (gradient=4v²). Be aware that in patients with significant tricuspid regurgitation that there can be functional tricuspid stenosis due to increase flow, and not due to anatomical tricuspid stenosis.

8.6.3.4 Through-Plane Phase Contrast: Quantification of Tricuspid Regurgitation

Patients with Ebstein's anomaly develop significant tricuspid regurgitation. In echocardiography, severe tricuspid regurgitation is determined by color jet size, vena contracta width >0.7 cm², and systolic reversal of flow in the hepatic veins. In CMR, there have not been established criteria for severe tricuspid regurgitation; however, in general, valvular regurgitant fraction >40 % is considered severe. Unlike the aortic and pulmonic valves, the tricuspid annulus goes through significantly complex motion during systole, which renders direct measurements by through-plane phase contrast CMR

of the tricuspid valve difficult. For best results, a short-axis plane can be prescribed using 4 chamber cine SSFP to align the imaging plane with the valve annulus at end-systole. Additionally, the tricuspid regurgitant volume and regurgitant fraction can be measured indirectly from effective pulmonic flow and right ventricular stroke volume.

Effective pulmonary flow (Qp) can be obtained by ECG gated, free breathing, through-plane phase contrast imaging of the main pulmonary artery cross section above the pulmonic valve. Often, this prescription can be obtained from a perpendicular slice from the right ventricular outflow tract view (sagittal plane) above the pulmonic valve (Fig. 8.5) starting at VENC of 150 cm/s. The resultant velocity images should be immediately assessed for aliasing (low VENC setting) and repeated if necessary by increasing the VENC setting. Also check the magnitude images for appropriate vessel shape (arteries should be round) and phase wrap artifacts. Phase wrap does not significantly affect the precision of the measurements as long as wrap is not superimposed on the vessel of interest. Right ventricular stroke volume (RVSV) is obtained by subtracting the right ventricular end-systolic volume (RVESV) from the right ventricular end-diastolic volume (RVEDV). RVESV and RVEDV are obtained from either the short axis stack or axial stack SSFP cine images. Tricuspid regurgitant volume (RV_{TR}) can then be calculated by:

$$RV_{TR} = Qp - (RVEDV - RVESV) = Qp - RVSV$$

Regurgitant fraction (RF) can be obtained by:

$$RF\% = (RV_{TR} / RVSV) \times 100\%$$

This method can only be used if there is no interventricular shunt.

Without phase contrast flow measurements, RV_{TR} can also be calculated by:

$$RV_{TR} = RVSV - (LVEDV - LVESV) = RVSV - LVSV$$

This can only be performed if there are no other significant valvular regurgitations (aortic, mitral or pulmonic) or interventricular shunt.

8.6.3.5 Through-Plane Phase Contrast: Quantification of Shunt Ratio

Since patients with Ebstein's anomaly frequently have associated atrial or ventricular septal defects, shunt ratio quantification (Qp/Qs) can be helpful in determining need for closure of these defects. Shunt ratio quantification should be obtained from through-plane phase contrast.

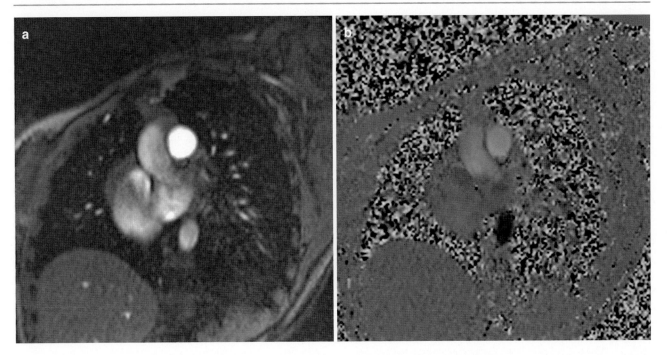

Fig. 8.5 Still frame of the main pulmonary artery just above the pulmonic valve for effective pulmonary flow (Qp) quantification. (**a**) Magnitude image for anatomy and (**b**) is corresponding phase image. Vessel of interest should be circular to quantify flow

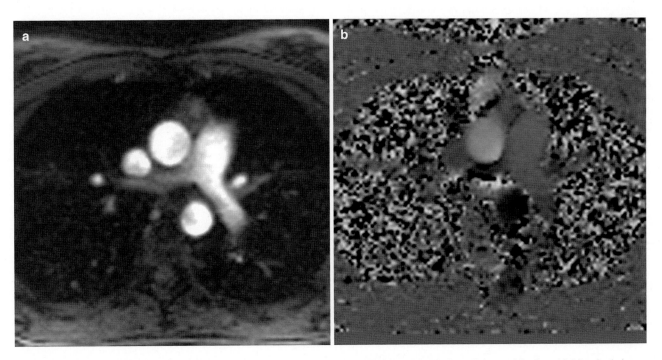

Fig. 8.6 Still frame of the ascending aorta at pulmonary artery bifurcation for effective systemic flow (Qs) quantification. (**a**) Magnitude image for anatomy and (**b**) is corresponding phase image. Vessel of interest should be circular to quantify flow

Qp prescription has been described above. Through-plane phase contrast of an appropriate axial slice above the aortic valve can be obtained for effective systemic flow (Qs) (Fig. 8.6). The encoding velocity for flow measurement in ascending aorta is usually set at 200 cm/s.

With phase contrast imaging, flow acquisition can be erroneous due to background phase off-set errors from non-compensated eddy currents [10]. This error can be corrected by obtaining phase contrast images from static gel phantoms post-acquisition with heart rate simulator simulating a heart rate similar to the time of Qp and Qs acquisition. The correction should then be used to adjust the original data. It's important to note that the table position should not be reset prior to obtaining the phantom images, as this can cause positioning errors in finding the original flow positions and acquisition of the correct background phase off-set errors.

8.6.4 Contrast Enhanced Magnetic Resonance Angiography

Patients with Ebstein's anomaly can have associated pulmonary artery or aortic anomalies. Contrast enhanced MRA can provide a three-dimensional view to detect hypoplastic pulmonary arteries, coarctation of the aorta, and transposition of the great arteries. It can also provide accurate vascular measurements for planning surgical treatment of these anomalies.

8.6.5 Late Gadolinium Enhancement Imaging

Late gadolinium enhancement imaging has been quite useful in detecting scar or fibrosis in patients with myocardial infarction and various cardiomyopathies. In patients with Ebstein's anomaly, late gadolinium enhancement can be used to identify fibrotic changes of the atrialized ventricular wall [11]. In patients with tricuspid stenosis or right ventricular dysfunction, late gadolinium enhancement can also identify right atrial and right ventricular thrombus.

8.7 Discussion

Echocardiography remains the primary method of diagnosing Ebstein's anomaly and identifying tricuspid leaflet deformities for possible surgical correction. Due to the higher spatial resolution, the tethering of the tricuspid leaflet can be more easily identified. Doppler echocardiography can also be helpful in evaluation of tricuspid regurgitation severity. However, in cases where there are limited acoustic windows and/or poor spatial resolution in deep structures, CMR is helpful in providing essential information. Since structures are more clearly defined and volumetric measurements are more reliable and reproducible than echocardiography, CMR is important in serial imaging to follow patients with established diagnosis of Ebstein's anomaly. Since patients with Ebstein's anomaly may have various associated vascular anomalies, CMR can help identify these other findings that may have been missed on echocardiography.

With the development of multi-slice computed tomography (CT) with electrocardiographic gating, CT scan has also become useful in evaluation of congenital heart disease. Since cardiac CT can provide excellent spatial resolution, complete volumetric coverage and functional analysis, it can be a valuable tool when echocardiography and CMR cannot be performed adequately. This can be due to inadequate acoustic windows or suboptimal right ventricular visualization for echocardiography, contraindication to CMR due to metallic implants, patients unable to lay flat for prolonged periods of time, or unable to hold their breaths repeatedly. However, at this time, cardiac CT cannot adequately calculate tricuspid regurgitation unless there is no other concomitant valvular regurgitation from RVSV and LVSV as described above. Since cardiac function evaluation with CT requires high doses of radiation, this should be limited to a last resort especially in young patients or women of childbearing age.

8.8 Limitations and Common Pitfalls

For patients with Ebstein's anomaly who are referred for CMR imaging, prior imaging studies should be reviewed to develop a plan of scanning to reduce scanning time. One of the limitations of CMR is that image acquisition can take a prolonged period of time. Some patients are unable to tolerate such prolonged scans due to claustrophobia, fatigue, back pain or other issues. If a patient has known atrial septal defect that has been adequately evaluated by echocardiography, one can consider skipping the 4-chamber cine stack. If a patient does not have RVOT or LVOT obstruction on Doppler echocardiography, one can consider skipping these imaging planes to reduce acquisition time.

Other limitations include patient cooperation in following breathing commands, which can limit the clarity in the SSFP cine images and late gadolinium enhancement images. The spatial resolution limits visualization of the tricuspid valve leaflet as clearly as echocardiography. Despite the common use of phase contrast for flow measurements, it is important to perform background offset error correction with static gel phantoms to obtain more accurate flow quantification data.

8.9 Other Tricuspid Valve Anomalies

Isolated congenital tricuspid stenosis is an extremely rare congenital heart malformation. The condition is a result of hypoplasia and thickening of the tricuspid valve, deformity of the chordae, or malformation of the entire subvalvular apparatus including parachute valve [12]. It is commonly associated with perforated foramen ovale or atrial septal defect [13–15]. They are also associated with right sided

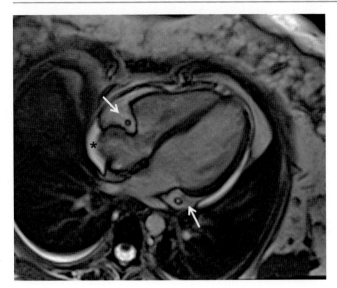

Fig. 8.7 Still frame of 4 chamber SSFP cine demonstrating small tricuspid valve annulus. There is small pericardial effusion (*asterisk*) and prominent intrapericardial fat (*arrows*)

hypoplasia including right ventricular hypoplasia and pulmonic stenosis or atresia. SSFP cine in the long axis views of the right atrium/right ventricle can be helpful in identifying the cause of tricuspid stenosis (Fig. 8.7 and Movie 8.5). The tricuspid gradient can be identified by ECG gated, free breathing, in-plane phase contrast imaging in the long axis through the tricuspid valve as described above. Due to the tricuspid annular plane systolic excursion, multiple cross sections through the tricuspid valve with no skip may be required to obtain a planimetry of the valve opening and optimal through-plane phase contrast to obtain the maximal gradient through the valve. A short-axis plane using 4-chamber cine SSFP to align the imaging plane with the valve annulus at end-systole usually provides the best result for gradient estimation.

Congenital tricuspid regurgitation is generally due to Ebstein's anomaly. Isolated congenital tricuspid regurgitation is even less common. The valvular insufficiency can be caused by tricuspid leaflet prolapse, hypoplastic or cleft leaflets, absence of papillary muscle or chordae, or annular dilation [16–18]. Functional causes include right ventricular outflow tract obstruction or right ventricular dysfunction [12]. In these patients, CMR can be used to calculate regurgitant volume and fraction similar to the methods mentioned in Ebstein's anomaly. SSFP cine imaging of the tricuspid valve in long axis views can be helpful in identifying tricuspid valve prolapse and other causes of tricuspid regurgitation. Right ventricular volumes can also be followed over time.

The role of CMR in these cases is similar to patients with Ebstein's anomaly. In patients who do not have optimal acoustic windows for echocardiography, the need to evaluate other associated anomalies or serial follow up of right sided volumes, CMR can be beneficial.

Conclusions

Ebstein's anomaly and congenital tricuspid anomalies are rare congenital heart defects that affect less than 1 % of all congenital heart diseases. Although echocardiography is the primary modality for diagnosis of these rare anomalies, it is limited in evaluation of the right ventricular size and function. Adult patients who present with little to no symptoms would need to be followed for years prior to the necessary surgical correction due to right ventricular enlargement and failure. CMR not only provides the capability to diagnose these rare anomalies, but can also provide accurate serial measurements of right ventricular volume and function and severity of tricuspid regurgitation. Many of these patients also present with various associated anomalies that can be detected readily by a comprehensive CMR study. In patients with associated shunts, quantification of pulmonary artery to aorta flow ratio (Qp/Qs) can be performed to assess the severity of these shunts.

8.10 Practical Pearls

- Review of prior imaging studies (especially echocardiographic images) is extremely helpful in planning scanning protocol to minimize scan time
- Echocardiography is usually the first line imaging modality for the diagnosis of Ebstein's anomaly. CMR has a complimentary role for the evaluation of right ventricle and other associated anomalies.
- CMR can be used to evaluate apical displacement of the tricuspid valve, tricuspid valvular regurgitation/stenosis, accurate measurements of right and left ventricular size and function, associated anomalies such as septal defects and great vessel abnormalities and quantification of shunt ratio.
- Serial CMR imaging for assessment of right ventricular size and function should be performed in the same orientation as the initial study (short axis stack or axial plane stack cines).
- Interatrial and interventricular communication can be difficult to see on SSFP cine images. ECG gated, free breathing, in-plane phase contrast flow imaging is helpful in these situations.
- 3D Contrasted MRA can be helpful in defining any aortic or pulmonary artery abnormalities.
- Flow quantification for Qp, Qs and tricuspid regurgitation measurements should be carefully planned.

References

1. Attenhofer Jost CH, et al. Ebstein's anomaly. Circulation. 2007;115(2):277–85.
2. Ebstein W. Ueber einen sehr seltenen Fall von insufficienz der valvula tricuspidatis, bedingt durch eine angeborene hochgradige Missbildung derselben. Arch Anat Physiol. 1866;33:238–54.
3. Soloff LA, Stauffer HM, Zatuchni J. Ebstein's disease: report of the first case diagnosed during life. Am J Med Sci. 1951;222(5):554–61.
4. Shiina A, et al. Two-dimensional echocardiographic spectrum of Ebstein's anomaly: detailed anatomic assessment. J Am Coll Cardiol. 1984;3(2 Pt 1):356–70.
5. Edwards WD. Embryology and pathologic features of Ebstein's anomaly. Prog Pediatr Cardiol. 1993;2(1):5–15.
6. Carpentier A, et al. A new reconstructive operation for Ebstein's anomaly of the tricuspid valve. J Thorac Cardiovasc Surg. 1988;96(1):92–101.
7. Celermajer DS, et al. Ebstein's anomaly: presentation and outcome from fetus to adult. J Am Coll Cardiol. 1994;23(1):170–6.
8. Grothues F, et al. Interstudy reproducibility of right ventricular volumes, function, and mass with cardiovascular magnetic resonance. Am Heart J. 2004;147(2):218–23.
9. Alfakih K, et al. Comparison of right ventricular volume measurements between axial and short axis orientation using steady-state free precession magnetic resonance imaging. J Magn Reson Imaging. 2003;18(1):25–32.
10. Holland BJ, Printz BF, Lai WW. Baseline correction of phase-contrast images in congenital cardiovascular magnetic resonance. J Cardiovasc Magn Reson. 2010;12:11.
11. Nakamura I, et al. Ebstein anomaly by cardiac magnetic resonance imaging. J Am Coll Cardiol. 2009;53(17):1568.
12. Dearani JA, Danielson GK. Congenital heart surgery nomenclature and database project: Ebstein's anomaly and tricuspid valve disease. Ann Thorac Surg. 2000;69(4 Suppl):S106–17.
13. Chuah SY, Hughes-Nurse J, Rowlands DB. A successful pregnancy in a patient with congenital tricuspid stenosis and a patent oval foramen. Int J Cardiol. 1992;34(1):112–4.
14. Khan AN, Boatman J, Anderson AS. Management of new-onset congestive heart failure in a patient with complex congenital heart disease. Congest Heart Fail. 2002;8(1):54–6.
15. Krishnamoorthy KM. Balloon dilatation of isolated congenital tricuspid stenosis. Int J Cardiol. 2003;89(1):119–21.
16. Kobza R, et al. Aberrant tendinous chords with tethering of the tricuspid leaflets: a congenital anomaly causing severe tricuspid regurgitation. Heart. 2004;90(3):319–23.
17. Motoyoshi N, et al. Cleft on tricuspid anterior leaflet. Ann Thorac Surg. 2001;71(4):1350–1.
18. Katogi T, et al. Surgical management of isolated congenital tricuspid regurgitation. Ann Thorac Surg. 1998;66(5):1571–4.

Puja Banka and Tal Geva

9.1 Introduction

Congenital abnormalities of left ventricular inflow and outflow include abnormalities of the left atrium, mitral valve (supravalvar, valvar, and subvalvar), and abnormalities of the left ventricular outflow tract, the aortic valve, and supravalvar area. Cardiac magnetic resonance imaging (CMR) has become an important adjunctive tool in evaluating and following patients with this group of anomalies. This chapter reviews the role of CMR in the care of patients with congenital abnormalities of left ventricular inflow and outflow. In addition to describing the morphologic abnormalities and their clinical presentations, the indications and limitations of CMR in each condition are discussed and a suggested CMR examination protocol is provided.

9.2 Abnormalities of Left Ventricular Inflow

9.2.1 Left Atrium

9.2.1.1 Definitions

Abnormalities of the left atrium include congenital left atrial aneurysm and cor triatriatum. The former is characterized by intrinsic left atrial enlargement out of proportion to the hemodynamic load on the left atrium. The latter is characterized

P. Banka, M.D. (✉)
Department of Cardiology, Harvard Medical School,
Boston, MA, USA

Department of Cardiology, Boston Children's Hospital,
300 Longwood Avenue, Boston, MA 02115, USA
e-mail: puja.banka@cardio.chboston.org

T. Geva, M.D.
Harvard Medical School, Boston, MA, USA

Department of Cardiology,
Children's Hospital Boston,
300 Longwood Avenue, Boston, MA 02115, USA
e-mail: tal.geva@cardio.chboston.org

by a dividing "membrane" within the left atrium resulting in a proximal pulmonary venous chamber and a distal supramitral chamber containing the appendage.

9.2.1.2 Congenital Left Atrial Aneurysm

Morphologic and Functional Abnormalities
Congenital left atrial aneurysm is a rare anomaly associated with dysplasia of the left atrial myocardium [1]. This anomaly, also called giant left atrium, is characterized by a markedly dilated left atrium with thinning or partial absence of the myocardium. The left atrial enlargement is out of proportion to its hemodynamic load. The diagnosis is made in the absence of an inflammatory or degenerative process [2].

Associated Anomalies
The etiology and morphogenesis of congenital left atrial aneurysm are poorly understood. This lesion is generally found as an isolated condition, and the presence of associated cardiac anomalies that can cause left atrial dilation usually exclude it from the differential diagnosis.

Clinical Presentation
Congenital left atrial aneurysm often presents as an incidental finding on radiographic imaging done for other reasons [3]. In some cases, however, patients present with tachyarrhythmias, cardiac arrest, pericardial tamponade from rupture of the aneurysm, systemic embolization of atrial thrombi, respiratory distress, or heart failure [2, 4]. Since the aneurysm can increase in size over time, long-term follow-up is generally recommended to monitor its size and associated complications. Surgical resection may be considered, especially in symptomatic patients [2].

Electronic supplementary material The online version of this chapter (doi:10.1007/978-1-4471-4267-6_9) contains supplementary material, which is available to authorized users.

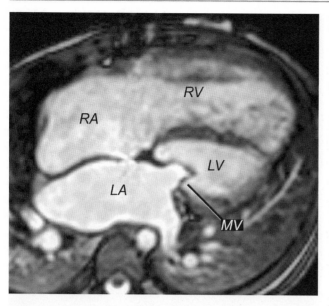

Fig. 9.2 Congenital mitral stenosis. Cine SSFP image in a 4-chamber plane showing a hypoplastic mitral valve annulus with thickened leaflets and restricted leaflet motion (*MV*). The left ventricle (*LV*) is also hypoplastic. *LA* left atrium, *RA* right atrium, *RV* right ventricle

anatomic abnormality of one or more components of the valve anatomy leading to narrowing of left ventricular inflow. Abnormalities at any level of the valve apparatus can result in obstruction to left ventricular inflow.

- *Supramitral stenosis*: In this anomaly, fibrous tissue develops on the left atrial aspect of the mitral annulus and leaflets, resulting in a restricted inflow orifice and thickened, poorly mobile leaflets [10, 11]. The fibrous tissue often adheres to the atrial surface of the valve leaflets, and the location of the effective flow orifice varies between the annular plane and the leaflet tips.
- *"Typical" congenital mitral stenosis*: This anatomic variant involves the valve leaflets, chordae tendineae, and papillary muscles. The leaflets are thickened and can be myxomatous, the leaflet margins are rolled, the chordae tendineae are short (in some cases the leaflets insert directly onto the papillary muscles), the interchordal spaces are narrowed, and the papillary muscles are closely spaced and can be displaced towards the base of the ventricle (Fig. 9.2, Movie 9.2) [11, 12].
- *Parachute mitral valve*: All chordae tendineae insert into a single papillary muscle head, forming a parachute-like deformity (Fig. 9.3) [12]. A second, usually hypoplastic, papillary muscle may be present but does not receive chordae tendineae. In patients without an AV canal defect, the postero-medial muscle usually receives the chordae tendineae and the antero-lateral papillary muscle is either absent or underdeveloped. In patients with an AV canal defect the antero-lateral papillary muscle is usually dominant [11].
- *Mitral arcade*: This rare anomaly consists of short, thick, and poorly differentiated chordae tendineae with fusion

between the papillary muscles and the thickened, myxomatous, and rolled leaflet margins. The interchordal spaces are either completely or nearly completely obliterated with a bridge of fibrous tissue between the papillary muscles [13–15]. The valve annulus size is usually normal. The mitral valve in this anomaly has also been described as "hammock valve."

- *Double-orifice mitral valve*: An abnormal tensor apparatus can result in two or more functional orifices of the mitral valve. This anomaly is often associated with common AV canal but can be seen in isolation or with other congenital heart defects. The hemodynamic implications of double-orifice mitral valve are variable, depending on associated abnormalities of the valve and its tensor apparatus [16]. In some patients, this is an incidental finding with no mitral stenosis or regurgitation.

Associated Anomalies

Mitral stenosis is seldom an isolated anomaly. Although it has been reported in association with almost any other cardiac anomaly, mitral stenosis is most often accompanied by other left heart obstructive lesions, including left ventricular outflow tract obstruction, aortic stenosis, coarctation, and left ventricular hypoplasia [11].

Clinical Presentation

The clinical presentation and course of congenital mitral stenosis are highly variable and depend on the degree of obstruction and the presence, type, and severity of associated cardiovascular anomalies [9]. Patients with mild congenital mitral stenosis may be asymptomatic and the lesion may not progress. Patients with moderate or severe mitral stenosis exhibit signs and symptoms of left atrial and pulmonary hypertension, including tachypnea and dyspnea, pulmonary edema, and poor growth. Manifestations of long-standing mitral stenosis include hemoptysis, supraventricular tachyarrhythmias, and right heart failure related to severe pulmonary hypertension. When present, associated left heart obstructive lesions such as left ventricular outflow obstruction, coarctation of the aorta, left ventricular hypoplasia, and endocardial fibroelastosis play an important role in determining the clinical course and prognosis.

CMR of Mitral Stenosis

Echocardiography is the primary diagnostic tool in the evaluation of congenital mitral stenosis. The benefit of CMR is as an adjunctive technique, particularly in patients with poor acoustic windows, to assess valve morphology [17], evaluate the hemodynamic burden on the atria and ventricles, assess associated anomalies, and for longitudinal follow-up. There is also some experience in adults in using CMR to assess the severity of mitral stenosis. One report utilized CMR for mitral valve planimetry in patients with

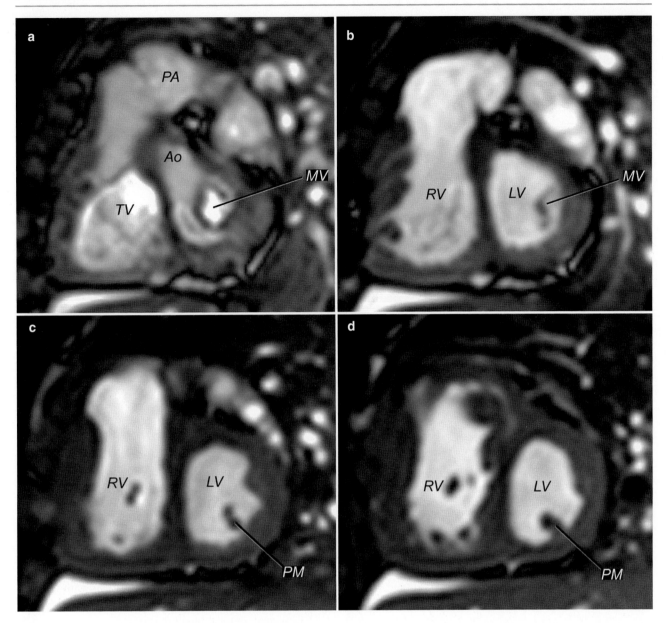

Fig. 9.3 Parachute mitral valve. Contiguous slices (**a–d**) from a cine SSFP ventricular short-axis stack showing a hypoplastic mitral valve (*MV*) with attachments to a single, dominant postero-medial papillary muscle (*PM*). The antero-lateral papillary muscle is poorly developed. *Ao* aorta, *LV* left ventricle, *PA* pulmonary artery, *RV* right ventricle, *TV* tricuspid valve

rheumatic heart disease [18]. Another report found good correlation between velocity encoded cine phase contrast flow and Doppler echocardiography in the assessment of transmitral peak velocity [19]. Published data in patients with congenital mitral stenosis are limited [17], and these techniques have not yet been validated for infants and children. Small structures, multilevel obstructions, and fast heart rates are some of the challenges in the pediatric age group.

The goals of CMR in patients with congenital mitral stenosis include detailed evaluation of mitral valve morphology (annulus, leaflets, chordae tendineae, and papillary muscles), mitral valve function (stenosis and regurgitation), left

atrial size, left ventricular size and function, presence and severity of associated anomalies (e.g., subvalvar aortic stenosis, coarctation, endocardial fibroelastosis), degree of pulmonary hypertension, and right ventricular size and function. These objectives can be realized with the following CMR examination protocol:

- ECG-triggered, breath-hold cine SSFP in the following planes:
  - LV 2-chamber (vertical long-axis)
  - RV 2-chamber (vertical long-axis)
  - Extended 4-chamber covering the entire mitral valve
  - LV 3-chamber view parallel to the left ventricular outflow

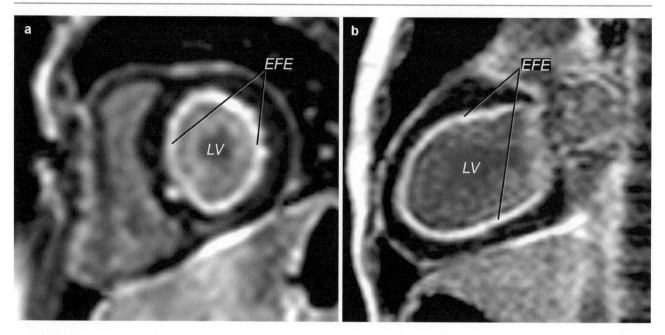

Fig. 9.4 Endocardial fibroelastosis. Late gadolinium enhancement (LGE) imaging in a ventricular short-axis (**a**) and left ventricular 2-chamber (**b**) planes showing hyperenhancement along the entire endocardial surface of the left ventricle (*LV*) consistent with endocardial fibroelastosis (*EFE*)

- Ventricular short-axis stack to evaluate ventricular volumes and function
- Gadolinium-enhanced 3D MRA to assess for coarctation of the aorta and other associated anomalies
- ECG-triggered, free-breathing cine phase contrast flow measurements in the AV valves, proximal ascending aorta, and main pulmonary artery. In-plane flow velocity mapping in the ventricular long-axis plane across the mitral valve can provide additional information about location of flow acceleration within the mitral valve
  - Flow velocity mapping in a short-axis plane of the mitral valve is hampered by through-plane annular motion in the base-to-apex direction. For best results, we prescribe the short-axis plane using a four-chamber cine SSFP to align the imaging plane with the valve annulus at end-systole
- Optional sequences:
  - ECG-triggered, breath-hold turbo (fast) spin echo sequence with blood suppression in patients with metallic artifacts from implanted devices and to visualize supramitral stenotic tissue
  - ECG-triggered, respiratory navigated, free breathing 3-dimensional isotropic SSFP for evaluation of the coronary arteries
  - In patients with suspected endocardial fibroelastosis (Fig. 9.4), LGE imaging in the ventricular short-axis, 4-chamber, and LV 2- and 3-chamber planes

9.2.2.3 Mitral Regurgitation

Morphologic and Functional Abnormalities

Isolated congenital mitral regurgitation is rare. In the majority of cases, mitral regurgitation is found in association with other congenital or acquired cardiovascular anomalies. As with obstructive lesions, mitral regurgitation can result from abnormalities at any level of the valve apparatus.

- *Annular dilatation*: This is a common mechanism contributing to mitral regurgitation in patients with left ventricular dilatation due to chronic volume load (e.g., left-to-right shunt through a ventricular septal defect or patent ductus arteriosus, aortic regurgitation) or dilated cardiomyopathy. In addition to preventing systolic coaptation between the anterior and posterior leaflets, left ventricular dilatation also causes displacement of the papillary muscles, which further contributes to mitral regurgitation.
- *Congenital perforation*: This rare anomaly comprises a congenital defect within one of the leaflets of the mitral valve resulting in regurgitation [20].
- *Mitral arcade*: As described in the section on mitral stenosis, mitral arcade can also result in regurgitation [15].
- *Cleft mitral valve*: A cleft refers to a split anterior leaflet with each component of the leaflet attaching to a different papillary muscle group (Fig. 9.5, Movie 9.3) [21]. It is differentiated from a commissure in that the latter is defined as a split between leaflets with both leaflets attaching to

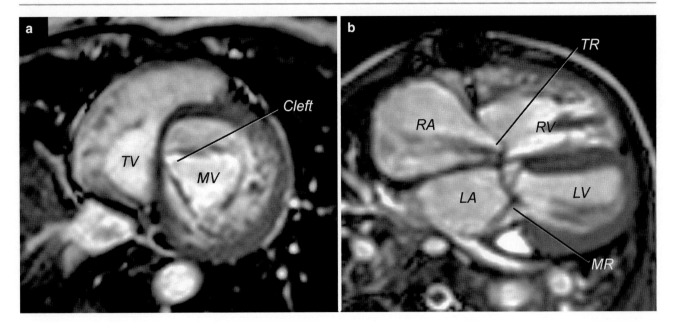

Fig. 9.5 Cleft mitral valve. Cine SSFP images in a ventricular short-axis plane (**a**) showing a cleft in the anterior leaflet of the mitral valve extending to the ventricular septum. On 4-chamber views (**b**) in a patient after atrioventricular canal defect repair, there is a posteriorly directed mitral regurgitation jet (*MR*) through a residual cleft and a medial tricuspid regurgitation jet (*TR*). *LA* left atrium, *LV* left ventricle, *MV* mitral valve, *RA* right atrium, *RV* right ventricle, *TV* tricuspid valve

the same papillary muscle. Although, in most cases, cleft anterior mitral leaflet is associated with one of several types of common AV canal (e.g., primum atrial septal defect, complete common AV canal), it can rarely present either as an isolated anomaly or in association with cardiac defects other then AV canal (e.g., conotruncal anomalies) [21]. Regurgitation typically emanates from the region of the cleft itself.

- *Mitral valve prolapse*: Although mitral valve prolapse usually presents in adolescents and adults, it can infrequently manifest in infancy and childhood [22]. In most cases, mitral valve prolapse is associated with one of several forms of connective tissue disorder (e.g., Marfan syndrome, Ehlers-Danlos syndrome). Elongated chordae tendineae and redundant, myxomatous leaflets characterize mitral valve prolapse (Fig. 9.6, Movie 9.4). Regurgitation results from ineffective coaptation between the anterior and posterior leaflets. In severe cases, ruptured chordae result in a flail leaflet and severe regurgitation.
- *Papillary muscle dysfunction*: Mitral regurgitation can result from papillary muscle dysfunction due to myocardial ischemia or infarction. Examples include congenital anomalies such as anomalous origin of the left coronary artery from the main pulmonary artery [23] and acquired conditions such as coronary insufficiency due to complications of Kawasaki disease [24].

- *Straddling mitral valve*: This anomaly is defined as having attachments of the mitral valve chords to both sides of the interventricular septum (Fig. 9.7). The mitral valve straddles the ventricular septum through an anterior, outlet ventricular septal defect, usually a conoventricular-type defect. The straddling portion of the valve attaches to the infundibular portion of the right ventricle [25]. Frequently, the anterior leaflet is divided by an accessory commissure [25]. The degree of mitral regurgitation is usually mild.

In addition to congenital anomalies of the mitral valve, mitral regurgitation can complicate the course of acquired heart disease in children. Examples include endocarditis, systemic lupus erythematosus, and drug-induced valvulitis.

Associated Anomalies

Cleft mitral valve is usually associated with primum atrial septal defect or other forms of common AV canal defect, a topic covered elsewhere in this book. Straddling mitral valve is associated with conotruncal anomalies such as transposition of the greater arteries or double-outlet right ventricle. It is also found in complex anomalies in which the ventricles are malposed, resulting in superior-inferior ventricles with or without criss-cross atrioventricular relations [25, 26]. Fraisee et al. found dextrocardia in 6 of 46 cases of straddling mitral valve (13 %) [25].

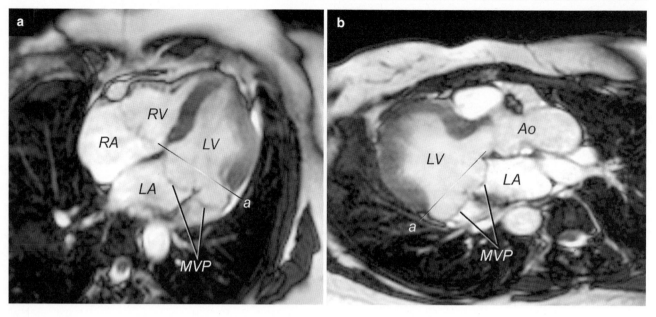

Fig. 9.6 Mitral valve prolapse. Cine SSFP images in 4-chamber (**a**) and ventricular 3-chamber (**b**) planes showing bileaflet mitral valve prolapse (*MVP*) past the plane of the annulus *AO* aorta, (*a*) and associ- ated jet of mitral regurgitation. *LA* left atrium, *LV* left ventricle, *RA* right atrium *RV* right ventricle

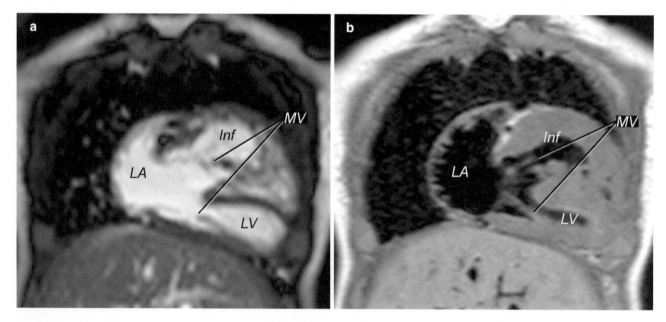

Fig. 9.7 Straddling mitral valve. Cine SSFP (**a**) and turbo (fast) spin echo (**b**) images in a coronal plane in a patient with superior-inferior ventricles and a horizontal ventricular septum. The mitral valve (*MV*) overrides the septum and has straddling attachments to the right ven- tricular infundibulum (*Inf*). *LA* left atrium, *LV* left ventricle

Clinical Presentation

The clinical manifestations of mitral regurgitation depend on the severity and duration of the regurgitation and on associ- ated anomalies. Patients with mild regurgitation may be asymptomatic with only a holosystolic high frequency mur- mur at the cardiac apex. Severe acute mitral regurgitation generally presents with signs and symptoms of acute left atrial hypertension such as pulmonary arterial hypertension and edema, dyspnea or respiratory failure, left ventricular dysfunction, and decreased cardiac output. With chronic mitral regurgitation, the symptoms are more gradual in onset, occurring once ventricular dysfunction and/or pulmonary hypertension occurs. Supraventricular tachyarrhythmias can also complicate the clinical course of patients with mitral regurgitation.

CMR of Mitral Regurgitation Lesions

CMR is a particularly useful tool for quantitative assessment of the degree of mitral regurgitation and the hemodynamic load on the left ventricle and atrium. The ability to measure flow rates and biventricular volumes allow CMR to provide quantitative information that is not readily or reliably available by echocardiography. In the absence of intracardiac shunts or additional regurgitant lesions, mitral regurgitation volume and fraction can be calculated either by comparison of ventricular stroke volumes, AV valve inflows (Fig. 9.8), mitral versus aortic or pulmonary valve flows, or a combination of these measurements. Assessment of mitral regurgitation volume and fraction by several methods is recommended so that results can be compared for consistency.

Although data in children are limited, studies in adults have shown that CMR derived mitral inflow and regurgitation values are highly reproducible [27, 28], and correlate well with other noninvasive [29] and invasive [30] measures of regurgitation. There has also been some interest in calculating anatomic regurgitant orifice for longitudinal follow-up using CMR flow mapping in adults [31], but the utility of this technique in pediatric patients has not been evaluated.

The goals of CMR in patients with mitral regurgitation include evaluation of valve morphology and function, measurements of the hemodynamic burden (mitral regurgitation volume and fraction, left ventricular size and function, left atrial size), and assessment of associated anomalies. These objectives can be realized with the following CMR examination protocol:

- ECG-triggered, breath-hold cine SSFP in the following planes:
  - LV 2-chamber (vertical long-axis)
  - Extended 4-chamber covering the entire mitral valve
  - LV 3-chamber view parallel to the left ventricular outflow
  - Ventricular short-axis stack to evaluate ventricular volumes and function
  - Additional cine SSFP acquisitions for evaluation of mitral valve leaflets or subvalvar support apparatus
- ECG-triggered, free-breathing cine phase contrast flow measurements in the AV valves, proximal ascending aorta, and main pulmonary artery. In-plane flow velocity mapping in the ventricular long-axis plane across the mitral valve can provide additional information about location of flow acceleration within a valve
  - Flow velocity mapping in a short-axis plane of the mitral valve is hampered by through-plane annular motion in the base-to-apex direction. For best results, we prescribe the short-axis plane using a four-chamber cine SSFP to align the imaging plane with the valve annulus at end-systole
- Optional sequences:
  - Gadolinium-enhanced 3D MRA to assess for associated anomalies of the great vessels and veins

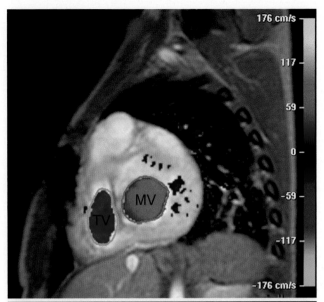

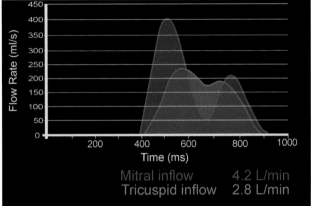

Fig. 9.8 Measurement of mitral regurgitation. *Top panel*: Cine phase contrast through-plane flow mapping perpendicular to the atrioventricular valve inflows. A region of interest is prescribed encompassing the mitral (*red*) and tricuspid (*green*) valve inflows. *Bottom panel*: For each AV valve, the area under the diastolic phase of the cardiac cycle represents the antegrade flow across that valve, in this case, 4.2 L/min across the mitral and 2.8 L/min across the tricuspid valve, respectively. Mitral regurgitation fraction is calculated as follows: (mitral inflow − tricuspid inflow) ÷ mitral inflow × 100 = 33 %. *MV* mitral valve, *TV* tricuspid valve

9.3 Abnormalities of Left Ventricular Outflow

9.3.1 Obstructive Lesions

9.3.1.1 Definition

Obstructive left ventricular outflow lesions include subaortic stenosis, aortic valve stenosis, and supravalvar aortic stenosis. Subaortic stenosis is defined as obstruction in the left ventricular outflow below the aortic valve annulus. Aortic valve stenosis occurs at the level of the annulus and leaflets. Supravalvar aortic stenosis involves the aortic sino-tubular junction and may extend to the ascending aorta.

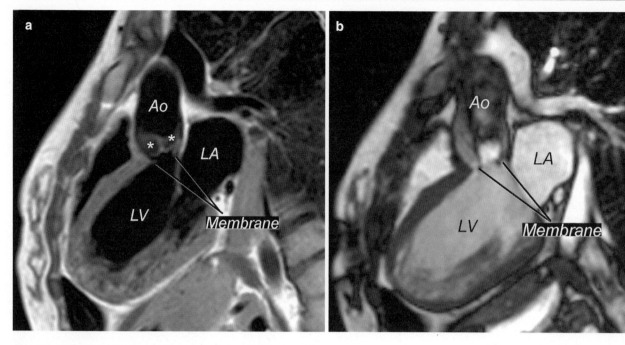

Fig. 9.9 Discrete subaortic stenosis. (**a**) Turbo (fast) spin echo sequence with blood suppression in a left ventricular 3-chamber plane parallel to the outflow tract demonstrating a discrete subvalvar membrane immediately below the aortic valve leaflets (*). (**b**) Cine SSFP image in the same plane as in panel A demonstrating systolic dephasing consistent with stenosis beginning at the level of the subaortic membrane. *Ao* aorta, *LA* left atrium, *LV* left ventricle

9.3.1.2 Morphologic and Functional Abnormalities

The left ventricular outflow tract includes the subaortic region, aortic valve, and supravalvar area. The subaortic outflow is bound by the membranous and infundibular segments of the ventricular septum and by the anterior leaflet of the mitral valve. In cross section, the geometry of the subaortic outflow is oval. The normal aortic valve consists of three pocket-like cusps, each approximately equal in size with dividing commissures, adhering to a crown shaped fibrous annulus. The normal aortic root, which contains the aortic valve, comprises three sinuses, named sinuses of Valsalva, with the left and right coronary arteries arising from their respective sinuses. The junction between the aortic root and ascending aorta is called the sino-tubular junction and is the site of supravalvar aortic stenosis. As with the mitral valve, structural abnormalities causing obstruction of the left ventricular outflow can occur at any level or in combination:

- *Discrete subaortic stenosis*: A fibromuscular "membrane" or "ridge" forms below the aortic valve, sometimes extending up and adherent to the ventricular surface of aortic and mitral valve leaflets (Fig. 9.9). The morphology of the left ventricular outflow is characterized by elongation of the aortic-mitral intervalvular fibrosa and an acute angle between the ventricular septum and proximal ascending aorta (called aorto-septal angle) [32]. The etiology of discrete subaortic stenosis is unknown but it has been speculated that the aforementioned abnormal geometry of the left ventricular outflow tract results in increased flow sheer stress, which can promote proliferation of obstructive fibrous tissue [33, 34].

- *Tunnel-type subaortic stenosis*: The left ventricular outflow tract is diffusely narrowed, usually due to septal hypertrophy, resulting in long-segment obstruction [35]. This lesion can be seen in patients with hypertrophic cardiomyopathy.

- *Subaortic stenosis due to posterior deviation of the conal septum*: In patients with a posterior malalignment conoventricular septal defect, the deviated conal septum protrudes into the subaortic outflow, causing subaortic obstruction [36]. This type of subvalvar aortic stenosis is typically found in patients with type B interrupted aortic arch [37].

- *Subaortic stenosis due to AV valve attachments*: Subvalvar aortic stenosis is seen in some patients with a common AV canal (usually primum atrial septal defect), isolated cleft mitral valve and transposition of the great arteries or double-outlet right ventricle, straddling mitral valve, and, rarely, straddling tricuspid valve.

- *Valvar aortic stenosis*: Decreased effective aortic valve flow area can result from annular hypoplasia, leaflet thickening, and commissural underdevelopment and/or fusion. In most cases of congenital aortic valve stenosis the mechanism of obstruction includes a combination of these abnormalities. Unicommissural or bicommissural aortic valve are common variants of congenital aortic stenosis (Fig. 9.10, Movie 9.5) [38–40].

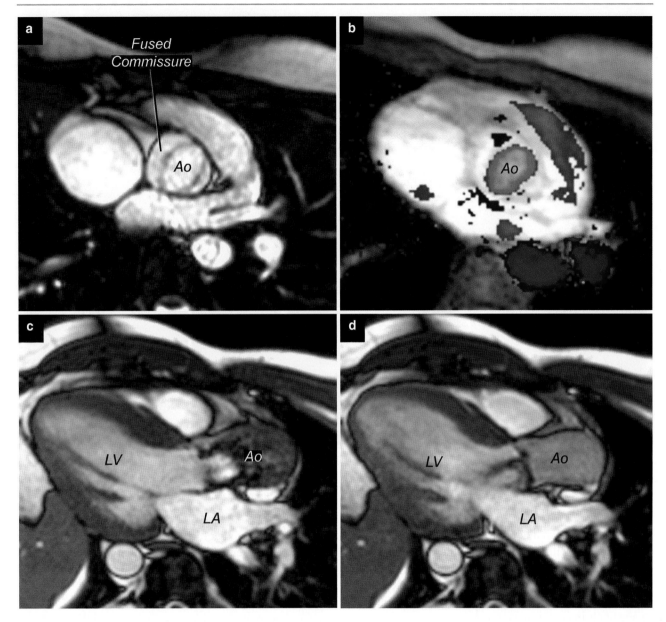

Fig. 9.10 Valvar aortic stenosis and regurgitation. (**a**) Cine SSFP image in a plane perpendicular to the aortic root demonstrating a bicuspid aortic valve with fusion of the right and noncoronary cusps. (**b**) Cine phase contrast through-plane flow mapping perpendicular to the aortic root demonstrating the eccentric antegrade flow jet across the bicuspid valve. (**c**) Systolic cine SSFP image in a left ventricular (*LV*) 3-chamber view parallel to the outflow tract showing a dephasing jet consistent with valvar aortic stenosis. (**d**) Diastolic cine SSFP image in a left ventricular 3-chamber view parallel to the outflow tract showing an aortic regurgitation jet. *Ao* aorta *LA* left atrium

- **Supravalvar aortic stenosis**: Supravalvar aortic stenosis is located above the level of the aortic valve, most commonly at the sino-tubular junction (Fig. 9.11, Movie 9.6) [41].

9.3.1.3 Associated Anomalies

Left ventricular outflow tract obstruction is often seen in conjunction with other left heart obstructive lesions such as mitral stenosis, coarctation, or Shone syndrome. Discrete subvalvar aortic stenosis is associated with aortic valve

stenosis (29 %), membranous ventricular septal defect (23 %), coarctation (14 %), double-chambered right ventricle (8 %), and interrupted aortic arch (3 %) [42]. Supravalvar aortic stenosis may be associated with Williams syndrome or with the autosomal dominant familial form of the disease [43, 44].

9.3.1.4 Clinical Presentation

The clinical presentation of obstructive lesions of the left ventricular outflow tract depends on the severity of obstruc-

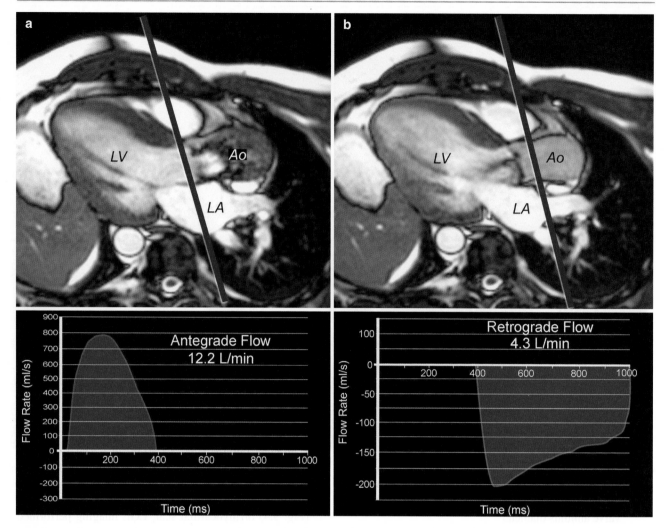

Fig. 9.13 Measuring aortic flow in mixed aortic valve disease (stenosis and regurgitation). (**a**) Antegrade flow across the left ventricular outflow is measured below the aortic valve. *Top panel*: The imaging plane (*LV* left ventricle, *LA* left atrium, *Ao* aorta) for subsequent cine phase contrast flow mapping is prescribed from cine SSFP systolic image in the ventricular 3-chamber plane. *Bottom panel*: The area under the systolic phase of the cardiac cycle represents the antegrade flow across the left ventricular outflow (12.2 L/min). (**b**) Retrograde flow in the aortic root is mea- sured above the aortic valve. *Top panel*: The imaging plane (*LV* left ventricle, *LA* left atrium, *Ao* aorta) for subsequent cine phase contrast flow mapping is prescribed from cine SSFP diastolic image in the ventricular 3-chamber plane. *Bottom panel*: The area under the diastolic phase of the cardiac cycle represents the retrograde flow in the aortic root (4.3 L/min; regurgitation volume). Net aortic flow is, therefore: antegrade flow – retrograde flow = 7.9 L/min. Aortic regurgitation fraction is calcu- lated as retrograde flow ÷ antegrade flow × 100 = 35%

9.3.2.2 Morphologic and Functional Abnormalities

Regurgitation at the level of the left ventricular outflow tract can result from several morphologic abnormalities.

- *Unicommissural or bicommissural aortic valve*: Although bicommissural aortic valve disease is often associated with stenosis, mixed lesions and pure aortic regurgitation are seen in a proportion of patients. In one large series of patients undergoing aortic valve surgery, 75 % had aortic stenosis, 13 % had regurgitation, and 10 % had mixed valve disease [56]. Regurgitation results from leaflet tissue deficiency, redundancy and prolapse, restriction of diastolic motion, and root dilatation [39, 57].

- *Aortic valve prolapse*: Prolapse of one or more leaflets of an otherwise normal tricommissural aortic valve can be seen in patients with conal septal (subpulmonary, outlet) ventricular septal defect and, less frequently, in membra- nous ventricular septal defect [58]. The prolapsing leaflet can create a windsock-like deformity and restrict or even close the ventricular septal defect.

- *Congenital leaflet perforation*: This is a rare congenital anomaly of the aortic valve resulting in severe regurgita- tion [59].

- *Iatrogenic aortic regurgitation*: The most common cause of iatrogenic aortic regurgitation in congenital heart dis- ease is due to transcatheter balloon dilatation of congeni-

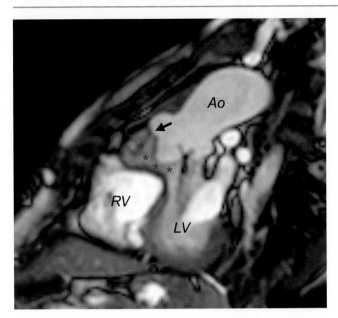

Fig. 9.14 Aortico-left ventricular tunnel. Cine SSFP image in an oblique sagittal plane parallel to the left ventricular outflow tract demonstrating a defect in the aortic wall (*arrow*) and the tunneling flow (*) into the left ventricle. *Ao* aorta, *LV* left ventricle, *RV* right ventricle

tal aortic stenosis [60]. A therapeutic tear in the anterior aspect of the stenotic valve is common, and the ensuing regurgitation may progress over time.

- **Acquired aortic regurgitation**: Bacterial endocarditis is a leading cause of acquired, non-iatrogenic aortic regurgitation in children. It is associated with bicommissural aortic valve and subvalvar aortic stenosis but can also occur with or without associated congenital heart disease [61].

- **Aortico-left ventricular tunnel**: This is a rare paravalvar communication between the aorta and the left ventricle (Fig. 9.14, Movie 9.7) [62]. The tunnel most commonly originates above the origin of the right coronary artery and courses posterior to the right ventricular outflow tract to enter the left ventricle immediately below the aortic valve [62].

9.3.2.3 Clinical Presentation

As with mitral regurgitation, the clinical presentation of aortic regurgitation in children depends on the severity and duration of the lesion as well as associated anomalies. Patients who develop acute severe aortic regurgitation can present with signs and symptoms of heart failure. Patients with chronic or slowly progressing aortic regurgitation may be asymptomatic until the compensatory mechanisms of the left ventricle fail and systolic dysfunction occurs.

9.3.2.4 CMR of Aortic Regurgitation

The primary goals of CMR include quantification of the regurgitation volume and fraction, assessment of the hemo-

dynamic burden on the left ventricle, and visualization of the mechanism of valve dysfunction. Although cases of aortico-left ventricular tunnel have typically been diagnosed by echocardiography and conventional x-ray angiography, Humes et al. reported on CMR diagnosis of this rare anomaly [63]. More frequently, however, CMR has been used to quantify aortic regurgitation in children and adults [64–66]. Several studies found good correlation between CMR and other noninvasive [29, 66] and invasive [67] measures of aortic regurgitation as well as good reproducibility [68]. As noted previously, there are also published data demonstrating the ability of CMR to assess valve morphology [46–48], although studies evaluating the ability of CMR to delineate the mechanism of valve regurgitation are limited.

The CMR protocol for evaluation of aortic regurgitation is essentially identical to that of obstructive lesions in the left ventricular outflow. In patients with both stenosis and regurgitation in the left ventricular outflow, flow measurements should be performed both below and above the areas of turbulent flow (Fig. 9.13). In this circumstance, antegrade flow is measured from the systolic phase of the cardiac cycle obtained in the left ventricular outflow below the aortic valve. The retrograde (regurgitation) flow is measured from the diastolic phase of the cardiac cycle obtained at the level of the sinotubular junction. In the absence of mitral regurgitation or ventricular septal defect, the antegrade flow can also be obtained by measurement of left ventricular stroke volume from end-diastolic and end-systolic volumes. The phase contrast and volumetric measurements can then be compared for consistency.

9.4 Abnormalities of Combined Left Ventricular Inflow and Outflow

9.4.1 Definitions

Multiple left heart obstructions encompass a wide range of congenital anomalies affecting the mitral valve, left ventricle, left ventricular outflow tract, and thoracic aorta. Schwartz et al. defined multiple left heart obstructive lesions as having two or more of the following areas of obstruction or hypoplasia: (1) **mitral valve**: mitral stenosis (mean gradient >3 mmHg), mitral annulus hypoplasia, or parachute mitral valve; (2) **left ventricular outflow tract**: subaortic stenosis or diameter less than normal aortic annulus; (3) **aortic valve**: aortic valve stenosis (maximum instantaneous Doppler gradient ≥20 mmHg) or aortic valve annulus hypoplasia; (4) **aortic arch**: aortic arch hypoplasia, isthmic hypoplasia, coarctation, or interrupted aortic arch; or (5) **left ventricle**: left ventricular-to-right ventricular long-axis ratio <0.8 or subnormal LV end-diastolic volume. Hypoplasia for each

Fig. 9.15 Shone syndrome. Schematic representation of Shone syndrome depicting a supramitral membrane, parachute mitral valve with a single papillary muscle, discrete subaortic stenosis, and coarctation of the aorta *Ao* aorta, *LA* left ventricle, *LV* left ventricle, *RA* right atrium, *RV* right ventricle

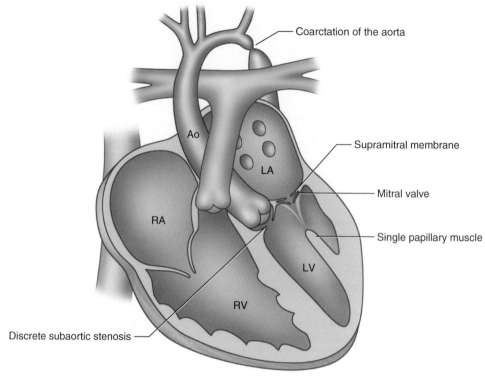

parameter was defined by a measurement with a Z-score smaller than −2.0 [69].

- *Morphologic and Functional Abnormalities*

  Several patterns of multiple left heart obstructive lesions are recognized:

- *Hypoplastic left heart syndrome*: This most severe form of multiple left heart obstructions is characterized by severe hypoplasia or atresia of the mitral and/or aortic valves and marked hypoplasia of the left ventricle, often with endocardial fibroelastosis.

- *Shone Syndrome*: Shone syndrome consists of the following four anatomic obstructions (Fig. 9.15): (1) supramitral membrane; (2) parachute mitral valve; (3) discrete subaortic stenosis; and (4) aortic coarctation. It is worth noting that in Shone's original report not all patients exhibit all four lesions [70].

- *Multiple left heart obstructive lesions*: Included in this category are the many patients with more than one level of left heart obstruction as defined above but not fulfilling criteria for Shone syndrome [69].

9.4.1.1 Clinical Presentation

The clinical presentation, course, and prognosis of patients with obstructions at multiple levels of left ventricular inflow and outflow vary considerably. The location and severity of the obstructive lesions as well as associated defects, such as patent ductus arteriosus and atrial septal defect, are important determinants of initial clinical course. At one end of the clinical spectrum are newborns with hypoplastic left heart syndrome presenting with cyanosis and cardiovascular collapse as the patent ductus arteriosus closes. At the other end of the spectrum are asymptomatic patients with slowly progressing coarctation of the aorta, mild mitral or aortic valve stenosis, and normal left ventricular size and function. Prematurity and associated genetic and major non-cardiac congenital defects adversely affect prognosis.

9.4.1.2 CMR Evaluation of Combined Left Ventricular Inflow and Outflow Obstructions

CMR offers important advantages in the evaluation of patients with multiple left heart obstructive lesions, Shone syndrome, and hypoplastic left heart syndrome. As noted above in the sections on individual lesions, CMR allows for visualization of mitral and aortic valve morphology and quantification of valve function, assessment of the hemodynamic burden, and evaluation of any associated lesions.

Of particular importance in this group of patients is the ability of CMR to aid in clinical decision making with regard to single versus biventricular management strategies. Although echocardiography has been used effectively to predict a successful biventricular outcome in patients with aortic stenosis [71] and with multiple left heart obstructive lesions [69], its ability to accurately measure the size and function of the hypoplastic, abnormally shaped left ventricle has been questioned [72]. CMR has particular strengths in quantitative evaluation of left ventricular volumes, mass, ejection fraction, and stroke volume. Additional important information provided by CMR includes evaluation of endocardial fibroelastosis, flow measurements through the left heart, and assessment of associated anomalies [72]. Therefore, the goals of the preoperative CMR examination in the infant with a borderline left ventricle include measurements of biventricular size and function, visualization of valve anatomy, quantification of valve flow and regurgitation on both sides of the heart, and assessment of associated anomalies. These objectives can be realized with the following CMR examination protocol:

- ECG-triggered, breath-hold cine SSFP in the following planes:
  - LV and RV 2-chamber (vertical long-axis)
  - 4-chamber stack covering the left ventricular inflow and outflow
  - LV 3-chamber view parallel to the left ventricular outflow for visualization of the subvalvar area and aortic valve.
  - Oblique coronal plane parallel to the left ventricular outflow (optional)
  - Short-axis stack perpendicular to the aortic root for assessment of aortic valve morphology
  - Ventricular short-axis stack for measurements of biventricular size, function, and mass
- ECG-triggered, breath-hold turbo (fast) spin echo sequence with blood suppression for evaluation of the aortic arch (optional)
- Gadolinium-enhanced 3D MRA to assess for coarctation of the aorta and other associated thoracic vascular anomalies
- ECG-triggered, free-breathing cine phase contrast flow measurements in the proximal ascending aorta, main pulmonary artery, and AV valves
- LGE imaging performed 10–20 min after contrast administration in the ventricular short-axis, 4-chamber, and LV 2- and 3-chamber planes.
- Optional sequences:
  - ECG-triggered, breath-hold turbo (fast) spin echo sequence with blood suppression for evaluation of intra- or extracardiac anomalies not clearly seen by cine SSFP
  - Additional flow measurements (case-specific). Examples include differential pulmonary blood flow in patients with pulmonary artery or pulmonary vein anomalies or measurements of systemic-to-pulmonary collateral flow.

9.5 Practical Pearls

- Anatomic and physiologic evaluations by CMR are inseparable in patients with abnormalities of left ventricular inflow and outflow.
- Measurements of left and right ventricular volumes and function, as well as flow across the atrioventricular and semilunar valves are essential in most patients.

- The CMR protocol should be designed to allow internal validation of shunts and valve regurgitation fractions. For example, in patients with mitral regurgitation, the CMR protocol should allow quantification of the degree of regurgitation by both ventricular stroke volume differential and by comparison of mitral inflow to net aortic outflow.
- Due to through-plane annular motion of the atrioventricular valves in the base-to-apex direction, assessment of atrioventricular valve inflows is best prescribed using horizontal and vertical ventricular long-axis views, with the plane aligned with the valve annulus at end-systole.
- In patients with mixed aortic valve disease (aortic stenosis and regurgitation), flow measurements should be obtained both below the level of stenosis and above the valve for accurate determination of valve function
- Myocardial delayed enhancement imaging is particularly important in patients with left ventricular outflow tract obstruction and borderline left ventricular size for identification of endomyocardial fibrosis.

References

1. Victor S, Nayak VM. Aneurysm of the left atrial appendage. Tex Heart Inst J. 2001;28:111–8.
2. Chowdhury UK, Seth S, Govindappa R, Jagia P, Malhotra P. Congenital left atrial appendage aneurysm: a case report and brief review of literature. Heart Lung Circ. 2009;18:412–6.
3. Park JS, Lee DH, Han SS, Kim MJ, Shin DG, Kim YJ, Shim BS. Incidentally found, growing congenital aneurysm of the left atrium. J Korean Med Sci. 2003;18:262–6.
4. Wang D, Holden B, Savage C, Zhang K, Zwischenberger JB. Giant left atrial intrapericardial aneurysm: noninvasive preoperative imaging. Ann Thorac Surg. 2001;71:1014–6.
5. Van Praagh R, Corsini I. Cor triatriatum: pathologic anatomy and a consideration of morphogenesis based on 13 postmortem cases and a study of normal development of the pulmonary vein and atrial septum in 83 human embryos. Am Heart J. 1969;78:379–405.
6. Rumancik WM, Hernanz-Schulman M, Rutkowski MM, Kiely B, Ambrosino M, Genieser NB, Naidich DP. Magnetic resonance imaging of cor triatriatum. Pediatr Cardiol. 1988;9:149–51.
7. Locca D, Hughes M, Mohiaddin R. Cardiovascular magnetic resonance diagnosis of a previously unreported association: Cor triatriatum with right partial anomalous pulmonary venous return to the azygos vein. Int J Cardiol. 2009;135:e80–2.
8. McElhinney DB, Sherwood MC, Keane JF, del Nido PJ, Almond CSD, Lock JE. Current management of severe congenital mitral stenosis: outcomes of transcatheter and surgical therapy in 108 infants and children. Circulation. 2005;112:707–14.
9. Selamet Tierney ES, Graham DA, McElhinney DB, Trevey S, Freed MD, Colan SD, Geva T. Echocardiographic predictors of mitral stenosis-related death or intervention in infants. Am Heart J. 2008;156:384–90.
10. Toscano A, Pasquini L, Iacobelli R, Di Donato RM, Raimondi F, Carotti A, Di Ciommo V, Sanders SP. Congenital supravalvar mitral ring: an underestimated anomaly. J Thorac Cardiovasc Surg. 2009;137:538–42.
11. Ruckman RN, Van Praagh R. Anatomic types of congenital mitral stenosis: report of 49 autopsy cases with consideration of diagnosis and surgical implications. Am J Cardiol. 1978;42:592–601.

12. Marino BS, Kruge LE, Cho CJ, Tomlinson RS, Shera D, Weinberg PM, Gaynor JW, Rychik J. Parachute mitral valve: morphologic descriptors, associated lesions, and outcomes after biventricular repair. J Thorac Cardiovasc Surg. 2009;137:385–93. e384.

13. Collins 2nd RT, Ryan M, Gleason MM. Images in cardiovascular medicine. Mitral arcade: a rare cause of fatigue in an 18-year-old female. Circulation. 2010;121:e379–83.

14. Layman TE, Edwards JE. Anomalous mitral arcade: a type of congenital mitral insufficiency. Circulation. 1967;35:389–95.

15. Losada E, Moon-Grady AJ, Strohsnitter WC, Wu D, Ursell PC. Anomalous mitral arcade in twin-twin transfusion syndrome. Circulation. 2010;122:1456–63.

16. Baño-Rodrigo A, Van Praagh S, Trowitzsch E, Van Praagh R. Double-orifice mitral valve: a study of 27 postmortem cases with developmental, diagnostic and surgical considerations. Am J Cardiol. 1988;61:152–60.

17. Hamilton-Craig C, Anscombe R, Platts D, Burstow D, Slaughter R. Congenital mitral stenosis by multimodality cardiac imaging. Echocardiography. 2009;26:284–7.

18. Lanjewar C, Ephrem B, Mishra N, Jhankariya B, Kerkar P. Planimetry of mitral valve stenosis in rheumatic heart disease by magnetic resonance imaging. J Heart Valve Dis. 2010;19:357–63.

19. Søndergaard L, Ståhlberg F, Thomsen C. Magnetic resonance imaging of valvular heart disease. J Magn Reson Imaging. 1999;10: 627–38.

20. Stos B, Hatchuel Y, Bonnet D. Mitral valvar regurgitation in a child with Sweet's syndrome. Cardiol Young. 2007;17:218–9.

21. Van Praagh S, Porras D, Oppido G, Geva T, Van Praagh R. Cleft mitral valve without ostium primum defect: anatomic data and surgical considerations based on 41 cases. Ann Thorac Surg. 2003; 75:1752–62.

22. Geva T, Sanders SP, Diogenes MS, Rockenmacher S, Van Praagh R. Two-dimensional and Doppler echocardiographic and pathologic characteristics of the infantile Marfan syndrome. Am J Cardiol. 1990;65:1230–7.

23. Ben Ali W, Metton O, Roubertie F, Pouard P, Sidi D, Raisky O, Vouhe PR. Anomalous origin of the left coronary artery from the pulmonary artery: late results with special attention to the mitral valve. Eur J Cardiothorac Surg. 2009;36:244–8. discussion 248-249.

24. Takao A, Niwa K, Kondo C, Nakanishi T, Satomi G, Nakazawa M, Endo M. Mitral regurgitation in Kawasaki disease. Prog Clin Biol Res. 1987;250:311–23.

25. Fraisse A, del Nido PJ, Gaudart J, Geva T. Echocardiographic characteristics and outcome of straddling mitral valve. J Am Coll Cardiol. 2001;38:819–26.

26. Milo S, Siew Yen H, Macartney FJ, Wilkinson JL, Becker AE, Wenink ACG, De Groot ACG, Anderson RH. Straddling and overriding atrioventricular valves: morphology and classification. Am J Cardiol. 1979;44:1122–34.

27. Fujita N, Chazouilleres AF, Hartiala JJ, O'Sullivan M, Heidenreich P, Kaplan JD, Sakuma H, Foster E, Caputo GR, Higgins CB. Quantification of mitral regurgitation by velocity-encoded cine nuclear magnetic resonance imaging. J Am Coll Cardiol. 1994;23: 951–8.

28. Hartiala JJ, Mostbeck GH, Foster E, Fujita N, Dulce MC, Chazouilleres AF, Higgins CB. Velocity-encoded cine MRI in the evaluation of left ventricular diastolic function: measurement of mitral valve and pulmonary vein flow velocities and flow volume across the mitral valve. Am Heart J. 1993;125:1054–66.

29. Gelfand EV, Hughes S, Hauser TH, Yeon SB, Goepfert L, Kissinger KV, Rofsky NM, Manning WJ. Severity of mitral and aortic regurgitation as assessed by cardiovascular magnetic resonance: optimizing correlation with Doppler echocardiography. J Cardiovasc Magn Reson. 2006;8:503–7.

30. Hundley WG, Li HF, Willard JE, Landau C, Lange RA, Meshack BM, Hillis LD, Peshock RM. Magnetic resonance imaging assess-ment of the severity of mitral regurgitation: comparison with invasive techniques. Circulation. 1995;92:1151–8.

31. Buchner S, Debl K, Poschenrieder F, Feuerbach S, Riegger GA, Luchner A, Djavidani B. Cardiovascular magnetic resonance for direct assessment of anatomic regurgitant orifice in mitral regurgitation. Circ Cardiovasc Imaging. 2008;1:148–55.

32. Kleinert S, Geva T. Echocardiographic morphometry and geometry of the left ventricular outflow tract in fixed subaortic stenosis. J Am Coll Cardiol. 1993;22:1501–8.

33. Cape EG, VanAuker MD, Sigfússon G, Tacy TA, del Nido PJ. Potential role of mechanical stress in the etiology of pediatric heart disease: septal shear stress in subaortic stenosis. J Am Coll Cardiol. 1997;30:247–54.

34. Leichter DA, Sullivan I, Gersony WM. "Acquired" discrete subvalvular aortic stenosis: natural history and hemodynamics. J Am Coll Cardiol. 1989;14:1539–44.

35. Suri RM, Dearani JA, Schaff HV, Danielson GK, Puga FJ. Long-term results of the Konno procedure for complex left ventricular outflow tract obstruction. J Thorac Cardiovasc Surg. 2006;132: 1064–71. e1062.

36. Suzuki T, Ohye RG, Devaney EJ, Ishizaka T, Nathan PN, Goldberg CS, Gomez CA, Bove EL. Selective management of the left ventricular outflow tract for repair of interrupted aortic arch with ventricular septal defect: management of left ventricular outflow tract obstruction. J Thorac Cardiovasc Surg. 2006;131:779–84.

37. Geva T, Hornberger LK, Sanders SP, Jonas RA, Ott DA, Colan SD. Echocardiographic predictors of left ventricular outflow tract obstruction after repair of interrupted aortic arch. J Am Coll Cardiol. 1993;22:1953–60.

38. Campbell M, Kauntze R. Congenital aortic valvular stenosis. Br Heart J. 1953;15:179–94.

39. Siu SC, Silversides CK. Bicuspid aortic valve disease. J Am Coll Cardiol. 2010;55:2789–800.

40. Mookadam F, Thota VR, Lopez AM, Emani UR, Tajik AJ. Unicuspid aortic valve in children: a systematic review spanning four decades. J Heart Valve Dis. 2010;19:678–83.

41. Williams JCP, Barratt-Boyes BG, Lowe JB. Supravalvular aortic stenosis. Circulation. 1961;24:1311–8.

42. Geva A, McMahon CJ, Gauvreau K, Mohammed L, del Nido PJ, Geva T. Risk factors for reoperation after repair of discrete subaortic stenosis in children. J Am Coll Cardiol. 2007;50: 1498–504.

43. Youn HJ, Chung WS, Hong SJ. Demonstration of supravalvar aortic stenosis by different cardiac imaging modalities in Williams syndrome. Heart. 2002;88:438.

44. Beitzke A, Becker H, Rigler B, Stein JI, Suppan C. Development of aortic aneurysms in familial supravalvar aortic stenosis. Pediatr Cardiol. 1986;6:227–9.

45. Brown DW, Dipilato AE, Chong EC, Gauvreau K, McElhinney DB, Colan SD, Lock JE. Sudden unexpected death after balloon valvuloplasty for congenital aortic stenosis. J Am Coll Cardiol. 2010;56:1939–46.

46. Gleeson TG, Mwangi I, Horgan SJ, Cradock A, Fitzpatrick P, Murray JG. Steady-state free-precession (SSFP) cine MRI in distinguishing normal and bicuspid aortic valves. J Magn Reson Imaging. 2008;28:873–8.

47. Buchner S, Hulsmann M, Poschenrieder F, Hamer OW, Fellner C, Kobuch R, Feuerbach S, Riegger GAJ, Djavidani B, Luchner A, Debl K. Variable phenotypes of bicuspid aortic valve disease: classification by cardiovascular magnetic resonance. Heart. 2010;96:1233–40.

48. Debl K, Djavidani B, Buchner S, Poschenrieder F, Heinicke N, Schmid C, Kobuch R, Feuerbach S, Riegger G, Luchner A. Unicuspid aortic valve disease: a magnetic resonance imaging study. Rofo. 2008;180:983–7.

49. Sing-Chien Y, van Geuns R-J, Meijboom FJ, Kirschbaum SW, McGhie JS, Simoons ML, Kilner PJ, Roos-Hesselink JW. A

simplified continuity equation approach to the quantification of stenotic bicuspid aortic valves using velocity-encoded cardiovascular magnetic resonance. J Cardiovasc Magn Reson. 2007;9: 899–906.

50. Pouleur A-C, Le Polain de Waroux J-B, Pasquet A, Vanoverschelde J-LJ, Gerber BL. Aortic valve area assessment: multidetector CT compared with cine MR imaging and transthoracic and transesophageal echocardiography. Radiology. 2007;244:745–54.

51. Valsangiacomo Büchel ER, DiBernardo S, Bauersfeld U, Berger F. Contrast-enhanced magnetic resonance angiography of the great arteries in patients with congenital heart disease: an accurate tool for planning catheter-guided interventions. Int J Cardiovasc Imaging. 2005;21:313–22.

52. Debl K, Djavidani B, Buchner S, Poschenrieder F, Schmid F-X, Kobuch R, Feuerbach S, Riegger G, Luchner A. Dilatation of the ascending aorta in bicuspid aortic valve disease: a magnetic resonance imaging study. Clin Res Cardiol. 2009;98:114–20.

53. Hope MD, Hope TA, Meadows AK, Ordovas KG, Urbania TH, Alley MT, Higgins CB. Bicuspid aortic valve: four-dimensional MR evaluation of ascending aortic systolic flow patterns. Radiology. 2010;255:53–61.

54. Barker A, Lanning C, Shandas R. Quantification of hemodynamic wall shear stress in patients with bicuspid aortic valve using phase-contrast MRI. Ann Biomed Eng. 2010;38:788–800.

55. den Reijer PM, Sallee D, van der Velden P, Zaaijer E, Parks WJ, Ramamurthy S, Robbie T, Donati G, Lamphier C, Beekman R, Brummer M. Hemodynamic predictors of aortic dilatation in bicuspid aortic valve by velocity-encoded cardiovascular magnetic resonance. J Cardiovasc Magn Reson. 2010;12:4.

56. Sabet HY, Edwards WD, Tazelaar HD, Daly RC. Congenitally bicuspid aortic valves: a surgical pathology study of 542 cases (1991 through 1996) and a literature review of 2,715 additional cases. Mayo Clin Proc. 1999;74:14–26.

57. Boodhwani M, de Kerchove L, Glineur D, Rubay J, Vanoverschelde J-L, Noirhomme P, El Khoury G. Repair of regurgitant bicuspid aortic valves: a systematic approach. J Thorac Cardiovasc Surg. 2010;140:276–84. e271.

58. Chiu S-N, Wang J-K, Lin M-T, Wu E-T, Lu FL, Chang C-I, Chen Y-S, Chiu I-S, Lue H-C, Wu M-H. Aortic valve prolapse associated with outlet-type ventricular septal defect. Ann Thorac Surg. 2005;79:1366–71.

59. Walley VM, Black MD. Erosion and perforation of a cusp by nodular calcification: an unusual cause of insufficiency in a congenital bicuspid aortic valve. Can J Cardiol. 1991;7:202–4.

60. Brown DW, Dipilato AE, Chong EC, Lock JE, McElhinney DB. Aortic valve reinterventions after balloon aortic valvuloplasty for congenital aortic stenosis: intermediate and late follow-up. J Am Coll Cardiol. 2010;56:1740–9.

61. McMahon CJ, Ayres N, Pignatelli RH, Franklin W, Vargo TA, Bricker JT, El-Said HG. Echocardiographic presentations of endocarditis, and risk factors for rupture of a sinus of valsalva in childhood. Cardiol Young. 2003;13:168–72.

62. Martins JD, Sherwood MC, Mayer Jr JE, Keane JF. Aortico-left ventricular tunnel: 35-year experience. J Am Coll Cardiol. 2004;44:446–50.

63. Humes RA, Hagler DJ, Julsrud PR, Levy JM, Feldt RH, Schaff HV. Aortico-left ventricular tunnel: diagnosis based on two-dimensional echocardiography, color flow Doppler imaging, and magnetic resonance imaging. Mayo Clin Proc. 1986;61:901–7.

64. Søndergaard L, Lindvig K, Hildebrandt P, Thomsen C, Ståhlberg F, Joen T, Henriksen O. Quantification of aortic regurgitation by magnetic resonance velocity mapping. Am Heart J. 1993;125: 1081–90.

65. Honda N, Machida K, Hashimoto M, Mamiya T, Takahashi T, Kamano T, Kashimada A, Inoue Y, Tanaka S, Yoshimoto N. Aortic regurgitation: quantitation with MR imaging velocity mapping. Radiology. 1993;186:189–94.

66. Ley S, Eichhorn J, Ley-Zaporozhan J, Ulmer H, Schenk JP, Kauczor HU, Arnold R. Evaluation of aortic regurgitation in congenital heart disease: value of MR imaging in comparison to echocardiography. Pediatr Radiol. 2007;37:426–36.

67. Sondergaard L, Lindvig K, Hildebrandt P, Thomsen C, Stahlberg F, Joen T, Henriksen O. Quantification of aortic regurgitation by magnetic resonance velocity mapping. Am Heart J. 1993;125: 1081–90.

68. Dulce MC, Mostbeck GH, O'Sullivan M, Cheitlin M, Caputo GR, Higgins CB. Severity of aortic regurgitation: interstudy reproducibility of measurements with velocity-encoded cine MR imaging. Radiology. 1992;185:235–40.

69. Schwartz ML, Gauvreau K, Geva T. Predictors of outcome of biventricular repair in infants with multiple left heart obstructive lesions. Circulation. 2001;104:682–7.

70. Shone JD, Sellers RD, Anderson RC, Adams Jr P, Lillehei CW, Edwards JE. The developmental complex of "parachute mitral valve," supravalvular ring of left atrium, subaortic stenosis, and coarctation of aorta. Am J Cardiol. 1963;11:714–25.

71. Colan SD, McElhinney DB, Crawford EC, Keane JF, Lock JE. Validation and re-evaluation of a discriminant model predicting anatomic suitability for biventricular repair in neonates with aortic stenosis. J Am Coll Cardiol. 2006;47:1858–65.

72. Grosse-Wortmann L, Yun T-J, Al-Radi O, Kim S, Nii M, Lee K-J, Redington A, Yoo S-J, van Arsdell G. Borderline hypoplasia of the left ventricle in neonates: insights for decision-making from functional assessment with magnetic resonance imaging. J Thorac Cardiovasc Surg. 2008;136:1429–36.

Anna N. Seale and Philip J. Kilner

10.1 Introduction

Fontan procedures are radical surgical reconstructions performed for children born with only one effective ventricle, or two that cannot be separated functionally. They entail the connection of the pulmonary vascular resistance downstream of the systemic vascular resistance, flow through both being delivered, in series, by the one ventricle, but at the cost of elevated systemic venous pressure (Fig. 10.1). This aims to eliminate shunting and the associated ventricular volume loading, and to achieve full pulmonary oxygenation.

There is a great range of morphology in congenital heart disease. Whenever possible the surgeon aims to achieve a repair dividing the heart into two sides with one side providing the systemic circulation and the other side providing the pulmonary circulation. However, in some instances morphological features may make this impossible or too high risk (Table 10.1); in these cases palliation by a Fontan procedure is considered.

10.2 Definition

In a Fontan circulation the systemic venous return is connected to the pulmonary arteries without the interposition of an adequate ventricle, and without residual shunting at venous, atrial, ventricular or arterial levels [1].

A.N. Seale, MB BChir, MRCP (✉)
Department of Paediatric Cardiology, Royal Brompton Hospital,
Sydney Street, London, SW3 6NP, UK

Cardiovascular Magnetic Resonance Unit,
Royal Brompton Hospital and Imperial College,
Sydney Street, London, SW3 6NP, UK
e-mail: a.seale@rbht.nhs.uk

P.J. Kilner, M.D., Ph.D.
Cardiovascular Magnetic Resonance Unit,
Royal Brompton Hospital and Imperial College,
Sydney Street, London, SW3 6NP, UK
e-mail: p.kilner@rbht.nhs.uk

As Fontan surgery is used on a vast range of patients, initial intervention depends on the presenting morphology. Typically preliminary palliative surgery is performed to limit (pulmonary artery banding) or supplement (Blalock-Tausig shunt) blood flow to the lungs. Sufficient intracardiac mixing is also important, with an atrial septostomy or surgical septectomy being required in the first few days of life.

With time as the child grows, pulmonary blood flow is insufficient and usually a bi-directional cavo-pulmonary artery (Glenn) anastomosis is performed to augment pulmonary blood flow. In this procedure the superior vena cava is anastomosed onto the pulmonary artery. Timing of this procedure is debated [2], but it appears that about 6 months of age is ideal. Most children will also outgrow this limited blood flow, with increasing cyanosis especially during exercise and be converted to a complete Fontan circulation.

Completion of the Fontan aims to eliminate shunting and the associated volume loading of the dominant ventricle and desaturation of the arterial blood. The procedure involves connection of the pulmonary arteries downstream of the systemic veins so that the single effective ventricle delivers flow through the systemic then the pulmonary resistances in series.

Elevated systemic venous and hepatic portal pressure is needed to propel the blood forward through the relatively low resistance of the pulmonary vessels (Fig. 10.2). The delivery of flow through the pulmonary as well as the systemic resistance adds only about 10–15 % to the ventricle's work load when maintaining a given output – less strenuous for the myocardium than the volume loading that would have been present prior to surgery. The most critical and unavoidable pathophysiological consequence of Fontan surgery, however, is the height of the systemic venous pressure and its effects on the micro vessels upstream.

Electronic supplementary material The online version of this chapter (doi:10.1007/978-1-4471-4267-6_10) contains supplementary material, which is available to authorized users.

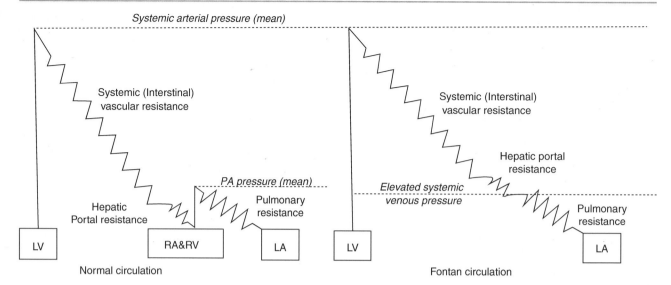

Fig. 10.1 Schematic diagrams indicating the relative vascular pressures and resistance of a normal biventricular circulation (*left*) compared to a Fontan circulation (*right*). Pressures (mean where pulsatile) are indicated by the *vertical heights*. Vascular resistances are represented by *zig-zag lines*. Because of the low pulmonary relative to systemic resistance, a Fontan circulation adds relatively little to the systemic ventricular afterload. The more critical issue is the height of the systemic venous pressure and its effect on the hepatic portal and systemic, notably intestinal, microvessels upstream. *LV* left ventricle; *RA* right atrium; *RV* right ventricle; *LA* left atrium

Table 10.1 Examples of types of congenital heart disease which may be palliated by the Fontan circulation

Ventricular septal defect
(a) with significant straddling of the atrioventricular valve chordal apparatus
(b) where there is almost the complete ventricular septal deficiency
Atrio-ventricular septal defect
(a) unbalanced defect
(b) where the ventricular component is very large
Pulmonary atresia with intact ventricular septum
Tricuspid atresia
Hypoplastic left heart syndrome
Mitral atresia
Double inlet left ventricle
Double outlet right ventricle
(a) with non-committed ventricular septal defect
(b) with mitral stenosis
Severe Ebstein's malformation (following over-sewing of the tricuspid valve)
Complex forms of congenital heart disease where there is only one good-sized ventricle
Complex forms of congenital heart disease where there are two ventricles but division into a biventricular circulation is too high risk

Fontan reconstruction should achieve nearly normal arterial saturation and avoids chronic volume overload, but at the cost of significant elevation of the systemic venous and hepatic portal pressure, typically to about 12–15 mmHg at rest. There is usually slightly decreased cardiac output at rest, and limited capacity to increase output on exercise.

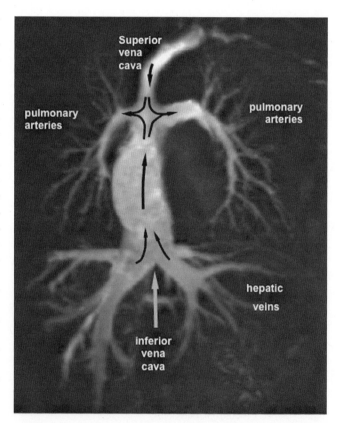

Fig. 10.2 The hepato-cavo-pulmonary flow paths after a lateral tunnel TCPC Fontan connection, illustrated by a magnetic resonance contrast angiogram. It is important that hepatic venous blood flows via the IVC pathway to both lungs as it carries a factor which prevents the formation of pulmonary arterio-venous malformations, a potential cause of desaturation (see Fig. 10.8b)

10.3   Preoperative Criteria

In order for a Fontan circulation to work successfully there are certain requirements:

1. Good ventricular function
2. Low (i.e. normal) pulmonary vascular resistance
3. No atrio-ventricular valve regurgitation
4. Unobstructed ventricular outflow
5. Good-sized branch pulmonary arteries without stenoses
6. Unobstructed pulmonary venous return
7. Absence of aorto-pulmonary collateral arteries

The more criteria met, one would expect a better outcome. However, this is not always the case.

10.4   Morphology of Different Fontan Circulations

Fontan operations have undergone several modifications and refinements in the decades since Fontan and Baudet published their initial results in humans in 1971 [3]. It is important when imaging a patient with a Fontan circulation, that details of what procedure has been performed are known.

Until the end of the 1980s, the right atrium was routinely included between the caval veins and the pulmonary arteries (Fig. 10.3a). Initially, atrial inflow and outflow valves were inserted, but they were not found to function satisfactorily (Fig. 10.4a). In patients with atrio-pulmonary Fontan connections, the right atrium tends to become dilated and subject to arrhythmias. The peaks of pressure caused by the contraction of a right atrium included in a Fontan circulation are propagated, detrimentally, upstream to the systemic and hepatic veins as well as beneficially downstream to pulmonary arteries. The work put into this part of the circulation by right atrial contraction not only fails to contribute usefully, the extra energy being largely dissipated in turbulent flow, but the turbulence itself slightly increases the local resistance to flow through the cavity and adjacent vessels. This was part of the rationale put forward by Marc de Leval and colleagues, for total cavo-pulmonary connection (TCPC) [4] (Fig. 10.3b) which has emerged as a superior technique.

This type of procedure also excludes part or all of the right atrial cavity from the elevated pressure of the cavo-pulmonary flow path, which may help to avoid the atrial distension which predisposes to arrhythmias, stagnation and thrombosis. It also allows the coronary sinus to drain to the low pressure part of the right atrium and then to the left atrium via an atrial septal defect. The superior caval vein is connected to the pulmonary artery (bidirectional

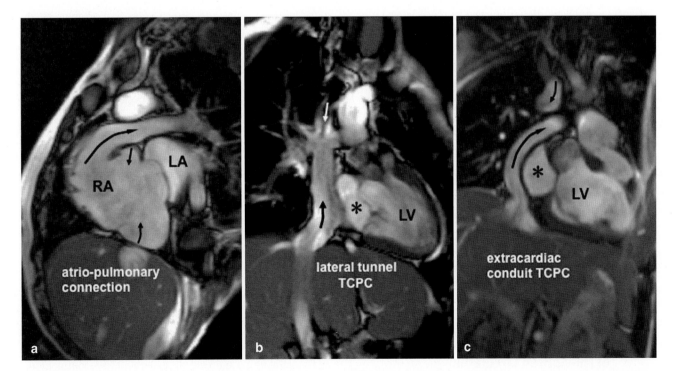

Fig. 10.3 Three types of Fontan connection illustrated by CMR cine images, (**a**) atrio-pulmonary connection, (**b** and Movie 10.1) lateral tunnel and (**c**) extracardiac conduit. **b** and **c** can both be called total cavo-pulmonary connection (*TCPC*). As a transitional stage to Fontan physiology, a limited residual shunt may be left in the form of a fenestration between the IVC pathway and the low-pressure atrial cavity to slightly alleviate systemic venous pressure. The TCPC avoids the progressive right atrial distension which can predispose to atrial arrhythmias, stagnation and thrombosis, and the coronary sinus drains to the low pressure part of the right atrium, which is marked*. *Arrows* show the direction of blood flow

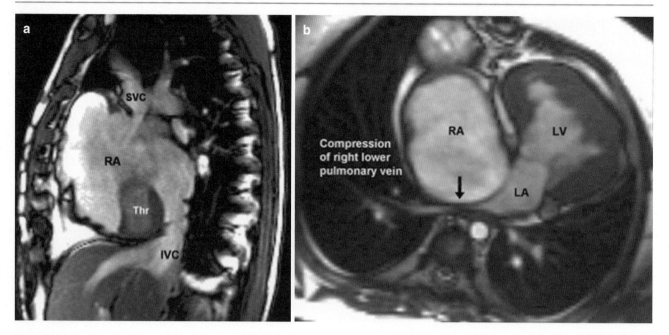

Fig. 10.4 Complications of early atrio-pulmonary Fontan procedures. (**a** and Movie 10.2) This sagittal cine image shows the dilated right atrium (*RA*) with a large thrombus attached to its floor. The solidified, ineffective leaflets of homograft atrial inflow valves can be seen in this case, mildly restricting inflow from the *SVC* and *IVC*. For this reason, atrial inflow valves were not included in later variants of the operation. (**b** and Movie 10.3) The dilated right atrium (*RA*) upstream of an atrio-pulmonary Fontan connection causing compression of the right lower pulmonary vein (*arrow*), which then tends to exacerbates right atrial pressure and distension. *SVC* superior vena cava; *Thr* thrombus; *IVC* inferior vena cava; *LV* left ventricle; *LA* left atrium

cavo-pulmonary anastomosis, glenn shunt). There are two variants to connect the inferior caval vein: the lateral tunnel (Fig. 10.3b) which consists of a prosthetic baffle and a portion of the lateral atrial wall and the extra cardiac conduit (Fig. 10.3c) consisting of a tube graft between the transsected inferior caval vein and the pulmonary artery.

Fenestration of a TCPC was a further modification introduced in 1990 as a transitional stage, slightly alleviating systemic venous congestion and augmenting filling of the systemic ventricle [5]. This aids in the postoperative course, maintaining cardiac output if pulmonary vascular resistance is labile. Usually a small fenestration may close spontaneously, or if the patient desaturates significantly on exercise, be closed by an occlusion device in the months following surgery. A small fenestration, however can be useful for the electrophysiologist providing access to the atria if electrophysiological procedures are needed in the future for arrhythmia.

10.5 Optimal Morphology of the Fontan Circulation

Marc de Leval and colleagues as well as other groups have gone on to apply computational fluid dynamic modelling to studies of the geometries and fluid dynamics of TCPC,

either by lateral tunnel or extra cardiac conduit [6]. There is little doubt that the dimensions and shapes of the connections matter. The factors likely to optimise cavo-pulmonary flow and minimise systemic venous congestion include:

1. Avoidance of stenosis. Each flow path (IVC and SVC to RPA and LPA) and the junctions between them must have adequate cross sectional area for the flow carried.
2. Avoidance of sharp angulations at the suture lines of the cavo-pulmonary anastomoses. Abrupt changes of direction predispose to flow separation and turbulence.
3. Avoidance of opposing or competing streams from the upward flowing IVC and the downward flowing SVC. In other words, they should not collide head on, but be slightly offset relative to one another. It is important, however, that hepatic venous blood contributes, via the IVC pathway, to both lungs as it carries a factor which prevents the formation of pulmonary arterio-venous malformations, a potential cause of progressive desaturation.
4. Minimisation of flow separation, flow disturbance, and regions of stagnation that might predispose to thrombosis by maintaining uniform diameters and smooth contours through the cavo-pulmonary flow paths.
5. The minimisation of energy dissipation, avoidance of potentially arhythmogenic and thrombogenic atrial scarring and distension.

10.6   Causes of Failure in the Fontan Circulation

With improvement in surgical technique and better selection of patients, the operative mortality for completion of Fontan is now less than 5 %. Patients, however frequently run into complications in the long term.

There are several factors that may contribute to failure of a Fontan circulation. They include:

1. **Elevated resistance of the cavo-(atrio)-pulmonary vasculature**, including stenosis at surgical connections, hypoplasia or stenosis of pulmonary arteries, thrombo-embolic obstruction, and pulmonary vein compression due to right atrial distension after atrio-pulmonary connection (Fig. 10.4b). In addition there may be abnormal microvasculature either due to high pulmonary blood flow earlier in life or intrinsic anomalies, there may be a role for sildenafil in some cases [7]

2. **Atrial arrhythmias** (sinus node dysfunction or atrial re-entry tachycardia) particularly late after atrio-pulmonary connection. It is important to establish whether there are any treatable haemodynamic lesions such as anastomotic or pulmonary arterial stenosis which may be exacerbating atrial distension and making the patient prone to arrhythmia.

3. **Thrombo-embolism.** Low velocity cavo-atrio-pulmonary flow causes patients to be susceptible to thromboembolism (Fig. 10.4a). Atrial arrhythmias increase this risk further. All Fontan patients should have anticoagulation [8]. Warfarinisation can be difficult in small children and sometimes a combination of aspirin +/− clopidogrel is used in this group. Unfortunately there are no randomised studies in the literature to guide the physician as to the best anticoagulation treatment.

4. **Ventricular dysfunction** The underlying congenital malformation, volume loading of the systemic ventricle prior to completion of Fontan reconstruction, the surgical procedure itself, and the abnormal pre-and after-loading of the ventricle following Fontan surgery, may all contribute to ongoing ventricular dysfunction. This may cause and be exacerbated by atrio-ventricular valve regurgitation. Outflow to the aorta via a ventricular septal defect/or an infundibulum can be subject to progressive obstruction and should be carefully assessed.

    Both systolic and diastolic ventricular function is important, and indeed it may be that diastolic dysfunction is responsible for poor outcome in some patients [9]. It is the author's preference that most patients with a Fontan circulation should be on an ACE inhibitor although there is little direct evidence to support this [10].

5. **Systemic venous and hepatic portal congestion** and complications following from these. Elevation of systemic venous pressure to near critical levels is an inevitable consequence of Fontan surgery and can have damaging consequences for the micro vessels and tissues of the organs upstream, notably the liver and the intestines. Ascites and hepatic edema, and less commonly, cirrhosis and hepatic carcinoma have been reported as sequel. Protein losing enteropathy is a further, relatively uncommon complication related to portal and lymphatic congestion. Plastic bronchitis, probably due to pulmonary lymphatic congestion and exudates is an uncommon, but potentially fatal complication.

6. **Shunts** can cause either cyanosis (blue blood mixing with pink blood) or exacerbate pulmonary congestion (pink blood mixing with blue blood). Unwanted shunts causing cyanosis may occur through a patch or baffle leak or through the development of pulmonary arterio-venous malformations or systemic vein to pulmonary vein collaterals. When the surgeons purposely leave a fenestration, they are effectively leaving such a shunt. Shunts that exacerbate pulmonary congestion include ventricular to right atrial leaks (in the atrio-pulmonary Fontan), or a residual or acquired systemic to pulmonary arterial shunt.

The technique used for Fontan completion is important, there are a particular group of problems associated with progressive right atrial dilatation following atrio-pulmonary connection, but the prevalence of complications in this patient group may be partly related to an earlier era of surgery, and more years of follow-up. In such patients, conversion from atrio-pulmonary to the potentially slightly more streamlined total cavo-pulmonary connection is an option to consider, combined with a right atrial maze procedure. However, such surgery is relatively high risk in most hands. It is therefore crucial to establish to what extent there is pathophysiology present which is likely to be alleviated by re-operation, as opposed to pathology that would not be alleviated but might exacerbate the risk.

10.7   Role of Cardiovascular Magnetic Resonance

Cardiovascular magnetic resonance (CMR) enables the non-invasive assessment of the anatomical structures without ionising radiation, and it enables ventricular functional assessment, quantification of flow, assessment of ventricular fibrosis and of myocardial viability.

In the Fontan patient, CMR can be used to help assess the suitability for the Fontan procedure to be performed in a particular patient, as well as having an important role in the assessment of the post-operative patient. Cine and 3D CMR acquisitions can be helpful in guiding interventions on Fontan patients, including those in the electrophysiology laboratory.

10.7.1 Assessment Pre-Fontan Completion

10.7.1.1 Goals of Imaging

As detailed above, there are certain requirements for a Fontan circulation to work. Imaging should be targeted to help answer whether the patient meets these criteria.

Important features which are shown fairly easily with CMR include:

- Ventricular function, and the relative volume and stroke volume of a second ventricle, if present.
- Atrio-ventricular valve regurgitation
- Ventricular outflow
- Branch pulmonary arteries
- Pulmonary venous return

It must be remembered that patients undergoing assessment pre-Fontan are usually less than 5 years old, and hence structures are small. This means sequences need to be modified appropriately, often necessitating smaller slice thickness on cine images, use of Turbo (fast) spin echo with blood suppression (TSE) or stacks of steady state free precession (SSFP) cines to image the pulmonary arteries and veins. Gadolinium enhanced CMR angiography can also be helpful when assessing small structures.

Features which are particularly difficult to assess in small children are:

- Aorto-pulmonary collateral arteries
- Transpulmonary gradient and pulmonary vascular resistance

Historically, children undergoing cavo-pulmonary anastomosis and completion of Fontan have had diagnostic cardiac catheterisation to detail anatomy and measure pulmonary artery pressure and transpulmonary gradient (pulmonary artery pressure minus left atrial pressure) prior to the procedure. In patients following cavo-pulmonary anastomosis, the pulmonary arteries are particularly difficult to see with echocardiography and collateral vessels and their course can not be clearly identified.

CMR has the ability to image the caval veins and pulmonary arteries clearly and allows assessment of flow down each vessel. In the absence of stenosis, pulmonary artery pressure can be measured by placing a small cannula into the jugular veins. Diagnostic alogorithms have been proposed [11] to avoid cardiac catheterisation in low-risk subjects before the Fontan operation. CMR has already been shown to be safe and effective and less costly alternative to routine catheterisation in the evaluation of selected patients before the bidirectional cavo-pulmonary anastomosis operation [12, 13].

Assessment of pulmonary vascular resistance has always been difficult, but CMR combined with catheter measurements of pressure have been used to evaluate pulmonary vascular resistance in patients with a left-to-right shunt [14]. In the future such techniques may be useful in the assessment of patients before the Fontan procedure.

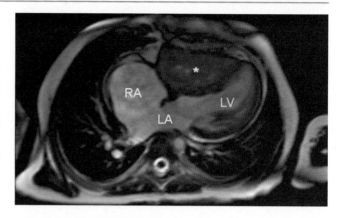

Fig. 10.5 CMR cine image acquired prior to a Fontan procedure in a 5 year old child with Ebstein's malformation. Previous Starne's procedure (over-sewing of the tricuspid valve) and atrial septectomy. Four chamber view shows thrombus in the right ventricle. The interatrial communication is widely patent. * thrombus in the right ventricle. *RA* right atrium; *LA* left atrium; *LV* left ventricle

Examples of CMR findings in the pre-operative Fontan patient are illustrated in Figs. 10.5 and 10.6.

10.7.2 Assessment Post-Fontan Completion

10.7.2.1 Goals of Imaging

As detailed above, there are several factors that may contribute to failure of a Fontan circulation. CMR can be used as a tool to assess for many of these [15].

1. **Elevated resistance of the cavo-(atrio)-pulmonary vasculature.**
   Assessment of:
   - the pulmonary arteries for anastomotic stenoses, branch pulmonary artery stenoses or hypoplasia
   - thrombosis in the Fontan pathways (Fig. 10.4a)
   - pulmonary vein compression and right atrial distension after atrio-pulmonary connection (Fig. 10.4b)
2. Thrombo-embolism
   - A stack of transaxial SSFP cines, for example 5 mm slice thickness with no gaps, is a good way to look for evidence of thrombus in cavo-atrio-pulmonary pathways, backed up by early gadolinium inversion recovery imaging of any suspected thrombus, which should then appear as dark signal void relative to bright blood signal.
3. Ventricular function
   - Volumetric measurement is performed from a short axis cine stack. If a second, usually small ventricle is present and communicating with the dominant ventricle, a decision must be made and recorded regarding separate or combined ventricular volume measurements.
   - Long axis cines should be acquired aligned with each ventricular inflow and outflow tract looking for evidence of regurgitation or stenosis which should be assessed further if found (Fig. 10.7).

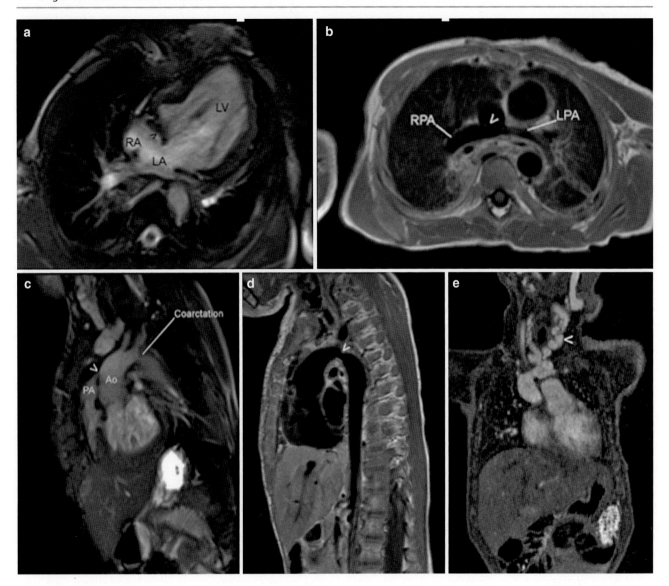

Fig. 10.6 Cardiac magnetic resonance scan pre-Fontan of a 2.5 year old child with tricuspid atresia, ventriculo-arterial discordance and interrupted aortic arch. Previous aortic arch repair and pulmonary artery banding, followed by Damus-Kaye Stansel procedure and right modified Blalock-Taussig shunt. Followed by bidirectional cavo-pulmonary anastomosis. (**a**) Four chamber view showing absent right connection (tricuspid atresia) and dominant left ventricle. The interatrial communication is widely patent. (**b**) Unobstructed cavo-pulmonary anastomosis (*arrowed*). The left pulmonary artery (*LPA*) is uniformly of lower caliber than the right (*RPA*). (**c**) Critical narrowing of the Damus-Kaye Stansel anastomosis (*arrowed*). (**d**) Residual *coarctation* of the aorta just distal to the left subclavian artery. (**e**) Varicose dilatation of the anterior jugular veins in the neck. *Ao* Aorta

4. Shunts

Assessment of:

- patch/baffle leak, (Fig. 10.8a) for example by a transaxial cine stack
- systemic vein to pulmonary vein collaterals (Fig. 10.8c)
- systemic to pulmonary arterial collaterals
- fenestrations

It must be remembered that patients undergoing post-Fontan assessment have usually undergone multiple previous procedures that may have involved coils, devices or stenting procedures in the cardiac catheterisation laboratory.

These can affect image quality, some earlier devices causing significant artefacts [16]. Sequences need to be changed appropriately, often necessitating increased use of Turbo (fast) spin echo with blood suppression (TSE) to image structures that have been stented.

Gadolinium enhanced MRA may be helpful assessing small structures such as collateral vessels and enabling manipulation of a three-dimensional data-set. However, the timing and distribution of contrast arrival in the pulmonary arteries and its dilution by non-opacified blood from inferior vena cava should be considered. Non contrast ECG and

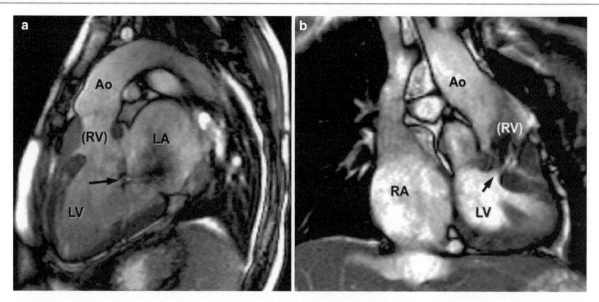

Fig. 10.7 Problems with the left ventricular inflow valve or the outflow tract after Fontan procedure. (**a**) Mitral regurgitation (*arrow*) contributes to back pressure in the pulmonary vessels and so back to the systemic veins. In this particular patient, who also had a pleural effusion, treatment of fluid retention alleviated the regurgitation. (**b**) Left ventricular outflow obstruction after Fontan operation caused by a moderately restrictive VSD and hypertrophy of the infundibulum of the rudimentary, sub aortic right ventricle

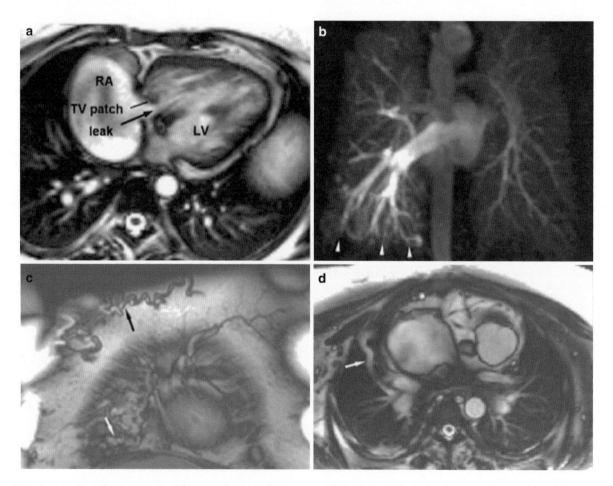

Fig. 10.8 Desaturating shunts in three different patients. (**a**, Movie 10.4) A diastolic leak through the detachment of a patch placed across the right atrio-ventricular valve of a patient with double inlet left ventricle and an atrio-pulmonary Fontan connection. (**b**) Magnetic resonance contrast angiogram showing evidence of right pulmonary arterio-venous malformations (*arrows*) in a patient after Kawashima operation in whom hepatic venous return was flowing to the left lung, but not the right. (**c**, **d**) Subcutaneous (*black arrow*) and intra-thoracic (*white arrows*) branches of systemic venous to pulmonary venous collateral veins

Table 10.2 Suggested imaging protocol for post-Fontan patient

Sequence		Technical notes
Multislice scouts	Transaxial, coronal and saggital multislice.	Bright blood SSFP is preferable for pulmonary vessels, plus one dark-blood stack to assist tissue characterisation.
Transaxial cine stack	Cover whole heart and mediastinum.	SSFP, 5 mm thickness, no gaps. All cines breath held and ECG gated.
Vertical long axis (VLA)	Cine (SSFP).	
Horizontal long axis (HLA)	Cine (SSFP).	
Short axis	Cine stack (SSFP).	
Four chamber	(If there are four!)	
Inflow valve(s) and outflow tract	Cines (SSFP). Oblique 'mitral stack' in 3 chamber orientation if inflow regurgitation is present.	
Oblique cavo-pulmonary cines	Align with all cavo-(atrio)-pulmonary pathways, cross cut where necessary.	
Aortic arch	Cine (SSFP)	
Flow velocity acquisitions	Through plane, breath hold acquisitions: slices chosen depend on individual patient anatomy	For accurate shunt calculations, post acquisition phantom correction may be needed.
Aortic flow	Velocity mapping	Venc 120–150 cm/s
SVC flow (optional)	Velocity mapping. Left SVC may be present	Venc 80 cm/s
IVC flow (optional)	Velocity mapping. At diaphragm to include hepatic flow if possible	Venc 80 cm/s
Branch pulmonary artery flows (RPA and LPA)	Velocity mapping. Individual anatomy needs consideration. Velocity above 1 m/s is likely to represent significant Fontan stenosis.	Venc 80 cm/s. Or 120 cm/s if at a suspected stenosis.
3D SSFP of whole heart and PAs	Free breathing, ecg gated, diaphragm navigated acquisition	
Possible CMR contrast angiography (optional)	But timing and dilution of bolus can be problematic	
Early gadolinium imaging (optional)	In selected slice(s) to confirm or exclude suspected thrombus	Inversion recovery
Late gadolinium enhancement (optional)	For possible ventricular fibrosis	Inversion recovery

Protocols must be individualized for each particular patient as the underlying anatomy and surgical technique may vary considerably

respiratory navigator gated 3D SSFP imaging, or injection of contrast from a leg, may be preferable.

Evaluation of myocardial fibrosis by *late gadolinium enhancement* may be informative in patients with impaired ventricular function. Myocardial fibrosis has been shown to be common in Fontan survivors and associated with adverse ventricular mechanics and a higher prevalence of non-sustained ventricular tachycardia [17].

Flow analysis is very helpful when assessing the postoperative Fontan patient. Differential flow in the right and left pulmonary arteries can be an indicator of stenoses, although be aware that there can be a marked variability of flow from the caval veins towards the right and left pulmonary arteries [15]. Variation from this can suggest pulmonary artery stenoses, but be wary there can be other explanations. Most current CMR systems are subject to background phase offset errors that can affect measurements of flow, particularly when areas of interest are further from the magnet iso-center, and in planes that depart from transaxial. Post-acquisition correction using an acquisition in a static phantom may be needed. Unilateral pulmonary venous obstruction can also result in differential pulmonary artery blood flow, with reduced pulmonary artery flow on the side with pulmonary venous obstruction.

Comparing the total flow in the branch pulmonary arteries to the total flow in the pulmonary veins can also be helpful and may help identify collateral flow [18]. These values should be equal, but if pulmonary venous flow is higher, it may suggest systemic-to-pulmonary collateral arteries. Of course, the values gained should be balanced against the quality of the imaging.

Protocols for CMR protocol assessment of the post-operative Fontan patient are outlined in Table 10.2

Examples of CMR findings in the post-operative Fontan patient are illustrated in Figs. 10.4, 10.7 and 10.8.

10.7.3 Cardiac Magnetic Resonance Imaging for Guiding Intervention in Fontan Patients

Patients following the Fontan procedure are at risk of developing atrial arrhythmias which can be particularly difficult to treat. They may require repeat electrophysiological interventions or repeat surgery. If no fenestration is left, access into the atrial mass is not possible at cardiac catheterisation without creation of a fenestration in the wall of the conduit/lateral tunnel.

CMR can have a role in identifying or excluding the presence of thrombus pre-procedure, and 3D CMR acquisitions, for example by SSFP, can allow a 'road map' of the cardiovascular pathways to be reconstructed which can be superimposed on the angiographic image to guide the interventionist.

10.8 Discussion, Limitations and Common Pitfalls

CMR's non-invasiveness and freedom from ionising radiation are particularly relevant as patients often now have completion of Fontan at 2–3 years of age, with a life-long need for serial assessment. Multiple procedures using ionising radiation can significantly increase the risk of malignancies later in life and should be avoided. In addition, CMR allows fairly easy quantification of ventricular function, flow analysis, fibrosis and myocardial viability.

However, patients may have intracardiac or pulmonary devices, stents or coils that can cause artefacts. They are also susceptible to arrhythmia, and some Fontan patients have pacing systems which exclude study by CMR.

Computed tomography (CT) offers excellent spatial resolution and relatively unrestricted access in much shorter acquisition times than CMR. This can be beneficial for children as there is no need for an anaesthetic, newer technology has greatly reduced ionizing radiation dose making CT angiography a more viable option for young children in specific cases.

Computed tomography is superior for imaging the epicardial coronary arteries and their relation to adjacent structures or conduits. As with CMR contrast angiography, the route of contrast passage relative to the cavo-pulmonary connections needs consideration. Given its high spatial resolution, CT angiography is likely to depict small vessels such as aorto-pulmonary collateral arteries more clearly. Angiography, similarly with direct injection into collateral vessels provides superior imaging of collateral vessels and their connections.

Transthoracic and/or transesophageal echocardiography still remains the first-line cardiovascular imaging modality in patients with congenital heart disease due to its availability and portability for bedside use. Although imaging is frequently very good in young patients, suboptimal acoustic access can be problematic in older patients particularly following cardiovascular surgery. Echocardiography is usually preferable to CMR for the identification of small baffle shunts, structural abnormalities of valve leaflets, and their suspensory apparatus, assessment of atrio-ventricular

valve regurgitation, assessment of gradients (when adequate Doppler angle gained) and infective endocardial vegetations.

Conclusion

The range of procedures known as Fontan operations are radical palliative procedures, not corrections, and there is no such thing as a 'perfect' Fontan operation. Patients invariably have complications at some point. Fontan surgery should, be undertaken only by experienced congenital cardiac surgical teams. Follow up needs to be life long, by cardiologists with specific knowledge of the peculiarities of Fontan pathophysiology. Expert imaging, including CMR, is an important aspect of assessment of the preoperative and post-operative Fontan patient. A potential cascade of complications underlines the importance of excellent pre-Fontan management and decision making, careful selection and planning for surgery, excellent surgical technique, and from then on, appropriate diagnostic follow up and management.

10.9 Practical Pearls

1. A contiguous stack of transaxial SSFP cines is an easy and informative way to start imaging a post Fontan patient. Cardiovascular structures and connections vary considerably between patients. Evidence of cavo-(atrio)-pulmonary stenosis, thrombosis or baffle leak can be sought on these cines. They also give preliminary information on the structure, function, inflow valve(s) and outflow tract of the ventricle(s).
2. Decide and record whether ventricular volume measurements of two communicating ventricular cavities are to be measured separately or in combination. When one is small, combined is recommended.
3. If performing contrast enhanced angiography, the unusual flow path and the potential dilution of contrast (given inflow from the IVC) should be considered. Non-contrast 3D whole-heart SSFP acquisition, or appropriately aligned cines, may be preferable.
4. Points to include in the report:
   I. Any Fontan pathway stenosis (SVC-PA and IVC-PA anastomoses)
   II. Branch pulmonary artery size and stenosis
   III. Fontan pathway thrombosis
   IV. Pulmonary vein narrowing
   V. Location and size of any baffle leak
   VI. Ventricular function
   VII. Any atrio-ventricular valve regurgitation
   VIII. Any aortic valve regurgitation
   IX. Any outflow tract +/− aortic arch obstruction

X. Presence of shunts (veno-venous, systemic-to-pulmonary collateral arteries, residual fenestration, patch leaks)

XI. Extra-cardiac anomalies (e.g. scoliosis, pleural effusions)

References

1. Gewillig M. The Fontan circulation. Heart. 2005;91(6):839–46.
2. Cleuziou J, Schreiber C, Cornelsen JK, Horer J, Eicken A, Lange R. Bidirectional cavopulmonary connection without additional pulmonary blood flow in patients below the age of 6 months. Eur J Cardiothorac Surg. 2008;34(3):556–61.
3. Fontan F, Baudet E. Surgical repair of tricuspid atresia. Thorax. 1971;26(3):240–8.
4. de Leval MR, Kilner P, Gewillig M, Bull C. Total cavopulmonary connection. J Thorac Cardiovasc Surg. 1989;97(4):636.
5. Bridges ND, Lock JE, Castaneda AR. Baffle fenestration with subsequent transcatheter closure. Modification of the Fontan operation for patients at increased risk. Circulation. 1990;82(5):1681–9.
6. Hsia TY, Migliavacca F, Pittaccio S, et al. Computational fluid dynamic study of flow optimization in realistic models of the total cavopulmonary connections. J Surg Res. 2004;116(2):305–13.
7. Reinhardt Z, Uzun O, Bhole V, et al. Sildenafil in the management of the failing Fontan circulation. Cardiol Young. 2010;20(5):522–5.
8. Seipelt RG, Franke A, Vazquez-Jimenez JF, et al. Thromboembolic complications after Fontan procedures: comparison of different therapeutic approaches. Ann Thorac Surg. 2002;74(2):556–62.
9. Akagi T, Benson LN, Green M, et al. Ventricular performance before and after Fontan repair for univentricular atrioventricular connection: angiographic and radionuclide assessment. J Am Coll Cardiol. 1992;20(4):920–6.
10. Kouatli AA, Garcia JA, Zellers TM, Weinstein EM, Mahony L. Enalapril does not enhance exercise capacity in patients after Fontan procedure. Circulation. 1997;96(5):1507–12.
11. Prakash A, Khan MA, Hardy R, Torres AJ, Chen JM, Gersony WM. A new diagnostic algorithm for assessment of patients with single ventricle before a Fontan operation. J Thorac Cardiovasc Surg. 2009;138(4):917–23.
12. Brown DW, Gauvreau K, Powell AJ, et al. Cardiac magnetic resonance versus routine cardiac catheterization before bidirectional Glenn anastomosis in infants with functional single ventricle: a prospective randomized trial. Circulation. 2007;116(23):2718–25.
13. Jones BO, Ditchfield MR, Cahoon GD, et al. Cardiac magnetic resonance imaging prior to bidirectional cavopulmonary connection in hypoplastic left heart syndrome. Heart Lung Circ. 2010;19(9):535–40.
14. Bell A, Beerbaum P, Greil G, et al. Noninvasive assessment of pulmonary artery flow and resistance by cardiac magnetic resonance in congenital heart diseases with unrestricted left-to-right shunt. JACC Cardiovasc Imaging. 2009;2(11):1285–91.
15. Kilner PJ, Geva T, Kaemmerer H, Trindade PT, Schwitter J, Webb GD. Recommendations for cardiovascular magnetic resonance in adults with congenital heart disease from the respective working groups of the European Society of Cardiology. Eur Heart J. 2010;31(7):794–805.
16. Garg R, Powell AJ, Sena L, Marshall AC, Geva T. Effects of metallic implants on magnetic resonance imaging evaluation of Fontan palliation. Am J Cardiol. 2005;95(5):688–91.
17. Rathod RH, Prakash A, Powell AJ, Geva T. Myocardial fibrosis identified by cardiac magnetic resonance late gadolinium enhancement is associated with adverse ventricular mechanics and ventricular tachycardia late after Fontan operation. J Am Coll Cardiol. 2010;55(16):1721–8.
18. Grosse-Wortmann L, Al-Otay A, Yoo SJ. Aortopulmonary collaterals after bidirectional cavopulmonary connection or Fontan completion: quantification with MRI. Circ Cardiovasc Imaging. 2009;2(3):219–25.

Joel R. Wilson and Mushabbar A. Syed

M.A. Syed, R.H. Mohiaddin (eds.), *Magnetic Resonance Imaging of Congenital Heart Disease*,
DOI 10.1007/978-1-4471-4267-6_11, © Springer-Verlag London 2012

175

J.R. Wilson, M.D.
Department of Cardiac Energetics, National Heart,
Lung and Blood Institute, National Institutes of Health,
Room B1D416, MSC 1061, 10 Center Drive, Bethesda, MD
20892-1061, USA

M.A. Syed, M.D., FACC (⊠)
Department of Medicine and Radiology, Stritch School of Medicine,
Loyola University Chicago, IL, USA

Cardiovascular Imaging, Heart and Vascular Institute,
Loyola University Medical Center, Maywood, IL, USA
e-mail: masyed@lumc.edu

Electronic supplementary material The online version of this chapter (doi:10.1007/978-1-4471-4267-6_11) contains supplementary material, which is available to authorized users.

11.1 Introduction

Transposition of the great arteries (TGA) is a form of conotruncal abnormalities in which the aorta arises from the morphological right ventricle and pulmonary artery arises from the morphological left ventricle (ventriculoarterial discordance). TGA encompasses two distinct defects, complete TGA and congenitally corrected TGA. Complete TGA has a prevalence of 0.24/1,000 live births [12] and represents ~5 % of all congenital heart disease [25]. It is the second most common congenital heart defect recognized in infancy [12]. Congenitally corrected TGA is rarer, recognized in 0.02–0.07 per 1,000 live births [15], or less than 1 % of congenital heart defects [25].

Whereas patients with congenitally corrected TGA can survive unrecognized into adulthood, patients with complete TGA present with varying degrees of cyanosis in infancy and almost always require early surgical intervention. Beginning in the late 1950s, surgical treatment for patients with complete TGA was revolutionized with the advent of the Senning and Mustard atrial shunt procedures. Although the arterial switch procedure was first described in 1976, it only became the corrective procedure of choice in the 1980s.

The role of cardiac magnetic resonance imaging (CMR) in these defects is dictated by the specific cardiac anatomy and by the reparative surgical interventions present (if any). In cases of congenitally corrected TGA, CMR can be instrumental in discriminating between the morphologic right and left ventricles, in characterizing abnormalities of viscero-atrial situs and in describing the associated cardiac anomalies that are nearly universally present. In the patients with complete TGA, almost all of whom will have had corrective surgery early in life, CMR can assess patency of conduits and baffles, and presence of residual defects. Furthermore, when the morphologic right ventricle (RV) is in the systemic position, it is prone to failure over time. Traditional methods of right ventricular function assessment are less accurate in this setting, and ventricular function and reserve may be better assessed by CMR in such cases.

11.2 Definitions and Morphology

11.2.1 Developmental Terms

• Bulboventricular looping: During normal embryologic development, the heart tube undergoes a bending and rightward rotation (dextro=D-looping). This normal D-looping indicates that the right ventricular inflow lies to the right of the left ventricle. L-looping (levo=L) is the abnormal leftward rotation of the heart tube, with the result that the right ventricular inflow becomes situated to the left of the left ventricle.

• Conotruncal development: In the primitive heart tube, the truncus arteriosus is the common origin for the aorta and pulmonary artery. Ventriculo-arterial connections are formed through growth or regression of muscular tissue, the conus, beneath each of the eventual semilunar valves. Growth of the conus beneath the pulmonic valve directs it anteriorly, while regression of conus beneath the aortic valve directs it posteriorly and creates fibrous continuity between the aortic and the mitral valve.

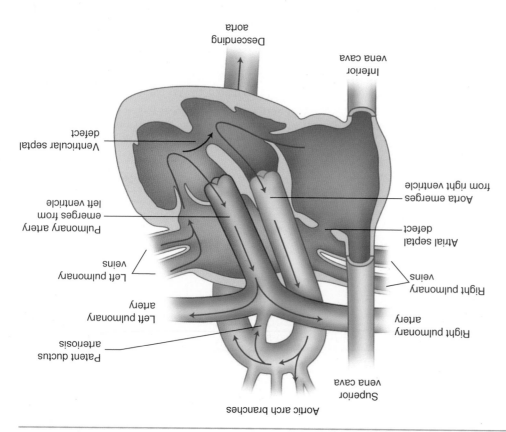

Fig. 11.1 Complete transposition of the great arteries (complete TGA, D-TGA). Schematic showing the arterial connections and flow of blood in the case of unrepaired complete TGA. The right atrium leads into the morphologic right ventricle and the left atrium into the morphologic left ventricle (atrioventricular concordance). The aorta arises from the morphologic (systemic) right ventricle, whereas the pulmonary artery originates from the morphologic left ventricle (ventriculoarterial discordance). In the unrepaired patient, the systemic and pulmonary circulations run in parallel. In order for blood in the systemic circulation to oxygenate, mixing must occur through one or more communications, such as a ventricular septal defect, atrial septal defect or patent ductus arteriosus

(Figure 11.1 labels: Descending aorta; Inferior vena cava; Ventricular septal defect; Pulmonary artery emerges from left ventricle; Left pulmonary veins; Left pulmonary artery; Patent ductus arteriosus; Aortic arch branches; Superior vena cava; Right pulmonary artery; Right pulmonary veins; Atrial septal defect; Aorta emerges from right ventricle)

11.2.2 Transposition of Great Arteries (TGA)

Transposition refers to ventriculoarterial discordance, when the morphologic RV leads to the aorta and the left ventricle to the pulmonary artery. The aorta is situated posterior and to the right in normal individuals. The direction of transposition (dextro- or levo-) refers to the rotation of the aorta relative to the pulmonary artery. By definition, the aorta follows the right ventricle in transposition syndromes.

- D-TGA or complete TGA (Fig. 11.1): Dextro-TGA signifies rightward rotation of the aorta and pulmonary artery (counterclockwise viewed from below). The aortic valve becomes displaced anteriorly and to the right of the pulmonic valve due to growth of conus tissue beneath the aortic valve and resorption of tissue beneath the pulmonic valve (Fig. 11.2). In most cases, the ventricles are d-looped, so atrioventricular concordance is preserved. The aorta overlies a systemic right ventricle (which lies to the right of the left ventricle) that is in turn connected to the right atrium. Systemic and pulmonary circulations are arranged in a parallel circuit with one another, thus a shunt, e.g. septal defect is required for mixing of oxygenated and deoxygenated blood.

- L-TGA or congenitally corrected TGA, ventricular inversion or double discordance – atrioventricular discordance and ventriculoarterial discordance (Fig. 11.3): Venous blood returns from the body into the right atrium then passes through the mitral valve into the morphological

left ventricle, also called subpulmonic ventricle. Blood then enters the lungs through the main pulmonary artery. Pulmonary venous blood returns to the left atrium and

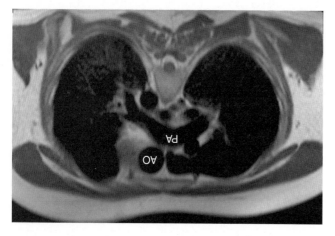

Fig. 11.2 Axial black blood image of a patient with complete transposition of the great arteries (complete TGA, D-TGA). In normal individuals, the aorta lies slightly posterior and to the right of the pulmonary artery. In most cases of complete TGA, the aorta is anterior and to the right of the pulmonary artery, however this spatial relationship is variable. This example, in which the aorta (*Ao*) lies anterior and to the left of the pulmonary artery (*PA*), demonstrates the variability in the relationship of the great arteries in transposition syndromes. The diagnosis of transposition should rely on the presence of ventriculoarterial discordance rather than on the position of the aorta

Fig. 11.3 Congenitally corrected transposition of the great arteries (congenitally corrected TGA, L-TGA). Schematic demonstrating the arterial connections and flow of blood in the case of congenitally corrected TGA. The right atrium leads into the morphologic left ventricle and the left atrium into the morphologic right ventricle (atrioventricular discordance). The aorta arises from the morphologic (systemic) right ventricle, whereas the pulmonary artery originates from the morphologic left ventricle (ventriculoarterial discordance). Because of the "double discordance," the systemic and pulmonary circulations are in series with one another, as in normal individuals, but the right ventricle becomes the systemic ventricle

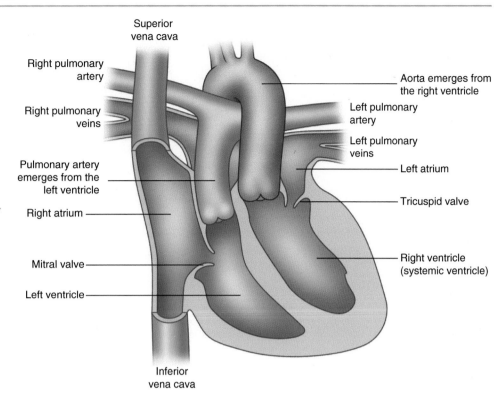

then through the tricuspid valve into the morphological RV, which acts as the systemic ventricle. Blood then exits through the aorta. The great arteries are typically arranged side-by-side in patients with congenitally corrected TGA, rather than anterior and posterior. Systemic and pulmonary circulations are arranged in a series circuit with one another, analogous to normal individuals.

11.2.3 Corrective Surgeries for Complete TGA

• Atrial baffle procedures (Senning and Mustard operation, also called atrial switch procedures, Fig. 11.4): Performed with either autograft (Senning) or synthetic (Mustard) baffle material, atrial baffle operations involve removal of the interatrial septum and creation of a partition which directs systemic venous return from the superior and inferior venae cavae into the left atrium and the pulmonary venous return into the right atrium. The baffle runs in an oblique coronal orientation and is roughly shaped like a pair of pants. One leg of the pants is in each of the venae cavae, and the waistband surrounds the non-systemic (mitral) atrioventricular valve. The excluded portions of the common atrium form the return pathway for the pulmonary veins to the systemic circulation through the morphologic RV.

• Arterial switch procedure (Jatene operation, Fig. 11.5): The aorta and main pulmonary arteries are transected at the level of the sinotubular junction. The coronary artery ostia with buttons are removed from the original aortic root and reimplanted in the previous main pulmonary artery root (the "neo-aorta"). The main pulmonary artery is brought forward and anastomosed to the previous aortic root, while the aorta is relocated posterior to the branch pulmonary arteries and anastomosed to the neo-aorta. As a result, the right pulmonary artery runs anterior to the ascending aorta in its new position.

• Rastelli procedure (Fig. 11.6): Used in the minority of patients (<10 %), who have pulmonary outflow tract stenosis and a ventricular septal defect, blood flow is directed from the left ventricle through the ventricular septal defect to the aorta. The normal flow of blood on the right side is reestablished by oversewing the pulmonary outflow tract and placing a conduit between the RV and the pulmonary artery.

11.3 Associated Anomalies

In contrast to other conotruncal abnormalities such as tetralogy of Fallot, chromosome 22q11.2 deletions are not seen in patients with complete TGA. Males are affected twice as often as females in both complete and congenitally corrected TGA [2, 12, 15]. There are no associated syndromes with TGA, nor is there a familial form [2, 12]. In both forms of TGA, there are few extracardiac anomalies reported, but associated cardiac anomalies are common (Table 11.1) [12, 25].

Fig. 11.4 Complete TGA with atrial baffle procedure (Mustard or Senning). This schematic illustrates the flow of blood in patients with complete TGA who have undergone repair with atrial baffle procedures. The interatrial septum is removed creating a single combined atrium. The systemic baffle (the shunt for blood returning from the systemic venous circulation) is shaped like a "pair of pants" with one "leg," or limb, connected to the superior vena cava and the other to the inferior vena cava. The "waist" of the pants is sutured to the mitral valve annulus. Blood returning from the pulmonary circulation enters the systemic right ventricle by flowing through the areas of the combined atria that are excluded by the systemic baffle

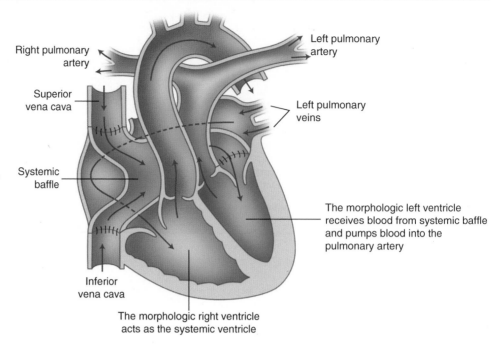

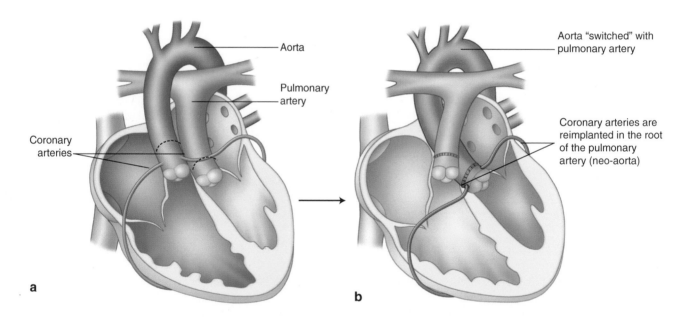

Fig. 11.5 Complete transposition of the great arteries with arterial switch procedure (Jatene operation). The arterial switch procedure is currently the favored approach for surgical correction of complete TGA. The coronary arteries and a cuff of aortic tissue surrounding the ostia are detached from the aorta and reimplanted in the root of the pulmonary artery. The aorta and pulmonary artery are transected and the pulmonary artery and the right main pulmonary artery are brought anterior to the aorta (see panel **a**). Note the new position of the right pulmonary artery in panel **b** is different than the normal anatomic position beneath the aortic arch. The pulmonary artery is anastomosed to the remaining rim of aortic tissue superior to the aortic valve. The aorta is anastomosed to the root of the pulmonary artery with the reimplanted coronary arteries, now termed the neo-aortic root. Residual shunts are repaired. The normal relationship of the pulmonary and systemic circulations is restored with the left ventricle in the systemic position. Blood returning from the lungs passes into the left atrium, through the mitral valve into the left ventricle, and out into the systemic circulation through the pulmonic valve and neo-aorta, which is now anastomosed to the aorta (panel **b**)

Fig. 11.6 Complete transposition of the great arteries (*TGA*) with Rastelli procedure. The Rastelli procedure is used as a primary surgical correction in the minority of patients with complete TGA who have a ventricular septal defect (*VSD*), and often stenosis in the pulmonary outflow. It involves patching and sometimes enlarging the VSD in such a manner as to create a left ventricular outflow through the VSD to reach the aorta. After resecting obstructions, the right ventricle is connected to the main pulmonary artery with a valved conduit. The morphologic left ventricle is now in the systemic position (correcting the ventriculoarterial discordance)

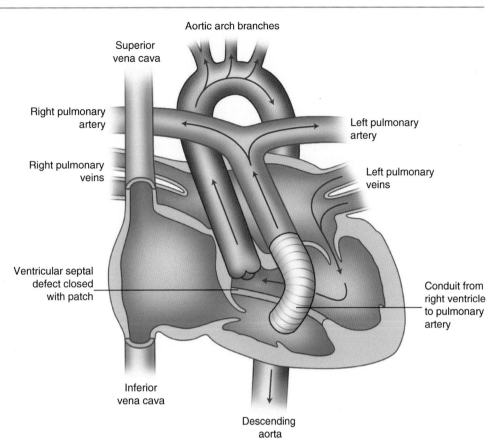

Table 11.1 Conditions associated with transposition syndromes

Complete TGA	Congenitally corrected TGA
Ventricular septal defect (VSD): 45–50 %	Ventricular septal defect (VSD): 70–80 % Typically perimembranous
Subpulmonic outflow tract obstruction: 25 %	Pulmonic/subpulmonic stenosis: 30–70 %
Patent ductus arteriosus.	Patent ductus arteriosus: 10 %
Anomalies of coronary artery origin and course: ~30 %.	Atrioventricular (AV) node and His bundles: abnormal position and course common. Presentation with heart block common. Those without heart block progress to AV block at ~2 %/year.
Coarctation of the aorta: ~5 %	Coarctation of the aorta: ~5 %
	Abnormalities of the systemic atrioventricular valve: 80–90 %, usually an apically displaced valve, but without other features of a typical Ebstein's anomaly.

11.4 Clinical Presentation

11.4.1 Complete TGA

Clinical presentation and age of presentation is usually determined by the presence or absence of a ventricular septal defect (VSD). In the absence of a VSD, newborns will present with cyanosis, either within the first day or as the ductus arteriosus closes during the first week [25]. In the remainder, the presenting signs and symptoms depend upon the degree of mixing between systemic and pulmonary blood pools. With VSD present, children may present between 4 and 8 weeks old with poor feeding, tachypnea and tachycardia, with cyanosis less prominent [19]. The presence of VSD with subpulmonic stenosis can mimic tetralogy of Fallot. In other cases, it may be difficult to distinguish complete TGA from double outlet right ventricle [12].

The majority of children with complete TGA will have undergone corrective surgery, since unrepaired there is a 90 % mortality in the first year of life. Dyspnea, fatigue and arrhythmias are common presenting complaints for late complications following corrective surgery. Arrhythmias may be poorly tolerated in patients with marginal hemodynamics. Exercise capacity is usually decreased due to a combination of factors, one of which is often sinus node dysfunction. Additionally, specific complications arise in association with the various corrective surgeries.

Long term survival after atrial baffle procedures (Mustard and Senning operations) in experienced centers is up to 77 % at 25 years [17]. In addition to systemic (morphologic RV) ventricular dysfunction and tricuspid valve regurgitation, subpulmonic obstruction or pulmonic stenosis may arise when enlargement of the systemic ventricle distorts these left-sided structures. Other important long-term sequelae include baffle leak or stenosis and pulmonary hypertension. Baffle stenosis, typically of the upper limb of the two-legged systemic baffle, presents with facial fullness, upper extremity edema, or subtle mental status changes mimicking a superior vena cava syndrome when severe. Stenosis of the lower limb of the systemic baffle may present as edema, ascites or hepatic dysfunction. When pulmonary return is compromised, pulmonary hypertension may develop. Hemodynamically significant baffle stenosis is relatively common and likely under recognized, although often managed without intervention [3].

First performed in 1976, the arterial switch procedure is the preferred surgical management in uncomplicated complete TGA infants. Survival following this procedure is around 90 % at 10 years, and quality of life scores are better for children who have undergone arterial switch procedures than those who have had atrial baffle procedures [25, 26]. The most common late complication following arterial switch operations is main pulmonary artery or branch pulmonary artery stenosis, sometimes as a result of neo-aortic root dilatation. Other complications include coronary insufficiency, coronary ostial narrowing, and coronary kinking leading to myocardial ischemia. Ventricular dysfunction, semilunar valve regurgitation and arrhythmias are also relatively common.

Survival following the Rastelli procedure is approximately 60 % at 20 years [6]. Late complications include left or right sided outflow tract or conduit obstruction, residual VSD, hypertrophy or chamber enlargement, aortic regurgitation and aortic root dilatation.

11.4.2 Congenitally Corrected TGA

Despite the fact that most (80–90 %) patients with congenitally corrected TGA have associated anomalies [2], in the majority of patients congenitally corrected TGA remains unrecognized until adulthood. Two-thirds of patients with associated abnormalities and one-quarter without will develop heart failure by age 45 [25]. Compromise of the systolic function of the systemic RV probably develops due to a combination of myocardial supply demand mismatch and regurgitation of the systemic atrioventricular valve. Other presenting features depend upon the associated abnormalities. Patients with subpulmonic/pulmonic stenosis and a VSD may present with variable degrees of cyanosis. Presentation with AV block or atrial tachyarrhythmia is common.

11.5   CMR Imaging

11.5.1   Indications and Goals of Imaging

Lifelong follow-up is needed as residual lesions and sequelae are common. The basic indications for CMR in patients with congenital heart disease are when the echocardiographic assessment is suboptimal or ambiguous. In infants presenting with complete TGA, echocardiography typically provides sufficient information and adjunctive CMR imaging is rarely required. However, surgeries for complete TGA are never curative. Thus, the primary indication for CMR is in long term follow-up after corrective surgery and in monitoring systemic right ventricular function, where routine surveillance is often indicated [21, 26]. CMR will often be obtained for further information when clinicians are contemplating surgical or catheter-based interventions and it is useful for imagers to be familiar with indications for reoperation procedures [26].

For patients with unrecognized congenitally corrected TGA presenting prior to diagnosis, CMR may be initially requested for further evaluation of ventricular dysfunction or dextrocardia. It is important for the imager to be familiar with the findings in transposition in order to make the diagnosis. Goals in this setting include establishing viscero-atrial situs, segmental cardiac anatomy, course of great vessels and quantifying ventricular function. Once the diagnosis of TGA has been established, the presence of associated anomalies, such as subpulmonic stenosis or stenosis of pulmonary valve, should be explored.

For the post-surgical patient, knowledge of the type of prior surgical procedures performed is critical to the imaging assessment. In patients with congenitally corrected TGA or complete TGA with atrial baffle operations, periodic assessment of the systemic right ventricular systolic function and the severity of systemic atrioventricular valve regurgitation are indicated. Systemic atrioventricular valve dysfunction in transposition represents an entity comparable to mitral valve regurgitation in patients without transposition syndromes. It is essential that tricuspid repair or replacement be performed before the ejection fraction of the systemic RV falls below 45 %. Competence of the surgically created baffles (after Mustard/Senning operations) and conduits (after Rastelli operations) should be assessed during follow-up. Shunts, whether from baffle leak or residual VSD, are another indication for intervention when the Qp:Qs is greater than 1.5:1, when they result in progressive dysfunction or chamber dilatation or when they cause symptoms. For patients with prior arterial switch operations, the presence of main pulmonary artery or branch pulmonary artery obstruction, as well as the size of the neo-aortic root, should be assessed during follow-up. Regurgitation of the semilunar valves should also be evaluated. Additionally, all adult patients should have the patency of the coronary arteries evaluated at least once [26], which may be accomplished by CMR in some cases or cardiac computed tomography.

Approximately 1 % of patients with prior atrial switch procedures will undergo heart transplantation [17]. As part of the evaluation prior to cardiac transplantation, CMR imaging goals include describing the atrio-visceral situs and venous return abnormalities, which complicate transplantation surgery. A large fraction of patients with transposition syndromes will require pacemaker implantation [17, 25]. In patients referred prior to pacemaker placement, the indication may be to assess the feasibility of a transvenous approach. Additionally, evaluation for small baffle leaks or residual VSD is indicated in this setting, as the presence of these increases the risks of paradoxical embolism during instrumentation.

Physiologic assessments such as stress tests are sometimes indicated for evaluation of symptoms like exercise intolerance or for evaluation for ischemia following arterial switch procedures. In patients with poor exercise tolerance, a dobutamine or exercise stress protocol can evaluate whether systolic function can be augmented. Because of the long term risks for coronary artery insufficiency following arterial switch procedures and because presentation can be clinically silent, intermittent surveillance for ischemia by CMR stress or other modalities has been suggested [22].

11.5.2 CMR Sequences and Imaging Protocols

As with clinical presentation and CMR indications, details of specific sequences will depend upon what form of TGA is present, which prior surgical procedures have been performed, if any, and the clinical setting. An example of CMR imaging protocol used in our institution is shown in Table 11.2.

11.5.2.1 Static Scout Images
Images obtained in the three anatomical reference planes allow for localization of structures, and are the images upon which further slice prescriptions are based. Coronal and sagittal SSFP scout images can be acquired in a single breath hold. Localizer imaging in the axial plane is often more extensive. A series of non-breath held axial images with close spacing of slices covering the entire thorax (slice thickness of 4.5–7 mm obtained every 4.5–10 mm, for example) provides sufficient detail to identify the relationship of the great vessels and to determine abdominal visceral situs. As an alternative to SSFP sequences, some centers prefer to use dark blood techniques for axial localizer images.

11.5.2.2 SSFP Cine Images
Cine sequences using SSFP-based sequences will typically be obtained in more than one imaging plane to sufficiently delineate the complex anatomy of TGA syndromes. Cine images are ECG-gated and should ideally be breath held, except in the assessment of ventricular interdependence.

Complete TGA Following Atrial Baffle Operation
Contiguous, axial or parallel 4 chamber cine stacks from the aortic arch to the lower heart border provides information on ventricular function, systemic atrioventricular valve competence and venous and arterial anatomy (Figs. 11.7 and 11.8, Movies 11.1 and 11.2). From these images or from the axial localizers, oblique coronal SSFP cines may be obtained to evaluate baffle function. These should be oriented parallel to the SVC and IVC plane. A contiguous stack of straight coronal and/or sagittal cines is an alternative initial approach [8, 14]. In the majority of cases, oblique sagittal or oblique coronal views optimally visualize the full extent of the systemic venous baffle, with double oblique views less frequently required, whereas axial or oblique coronal views are best for the pulmonary venous pathway [10]. A short axis stack should be obtained for quantification of the systolic function and chamber dimensions of the systemic RV. Short axis slices are usually obtained with 7 mm slice thickness and 3 mm inter-slice gap such that ~10 diastolic short axis slices can be obtained through the ventricle from base to apex. LV outflow tract cines should be obtained for evaluation of subpulmonic stenosis. Additional cine views include the 2 chamber/vertical long axis and right ventricular outflow tract cines for further qualitative assessment of ventricular and valvular function.

Complete TGA Following Rastelli Operation
As the pertinent post-surgical anatomy following the Rastelli operation is around the outflow tracts and pulmonary arteries, pulmonary artery cines to evaluate for stenosis in axial plane usually replace the oblique coronal cines. Each of the branch pulmonary arteries should have cine images prescribed parallel to blood flow and orthogonal to the axial scouts or cines. Pulmonary artery bifurcation is usually seen on axial cine. Cine of the prosthetic valve within the RVOT conduit should be obtained orthogonal to the RVOT views. More than one RVOT view (parallel RVOT views) may be needed to evaluate the RV to main pulmonary artery conduit (Movie 11.3). Similarly, parallel

Table 11.2 CMR protocol for imaging transposition of great arteries

Sequences Common to all transposition syndromes:

1. Localizer scout images

   (a) 3-Plane static steady state free precession (SSFP) images

   (b) 2 & 4 chamber scout SSFP images

   (c) Static axial localizer stack from lung apex through upper abdomen

2. Electrocardiogram (ECG) gated, expiratory breath-held SSFP cine images

   (a) 2 and 4 chamber views

   (b) Short axis stack from base to apex

      (i) 7 mm slice thickness with 3 mm interslice gap. Use the same spacing for late gadolinium enhancement.

   (c) Outflow views: Oblique sagittal and oblique coronal views of the systemic and subpulmonic outflow tracts ("right ventricular outflow tract" and "left ventricular outflow tract" or "3 chamber" views).

   (d) Contiguous axial (or parallel 4 chamber) SSFP cine stack from aortic arch to diaphragm

3. Isotropic whole heart diaphragm-navigated 3 dimensional SSFP imaging

4. Contrast magnetic resonance angiography (MRA)

   Bolus-timed MRA is typically used to study great vessels. High temporal resolution MRA images can track the bolus to evaluate abnormal connections (septal defects, baffle patency).

5. Phase contrast velocity encoded cines. In-plane images in 4 chamber, LVOT and RVOT orientations to assess valvular function.

6. Late gadolinium enhancement (LGE)

   (a) TI Scout: Use a mid-ventricular slice to acquire the correct TI time to null normal myocardium.

   (b) Inversion recovery LGE imaging in short axis and long axis planes (similar to cine images)

Additional sequences specific to clinical setting:

In complete TGA:

Following atrial baffle procedures:

1. SSFP cine images

   (a) Contiguous oblique coronal views parallel to the SVC and IVC to evaluate systemic baffle function.

   (b) Contiguous oblique sagittal views through the pulmonary baffle.

2. Phase contrast velocity-encoded cines

   (a) In-plane images in regions of suspected narrowing or flow acceleration on SSFP images, initial VENC of 100 cm/s is appropriate for baffle evaluation

   (b) Through-plane images to transect regions of suspected flow acceleration, increasing VENC by 50 cm/s until aliasing disappears.

   (c) If shunt or baffle leak suspected: Through-plane systemic and pulmonary flow assessments for shunt fraction quantification. Systemic flow obtained with through-plane images above the sinotubular junction. Pulmonary flow obtained with through-plane images transecting the main pulmonary artery.

Following Rastelli operation:

1. SSFP cine images

   (a) Contiguous oblique coronal and sagittal images parallel to the outflow tracts (parallel left and right outflow tract views).

   (b) Cine of the prosthetic valve within the RVOT conduit is obtained orthogonal to the RVOT views.

2. Phase contrast velocity-encoded cines

   (a) If residual VSD or other shunt is suspected, free breathing systemic and pulmonary flow images are obtained for shunt fraction quantification as described above.

   (b) If flow acceleration is suspected in the right ventricular outflow tract or pulmonary arteries from in-plane LVOT & RVOT images, then through-plane images are acquired oriented to transect confirmed flow accelerations. Initial VENC of 200 cm/s is appropriate for arterial flows, increasing by 50 cm/s until aliasing disappears.

Following arterial switch procedure:

1. Phase contrast velocity-encoded cines

   (a) In-plane images of the aortic root, main pulmonary artery and branch pulmonary arteries.

   (b) Through-plane images to transect regions of flow acceleration on in-plane images.

2. Isotropic diaphragm-navigated 3 dimensional SSFP coronary MRA to evaluate proximal vessels.

3. Pharmacologic stress testing with myocardial perfusion imaging, if ischemia suspected.

   Stress and resting first-pass perfusion imaging obtained in representative basal, mid and apical short axis slices.

In unoperated congenitally corrected TGA:

1. SSFP cine images

   (a) Contiguous coronal SSFP cine stack from anterior chest wall through descending aorta to delineate the relationship of the great vessels.

(continued)

Table 11.2 (continued)

2. Phase contrast velocity-encoded cines
    (a) In-plane images in regions of suspected VSD or stenosis on SSFP images.
    (b) If VSD is present, through-plane systemic and pulmonary flow assessments for shunt fraction quantification as described above.
3. If VSD suspected, GRE cine images with saturation bands can be helpful to localize VSD and characterize direction of jet. Care must be taken to orient saturation band to cover just one side of the heart.

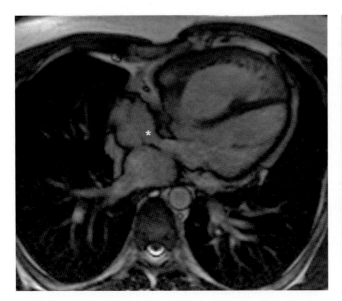

Fig. 11.7 Complete transposition of the great arteries following atrial baffle procedure. Still frame of an axial SSFP cine showing the systemic baffle to the left ventricle. The *asterisk* is located in the confluence of the superior and inferior limbs, which attach to the superior and inferior vena cavae, respectively (anastomoses not shown). The waist of the systemic baffle attaches to the mitral valve annulus

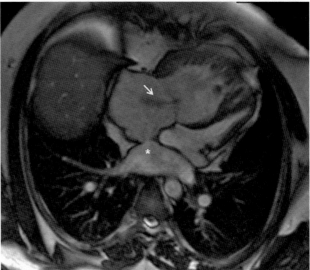

Fig. 11.8 Complete transposition of the great arteries following atrial baffle procedure. Still frame of a four chamber SSFP cine loop through the pulmonary baffle. Pulmonary veins can be seen draining into the posterior portion of the atrium, then through the pulmonary baffle (*asterisk*) to enter into the systemic right ventricle. The tricuspid valve is typically dysmorphic and is prone to regurgitation (*arrow*)

views may be needed to evaluate the LVOT as it tunnels through the repaired VSD (Movie 11.4). Contiguous parallel 4 chamber or axial cine stacks can assess qualitative evaluation of ventricular function and evaluate for residual VSD. The long axis views and short axis stack are obtained as above.

Complete TGA Following Arterial Switch Operation

Cine views should be obtained in several imaging planes, focusing primarily on the outflow tracts, neo-aortic root and pulmonary arteries. Contiguous axial cine stacks from the lower heart border or mid ventricle to the aortic arch, parallel 3 chamber (LVOT) cines and parallel RVOT cines allow for dynamic assessment surrounding the sites of surgical anastomoses. A cine view of the bifurcation of the main pulmonary artery should be obtained. Aortic valve cine should be obtained parallel to the aortic cusps to evaluate morphology. Assessment of ventricular function is obtained from short axis cine stack and 2 and 4 chamber views. A contiguous parallel coronal cine stack from the posterior aspect of

the sternum through the descending aorta is also recommended by some [16].

Congenitally Corrected TGA

The typical individual long axis cines (2, 3 and 4 chamber) and short axis cine stack should be obtained for qualitative and quantitative left ventricular function. Cines in a coronal orientation can demonstrate the parallel arrangement of the great vessels and provide additional information on semilunar valve function. A contiguous stack of cines oriented perpendicular to the line of coaptation of this valve can assess valvular morphology. Additional contiguous axial or parallel 4 chamber cine stacks allow for assessing regurgitation and for the presence of an associated ventricular septal defect. Coverage should extend through the outflow tracts, as most VSDs in congenitally corrected TGA are perimembranous. Right sided outflow tract and pulmonary artery cines are also indicated given the frequency with which pulmonic stenosis and subpulmonic obstructions are associated.

11.5.2.3 Phase Contrast (Velocity-Encoding) Imaging

Estimating Stenosis Severity

Volumetric coverage with SSFP cine images in more than one imaging plane allows for identification of regions of flow acceleration and anatomic narrowing and guide the acquisition of phase contrast imaging. This is particularly useful in exploring baffle stenosis, although other areas of flow acceleration may include the subpulmonic outflow tract, main pulmonary artery, branch pulmonary arteries, or along the ventricular septum at the site of a residual or unrecognized VSD. In-plane velocity encoded images, with the frequency encoding direction parallel to the jet or blood flow, can help to further localize the jet envelopes if not well seen on SSFP images.

Through plane phase contrast images should be obtained in a plane perpendicular to the jet or blood flow near the orifice. An initial VENC level of 100 cm/s is appropriate for evaluating baffles, increased in increments of 50 cm/s if aliasing exists. The estimated peak gradient across the defect, obtained using the modified Bernoulli's equation, will not exceed $4 \times (VENC)^2$ where the VENC is the level at which aliasing disappears. Flow curves in combination with peak velocity can provide additional useful information for estimating stenosis severity (Table 11.3).

For interrogating arterial or outflow tract stenosis, in-plane followed by through-plane phase contrast imaging with an initial VENC level of 200 cm/s is appropriate. Further characterization of gradients follows principles outlined above; perpendicularly transect the jet near the orifice and increase the VENC level on subsequent acquisitions if needed until aliasing disappears. In-plane and through-plane phase contrast imaging can be attempted for the valved conduit to assess for stenosis in patients with prior Rastelli operations; however susceptibility artifacts may compromise interpretation when stented bioprosthetic valves are used.

Flow Quantification

The ratio of pulmonary to systemic blood flow (Qp:Qs) is an important indicator of the need for surgical intervention in patients with TGA as in other conditions. An abnormal Qp:Qs may elucidate a need for further imaging for a VSD or baffle leak. A Qp:Qs of 1.5:1 or greater is an indication for repair of a baffle leak [2, 21, 24, 26]. Slice prescriptions for assessing pulmonary flows can be based off of RVOT or pulmonary artery images, and should be a cross section of the main pulmonary artery between the pulmonic valve and the bifurcation. Aortic flow measurement is obtained as a cross section of the aorta above the sinotubular junction, and can be prescribed from coronal views. Flow quantification measurements are usually non-breath held, ECG gated acquisitions with an initial velocity encoding (VENC) value in the through plane between 150 and 200 cm/s. Quantitative flows through the great vessels also provide estimates of regurgitant

Table 11.3 Estimating severity of baffle stenosis by characteristics of velocity-encoding images when anatomic narrowing is also present [14]

Estimated severity	Flow curve	Peak velocity (m/s)
Mild	Pulsatile, peaking in early diastole	<1
Moderate	Pulsatile	1–1.5
Severe	Damped curve, continuous flow	>1.5

These criteria must be interpreted in the clinical context

volumes across the semilunar valves. Subtracting stroke volume assessed by phase contrast from the stroke volume obtained by volumetric assessment of ventricular size provides another means of calculating atrioventricular valve regurgitant volumes and fractions.

11.5.2.4 Contrast Angiography (MRA)

Contrast enhanced MRA can provide a qualitative, 3 dimensional overview of complex anatomy. Contrast enhanced MRA acquisitions are usually bolus-timed to study specific anatomy. This technique is useful in the evaluation of main or branch pulmonary artery stenosis following arterial switch procedures, or in the setting of congenitally corrected TGA. Dynamic angiography, or 3-dimensional time resolved contrast enhanced MRA, is a 3 dimensional fast gradient echo sequence obtained once precontrast then repeated successively about every 5 s (high temporal resolution) during contrast administration. Since successive images are acquired as the contrast bolus moves through the circulation, it is potentially useful to detect shunt and baffle stenosis. However, mild stenosis may be missed by dynamic angiography and thus it is probably best used as an adjunct to other imaging sequences [14].

11.5.2.5 Noncontrast Angiography

Three dimensional non-contrast MRA is a bright blood SSFP-based sequence that is diaphragm-navigated and ECG-gated. The standard acquisition window covers the entire heart and mediastinum. It requires no breath holding or gadolinium contrast, but acquisition times are lengthy. There is potential utility in the assessment of all transposition syndromes. Since it is ECG-gated, it is more useful for measurements of the aortic root than non ECG-gated contrast enhanced MRA and should be considered for follow-up evaluations of patients after arterial switch procedures. It can be helpful in the assessment of pulmonary artery stenosis. While it can also be useful for assessing baffles, care must be taken to position the diaphragm navigator such that the saturation effect of the navigator band does not interfere with signal in the pulmonary venous pathways.

By including fat saturation, noncontrast diaphragm-navigated 3 dimensional acquisitions can also be modified for coronary angiography to assess for anomalies of coronary origins, and potentially rule out proximal stenoses or kinking in patients following arterial switch procedures [23].

11.5.2.6 Late Gadolinium Enhancement (LGE)

LGE has been evaluated in limited numbers of patients with transposition syndromes, and the significance of the finding in this population is debated [1, 11, 23]. Nonetheless, in patients who are receiving gadolinium-based contrast for other imaging sequences such as contrast MRA, LGE images should be obtained in the short and long axis orientations used for SSFP cine images. In patients with prior arterial switch procedures in whom coronary ostial narrowing and coronary kinking is a potential late complication, LGE may have some theoretic utility. In one small series, LGE was seen in 2 out of 16 pediatric patients who had prior arterial switch procedures. However, both of these patients had previously known or suspected peri-surgical myocardial infarctions, so it is unclear how LGE findings affected patient management [23]. The prognostic utility of LGE in patients with transposition syndromes awaits further study.

11.5.2.7 Stress Myocardial Perfusion Imaging

First pass myocardial perfusion imaging has established efficacy in patients being evaluated for atherosclerotic coronary artery disease. Typical protocols use vasodilator medications (regadenoson, adenosine, dipyridamole) for stress imaging. SSFP, echo planar and FLASH imaging sequences have been used. Stress and rest cine acquisitions are obtained in three representative short axis slices (base, mid and apex); gadolinium contrast is infused during both acquisitions. CMR stress protocols may be reasonable alternatives to nuclear stress testing in order to avoid repetitive radiation exposures over long term follow up, however at present they remain largely untested in this population [18].

11.5.3 CMR Findings

Abnormalities of atrio-visceral situs and ventricular orientation should be assessed in all patients with transposition syndromes (Figs. 11.9 and 11.10). Regurgitation of atrioventricular valves is common, more so when the morphologic RV is the systemic ventricle

11.5.3.1 Congenitally Corrected TGA, Unoperated

The trabecular pattern and position of the atrioventricular valve are features which help to distinguish the morphologic right from left ventricle. The morphologic RV has increased trabeculations. A moderator band may be visible. The tricuspid valve has a septal attachment that is apically displaced relative to the mitral valve, and the ventricles usually associate with their respective atrioventricular valve [25]. Fibrous continuity exists between the mitral valve and the semilunar valve in the morphologic left ventricle but not RV. Atrioventricular

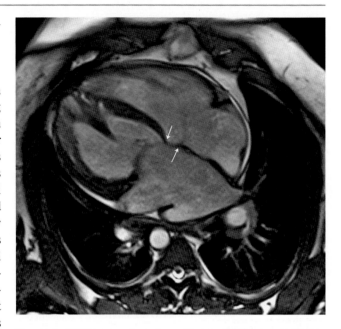

Fig. 11.9 SSFP image of a patient with congenitally corrected transposition of the great arteries and dextrocardia. The systemic right ventricle is posterior, with an eccentric jet of regurgitation through the systemic atrioventricular (tricuspid) valve directed posteriorly. Right ventricle is identified by its coarse trabecular pattern and its association with the morphologic tricuspid valve, demonstrated by the apical position of its septal attachment relative to the mitral valve (*arrows*)

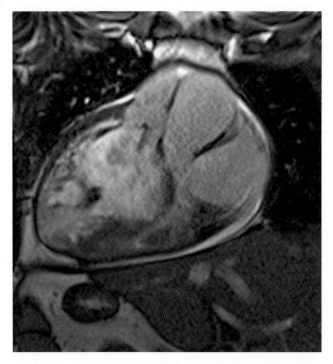

Fig. 11.10 Coronal view of a patient with congenitally corrected transposition of the great arteries (*TGA*), dextrocardia and situs inversus. The outflow tracts are seen in a side-by-side configuration, which is typical in congenitally corrected TGA. Regurgitation is seen in the systemic semilunar (aortic) valve. The liver is seen on the left

and semilunar valve regurgitation can be seen in many cases. By quantifying stroke volumes for both ventricles, the regurgitant

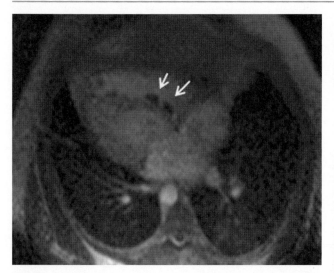

Fig. 11.11 Still frame of first pass perfusion imaging in a parallel four chamber orientation in patient with congenitally corrected TGA and situs inversus. Contrast enhancement of the nonsystemic ventricle outlines several non-enhancing masses consistent with thrombi along the base of the interventricular septum (*arrows*)

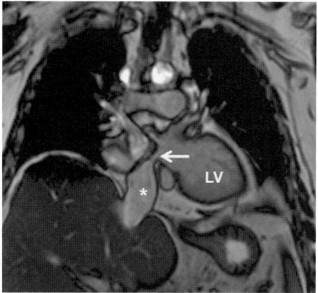

Fig. 11.12 Still frame of a coronal SSFP cine in a patient with complete transposition of the great arteries following an atrial baffle procedure. Anatomic narrowing of the inferior limb of the systemic baffle is seen (*arrow*) with concomitant dilation of the inferior vena cava (*asterisk*). *LV* left ventricle

fraction of a single regurgitant valve can be calculated by subtracting the ventricular stroke volumes from one another, divided by the stroke volume of the regurgitant ventricle. The typical orientation of the outflow tracts in congenital TGA is side-by-side (Movie 11.5). When ventricular function is abnormal, perfusion imaging can demonstrate coexisting pathologies (Fig. 11.11, Movie 11.6). Other associated abnormalities include malformations of the systemic atrioventricular valve, ventricular septal defect, left ventricular outflow tract obstruction and pulmonic stenosis (Movie 11.7). Abnormalities of coronary origin and course can also be seen.

11.5.3.2 Complete TGA, Unrepaired

Patients with complete TGA present early in infancy and the role for CMR in these patients is limited. Echocardiography is the main modality for evaluating these patients. The majority of newly diagnosed patients will undergo arterial switch procedures, however many adult patients will have undergone atrial switch operations.

11.5.3.3 Complete TGA Following Atrial Baffle Operations

Baffle leaks, fenestrations or stenosis can be identified by flow artifact on SSFP images or by anatomic narrowing on 3 dimensional imaging, and confirmed with velocity encoded images [3, 10]. While there is no standard definition of baffle stenosis, an internal dimension of <10 mm in either major or minor axis has been used by some to define anatomic narrowing [3] (Fig. 11.12). If present this finding should prompt

further investigation to determine hemodynamic significance, such as azygous vein dilation >5 mm or flow reversal in the azygous system on axial images (Fig. 11.13). The typical arrangement of the aorta is anterior and to the right of the pulmonary artery in patients with complete TGA (D-TGA).

11.5.3.4 Complete TGA Following Rastelli Operation

The course of the left ventricular outflow tract as it passes from the posterior morphologic left ventricle to the anteriorly displaced aortic valve can be traced (Fig. 11.14a). The left ventricular outflow tract may be stenotic. Residual VSD can be seen along the VSD patch/conduit. The RVOT conduit (Fig. 11.14b) can be incompetent, stenotic or aneurysmal. The native pulmonic valve may be present, or a valved conduit may have been used.

11.5.3.5 Complete TGA Following Arterial Switch Operation

During the arterial switch operation, the pulmonary artery is moved anterior to the aorta. In this position, the pulmonary arteries can be especially susceptible to obstruction, especially when there is enlargement of the neo-aortic root. The morphologic pulmonic valve remains attached to the left ventricle and therefore is vulnerable to regurgitation. Occasionally, stenosis of the coronary arteries or coronary kinking may be suspected by MRA.

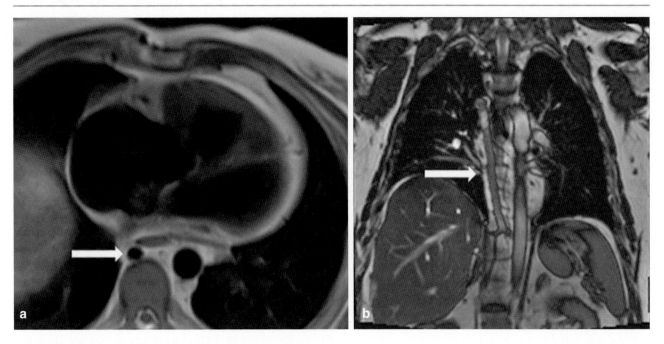

Fig. 11.13 Baffle stenosis in a patient with complete transposition of the great arteries. Axial black blood image (**a**) and coronal SSFP image (**b**) demonstrate a dilated azygous vein (*arrows*), suggesting baffle stenosis

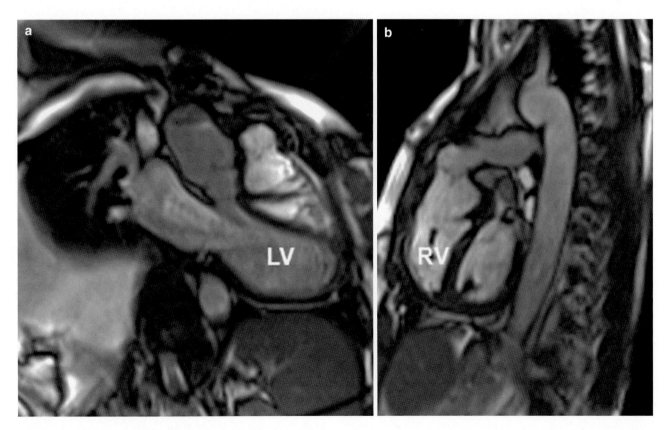

Fig. 11.14 SSFP images in a patient with complete transposition of the great arteries following a Rastelli operation. (**a**) The left ventricular outflow tract courses through a patched ventricular septal defect (*LV* indicates left ventricle). (**b**) The right ventricular outflow tract is formed by a conduit from the right ventricle (*RV*) to the main pulmonary artery

11.6 Discussion

While CMR has been considered adjunctive to echocardiography in the evaluation of transposition syndromes according to society guidelines [16, 21, 26], a more central role of CMR in the management of congenital heart disease is rapidly evolving. This is illustrated by the change in the European Society of Cardiology (ESC) guidelines for management of grown up congenital heart patients from 2003 to 2010. The 2003 ESC guidelines indicate that CMR is "rarely required if transesophageal echocardiography is available" in the evaluation of complete transposition following atrial baffle procedure [7]. In 2010, the ECS became the first major society to issue separate guidelines specific to the use of CMR in adults with congenital heart disease. In these guidelines, CMR should be employed in scenarios when it "usually informs management more effectively" such as in the evaluation of systemic and pulmonary veins, quantification of RV volumes and ejection fraction, shunt quantification, conduit function, and evaluation of the great vessels [16].

Echocardiography has several advantages relative to CMR, chiefly that it is portable, readily available and inexpensive. While availability is sometimes cited as an advantage of echocardiography relative to CMR, all patients with transposition syndromes should be followed at specialized centers, where CMR should also be available [26]. Periodic echocardiographic surveillance of systemic right ventricular function is a Class I indication by current ACC/AHA guidelines, generally every 1–2 years [4, 26]. At least one institution has implemented a combined approach to longitudinal monitoring of patients after atrial baffle procedures, using TTE routinely but with CT or MRI every 4–5 years adjunctively [3]. When initial transthoracic echocardiographic windows are suboptimal, echo contrast with either microbubbles or agitated saline can be employed, or the patient can be referred for further imaging with either transesophageal echocardiography (TEE), CMR or CT. There are no published data comparing efficacy or accuracy of TEE to CMR or CT to CMR in the management of transposition syndromes. The decision as to which modality to use when questions remain after TTE depends upon clinical setting and the discretion of the clinician.

CMR has been the gold standard in assessing ejection fraction in patients with systemic right ventricles in several studies. Accurate measurement of ventricular function is especially critical in patients with systemic right ventricles, as deterioration in function is a major source of morbidity and mortality. Echocardiography-derived measures of myocardial function, including myocardial performance index [20] and global longitudinal strain rate [5], correlate with right ventricular ejection fraction as assessed by CMR in patients with systemic right ventricles. However, it is not clear that this offers more prognostic information than ejection fraction alone. TTE-derived parameters have shown mixed efficacy to directly predict surrogates of clinical condition. While tricuspid annular peak systolic excursion and a *qualitative* assessment of global systemic right ventricular systolic function by TTE correlate with NYHA class, maximal exercise capacity and NT-proBNP levels, parameters such as peak systolic velocity, tissue Doppler derived strain and diastolic parameters did not [27].

There are important limitations to echocardiography. CMR is regarded to be superior to TTE and TEE in the assessment of great arteries and veins [26] and in the quantification of ventricular masses and volumes [2]. Inadequate sonographic windows has often been cited as a major limitation of TTE, but it is difficult to determine how often this is the case. One prospective study of echocardiography in adult patients with systemic RVs excluded 8 % of their initial sample because of inadequate transthoracic windows [27]. A retrospective study of 12 patients with prior atrial baffle procedures demonstrated limitations to viewing systemic baffles by TTE in most patients studied: there was inadequate visualization of the common baffle in 4 patients (33 %), of the SVC limb in 7 patients (58 %) and of the IVC limb in 8 patients (67 %) [9]. Finally, TTE with Doppler has been shown to be inferior to a combination of other modalities (75 % CMR, 15 % CT, 10 % invasive) in detecting superior limb baffle stenosis but the reasons for this discrepancy were not stated [3]. TEE were not performed in any of these studies, however.

Noninvasive CT coronary angiography may have an expanding role in imaging patients with complete TGA treated by arterial switch operations. Many of the patients treated with arterial switch operations are now adults, in whom assessment of coronary artery patency is warranted [26]. MRA of coronary arteries can be challenging and is generally best suited for evaluation of proximal vessels and anomalies of coronary origins. Given its high negative predictive value, noninvasive CT coronary angiography is an attractive alternative to invasive catheterization in patients who are otherwise low atherosclerotic risk and asymptomatic. Like CMR, it has the advantage of unhindered anatomic assessment of the great vessels and venous anatomy. Assessment of baffle leaks and baffle stenosis are also possible by CT angiography [3, 6]. However, CT may not be suitable for lifelong surveillance of congenital heart disease patients due to radiation effects.

11.6.1 Areas of Emerging Data

Patients with systemic RVs who are asymptomatic by self report often have dramatically decreased peak oxygen consumption and exercise tolerance, so clinical condition can be difficult to judge by history alone. Several studies have used dobutamine stress CMR protocols to unmask subclinical defects in patients with systemic RVs. The prognostic utility of such studies has not yet been described, however. Additionally, abnormal resting blood flow distribution in the main and branch pulmonary arteries as measured by CMR has been found to be correlated with poor cardiopulmonary response to exercise. The two exams have complementary information that may help to decide functional significance of stenoses in pulmonary arteries [13].

11.7 Limitations and Common Pitfalls

The frequency of contraindications to CMR is difficult to determine in patients with transposition syndromes. Long term follow-up of patients with prior atrial switch procedures indicate that around a third of patients will require permanent pacemaker implantation, most as adults [17]. In congenitally corrected patients, ~2 % per year will develop atrioventricular node dysfunction [25]; presumably a large fraction of those patients will require pacemaker implantation. One study of systemic right ventricular function excluded 34 % of enrolled patients from CMR analysis for unstated reasons. Furthermore, atrial dysrhythmias are common and may complicate ECG gating and image quality.

Evaluation for baffle leaks requires care and an understanding of phase contrast techniques, but reliance on one CMR method of assessing baffle function is not recommended. Atrial baffles generally have fairly low pressure gradients and care must be taken in selecting the VENC settings. Unrestricted baffle leaks may be missed if they generate too little turbulence and therefore dephasing to be identified on SSFP cine images. Reversal of azygous vein flow was only present in 53 % of patients with hemodynamically significant SVC baffle stenosis in one cohort [3]. Mild baffle stenosis is less well characterized by contrast MRA compared to the reference standard phase contrast mapping [14]. Similarly, while navigated 3D SSFP noncontrast MRA may be useful for assessing baffles, the saturation effect of the navigator band can potentially decrease signal in the pulmonary venous pathways. None of these techniques have been extensively evaluated against invasive methods.

Finally, for quantification of volumes and mass in the systemic right ventricular, extensive trabeculations may complicate delineation of muscle from cavity, and therefore potentially decrease reproducibility and accuracy.

Conclusion

Transposition of the great arteries (TGA) refers to ventriculoarterial discordance and encompasses two distinct entities, complete TGA and congenitally corrected TGA. Whereas the former is usually associated with cyanosis and therefore nearly always identified and surgically corrected in infancy, the latter may not be diagnosed until adulthood. Associated cardiac anomalies are common, but syndromic associations are absent. Three surgical procedures are commonly performed to correct complete TGA, and the method used informs the role of CMR in long-term follow-up. Periodic monitoring of systemic right ventricular function for patients with congenitally corrected TGA or complete TGA treated with atrial baffle procedures is required, with careful attention to the severity of regurgitation of the systemic atrioventricular valve. Stenosis or obstructions in the subpulmonic outflow tract through the branch pulmonary arteries can be seen in any form of TGA, but is especially common following arterial switch operations. CMR is especially useful following atrial baffle repairs and Rastelli procedures, where the complex, distorted anatomy can be especially challenging to evaluate by echocardiography. CMR exam should be performed under supervision of a physician familiar with imaging and interpretation of congenital heart disease in both pre-operative and post-operative settings.

11.8 Practical Pearls

- Consider the diagnosis of congenitally corrected TGA in the presence of dextrocardia with situs solitus.
- For the post-surgical patient, knowledge of the type of prior surgical procedures performed is critical to the imaging assessment.
- Multiple breath held sequences can be fatiguing, especially in patients who often have some degree of exercise intolerance or systolic function. The choice of which cine slice orientations to obtain first should be tailored to address the most pressing indication for a CMR study. For example, if systolic function is paramount, short axis cine stacks should be acquired early, whereas if a baffle stenosis is likely, coronal and axial stacks should be prioritized.
- Azygous vein enlargement (>5 mm) and flow reversal can be clues to the presence of baffle stenosis. Flow reversal indicates a superior baffle or vena cava obstruction [14]. These determinations usually do not require separate acquisitions as the azygous vein is frequently well seen on axial localizers and Qs phase contrast images.
- Aortic root measurements require ECG-gated imaging with either cine or 3D MRA protocols, for example following arterial switch operations.

References

1. Babu-Narayan SV, et al. Late gadolinium enhancement cardiovascular magnetic resonance of the systemic right ventricle in adults with previous atrial redirection surgery for transposition of the great arteries. Circulation. 2005;111(16):2091–8.
2. Baumgartner H, et al. ESC guidelines for the management of grown-up congenital heart disease (new version 2010): the task force on the management of grown-up congenital heart disease of the European Society of Cardiology (ESC). Eur Heart J. 2010; 31(23):2915–57.
3. Bottega NA, et al. Stenosis of the superior limb of the systemic venous baffle following a mustard procedure: an under-recognized problem. Int J Cardiol. 2010;154(1):32–7.
4. Cheitlin MD, et al. ACC/AHA guidelines for the clinical application of echocardiography. A report of the American College of Cardiology/American Heart Association Task Force on practice guidelines (Committee on Clinical Application of Echocardiography). Developed in collaboration with the American Society of Echocardiography. Circulation. 1997;95(6):1686–744.
5. Chow PC, et al. New two-dimensional global longitudinal strain and strain rate imaging for assessment of systemic right ventricular function. Heart. 2008;94(7):855–9.
6. Cook SC, et al. Usefulness of multislice computed tomography angiography to evaluate intravascular stents and transcatheter occlusion devices in patients with d-transposition of the great arteries after Mustard repair. Am J Cardiol. 2004;94(7):967–9.
7. Deanfield J, et al. Management of grown up congenital heart disease. Eur Heart J. 2003;24(11):1035–84.
8. Dorfman AL, Geva T. Magnetic resonance imaging evaluation of congenital heart disease: conotruncal anomalies. J Cardiovasc Magn Reson. 2006;8(4):645–59.
9. Fogel MA, Hubbard A, Weinberg PM. Mid-term follow-up of patients with transposition of the great arteries after atrial inversion operation using two- and three-dimensional magnetic resonance imaging. Pediatr Radiol. 2002;32(6):440–6.
10. Fogel MA, Hubbard A, Weinberg PM. A simplified approach for assessment of intracardiac baffles and extracardiac conduits in congenital heart surgery with two- and three-dimensional magnetic resonance imaging. Am Heart J. 2001;142(6):1028–36.
11. Fratz S, et al. Myocardial scars determined by delayed-enhancement magnetic resonance imaging and positron emission tomography are not common in right ventricles with systemic function in long-term follow up. Heart. 2006;92(11):1673–7.
12. Fulton DR, Flyer DC. D-transposition of the great arteries. In: Nadas' Pediatric Cardiology. 2nd ed. Philadelphia: Saunders; 2006.
13. Giardini A, et al. Effect of abnormal pulmonary flow distribution on ventilatory efficiency and exercise capacity after arterial switch operation for transposition of great arteries. Am J Cardiol. 2010; 106(7):1023–8.
14. Johansson B, et al. 3-Dimensional time-resolved contrast-enhanced magnetic resonance angiography for evaluation late after the Mustard operation for transposition. Cardiol Young. 2010;20(1):1–7.
15. Keane JF, Flyer D. Corrected' transposition of the great arteries. In: Nadas' pediatric cardiology. 2nd ed. Philadelphia: Saunders; 2006.
16. Kilner PJ, et al. Recommendations for cardiovascular magnetic resonance in adults with congenital heart disease from the respective working groups of the European Society of Cardiology. Eur Heart J. 2010;31(7):794–805.
17. Oechslin E, Jenni R. 40 Years after the first atrial switch procedure in patients with transposition of the great arteries: long-term results in Toronto and Zurich. Thorac Cardiovasc Surg. 2000;48(4): |233–7.
18. Prakash A, et al. Magnetic resonance imaging evaluation of myocardial perfusion and viability in congenital and acquired pediatric heart disease. Am J Cardiol. 2004;93(5):657–61.
19. Rao PS. Diagnosis and management of cyanotic congenital heart disease: part I. Indian J Pediatr. 2009;76(1):57–70.
20. Salehian O, et al. Assessment of systemic right ventricular function in patients with transposition of the great arteries using the myocardial performance index: comparison with cardiac magnetic resonance imaging. Circulation. 2004;110(20):3229–33.
21. Silversides CK, et al. Canadian Cardiovascular Society 2009 consensus conference on the management of adults with congenital heart disease: complex congenital cardiac lesions. Can J Cardiol. 2010;26(3):e98–117.
22. Skinner J, Hornung T, Rumball E. Transposition of the great arteries: from fetus to adult. Heart. 2008;94(9):1227–35.
23. Taylor AM, et al. MR coronary angiography and late-enhancement myocardial MR in children who underwent arterial switch surgery for transposition of great arteries. Radiology. 2005;234(2):542–7.
24. Therrien J, et al. Canadian Cardiovascular Society consensus conference 2001 update: recommendations for the management of adults with congenital heart disease part III. Can J Cardiol. 2001; 17(11):1135–58.
25. Warnes CA. Transposition of the great arteries. Circulation. 2006;114(24):2699–709.
26. Warnes CA, et al. ACC/AHA 2008 guidelines for the management of adults with congenital heart disease: a report of the American College of Cardiology/American Heart Association task force on practice guidelines (Writing Committee to develop guidelines on the management of adults with congenital heart disease). Developed in collaboration with the American Society of Echocardiography, Heart Rhythm Society, International Society for Adult Congenital Heart Disease, Society for Cardiovascular Angiography and Interventions, and Society of Thoracic Surgeons. J Am Coll Cardiol. 2008;52(23):e1–121.
27. Winter MM, et al. Echocardiographic determinants of the clinical condition in patients with a systemic right ventricle. Echocardiography. 2010;27(10):1247–55.

Sylvia S.M. Chen and Raad H. Mohiaddin

12.1 Introduction

Aortic congenital anomalies are common and comprised of a heterogenous group of conditions that may be due to either embryological or vessel wall architectural defects. Imaging is crucial for diagnosis, management, follow-up and reassessment after intervention of these conditions. Cardiovascular magnetic resonance (CMR) is a valuable non-invasive imaging method for providing detailed anatomical, functional and haemodynamic information on a wide spectrum of aortic anomalies and intra- and extracardiac associated abnormalities. The technique is radiation free and is ideally suited for diagnoses as well as serial follow-up pre and post interventions such as a dilated aortic root in Marfan syndrome and aortic coarctation. This chapter reviews the role of CMR in the management of a wide spectrum of congenital aortic anomalies and provides CMR scanning protocols and clinical reporting of the anomalies both in the native and post-repair states.

12.2 Aortic Anomalies

Aortic anomalies consist of a spectrum of conditions. The anomalies are usually due to either abnormality in embryological development or in the architecture of the vessel wall. Abnormal persistence or regression of the branchial arches during embryogenesis for example, may result in a double aortic arch and vascular ring [1]. Architectural defects due to

genetic mutations such as Marfan syndrome [2] or biochemical derangements as seen in the aortic matrix in the context of a bicuspid aortic valve [3] may result in aortic aneurysms that are susceptible to dissection or rupture. These aortic abnormalities may be associated with other cardiac defects that may also require treatment and follow up.

Diagnosis, instigation of treatment and subsequent follow up is therefore crucial. Definition of the anatomy is needed for diagnosis of the abnormality and its haemodynamic effects, its relationship to its surrounding structures and its associated cardiac anomalies. An important component of assessment is the impact on the heart, for example, what is the severity and therefore effect of a coarctation of the aorta (CoA) on the heart? Is there left ventricular hypertrophy and left ventricular impairment or is the dilated aortic root in Marfan syndrome causing aortic regurgitation? Detailed structural and functional information is vital not only for diagnosis, but to help guide management decisions, feasibility of a particular type of intervention, and in the post-repair phase, follow-up for residual defects, complications of repair, and recurrent disease.

12.2.1 CMR and Other Imaging Modalities for Aortic Anomaly Assessment

High quality and informative imaging is a valuable part of the process of diagnosis and management, and can be provided easily by cardiovascular magnetic resonance (CMR). Traditionally, chest X-ray (although rarely used for diagnosis alone), cardiac catheterisation and echocardiography were used to image the aorta. More recently, cardiac CT angiography (CTA) has become more available and is very useful for assessing the aorta.

CMR is perhaps the most ideal imaging technique as it is able to provide high quality and detailed examination of the

S.S.M. Chen, MBBS, M.D., FRACP (✉)
Cardiovascular Magnetic Resonance Unit, The Royal Brompton Hospital, Sydney Street, London, SW3 6NP, UK
e-mail: sylviasmchen@gmail.com

R.H. Mohiaddin, M.D., Ph.D., FRCR, PRCP, FESC
Cardiovascular Magnetic Resonance Unit, Royal Brompton Hospital and National Heart and Lung Institute, Imperial College London, Sydney Street, London, SW3 6NP, UK
e-mail: r.mohiaddin@imperial.ac.uk

Electronic supplementary material The online version of this chapter (doi:10.1007/978-1-4471-4267-6_12) contains supplementary material, which is available to authorized users.

anatomy and function of the entire aorta, its branches, relationship to the surrounding mediastinal structures and associated anomalies. It is non-invasive and does not use radiation or iodinated contrast agents, both of which, are ideal attributes for serial follow-up. Its ability to image in multiple planes is an advantage as it allows accurately aligned images to be obtained and therefore accurate depiction of the anomaly. The duration of study time is longer compared to other modalities, but may be shortened if the operator is experienced. The main contraindications for CMR are the presence of metallic devices, i.e. drug infusion pump, defibrillator, permanent pacemaker including biventricular pacing for cardiac resynchronisation therapy, or other metallic objects in particular regions of the body such as the eye. Several recent reports have described feasibility of safely performing CMR in selected patients with pacemakers and defibrillators. CMR compatible pacemaker models have recently become available, and therefore in the future, patients with these devices may be able to undergo routine CMR. Other potential difficulties may be overcome. Claustrophobia may be helped using partial sedation, or using alternative positioning for example entering the scanner feet first or using glasses that reflect out towards the control room. Careful counselling prior to scanning can be very valuable in alleviating anxiety. Similarly in our experience, children excluding the very young (<4 years old) may undergo CMR study without sedation or anaesthesia if they and their parents have been well prepared and counselled prior to study. Play therapists are extremely useful in the preparation including venous cannulation of these children. In the presence of impaired renal function or if venous cannulation was not possible, imaging that usually require contrast agent enhancement such as angiography, may be done using an alternative CMR sequence, 3D whole heart balanced steady-state precession with fat suppression (3D whole heart), done without the use of contrast agents.

In comparison, apart from echocardiography, other imaging modalities usually have the disadvantages of the need to use radiation, iodinated contrast agents, and/or are invasive. These modalities are:

- Chest X-ray: It is easily available and quick to perform. Widening of the mediastinum raises the suspicion of aortic dilatation, and evidence of a coarctation of the aorta (CoA) by the presence of rib notching or the '3 sign', the silhouette formed by a dilated left subclavian artery above and dilated distal descending aorta below the level of CoA [4] may be detected. However, specific diagnosis and detailed examination of all the various anomalies or serial follow up of an enlarging aneurysm cannot be achieved using X-ray alone.
- Cardiac catheterisation and aortography: Aortography allows examination of the structure and size of the thoracic aorta and its branches. Cardiac catheterisation's particular advantage over CMR and the other modalities is its ability to provide information of pressure gradients crucial

for example, in CoA. It also allows the opportunity to intervene at the same time if appropriate, for example, closing a patent ductus arteriosus (PDA) or stent implantation for CoA. However, although the coronary anatomy can be examined, other associated anomalies may not be easy to assess. Furthermore, it is invasive and may have complications of vascular injury, inducing ventricular arrhythmia, stroke or distal embolisation and should not be used alone for serial follow up.

- CTA: It is a quick study compared to CMR and therefore more suitable in acute settings such aortic dissection, and for children who may tolerate a short period of time in a CT scanner, but not the longer duration required to perform a CMR study. CTA is useful as an alternative to CMR for patients with pacemakers. As with CMR, CTA is able to provide detailed structural information of the aorta, its branches, its relationship to other structures in the mediastinum, other coexisting cardiac anomalies and the size and location of the defects (for example in CoA and PDA). Compared to CMR, the coronary anatomy, course and lumen are better visualised on CTA, as well as calcification, that is useful, for example in PDA, to know prior to surgery because calcification is associated with an increased risk of rupture during repair [5, 6]. An aortic stent can cause metallic artefacts on CMR and therefore detailed examination of the region is precluded. CTA is able to visualise the stented region better and assessment of the lumen within the stent easier. However, CTA is not the ideal modality for serial follow up for conditions such as aortic aneurysm because of the risk of complications from accumulative doses of radiation and iodinated contrast agents. Radiation may be reduced using prospective ECG-gated imaging which is good for structural assessment but not for functional analysis of the ventricles and valves, which may also be abnormal in aortic anomalies. Retrospective ECG-gating with higher doses of radiation, must be used instead. Temporal resolution is less than CMR, and therefore ventricular volume and function assessment is inferior in comparison [7]. Accurate shunt quantification is also not possible, and can only be estimated from volume analysis.
- Echocardiography: As with CMR, it is non-invasive, does not use radiation and highly informative on anatomy and function. It is more widely available, has a shorter duration of study time, bedside imaging is possible using portable machines, and should be used in most instances, as the first imaging modality of choice for diagnosis and follow up. Estimation of pulmonary vascular and right ventricular systolic pressure relevant in PDA assessment for example, can be done on echocardiography but not easily on CMR. However, compared to CMR, good quality imaging is dependent on an adequate echocardiographic window, patient's body habitus and presence of lung

Table 12.1 Suggested CMR protocol

Sequences	Parameters
Localizers: true fast imaging with steady-state precession	TR 337.1, TE 1.16, slice thickness 8 mm, matrix 2.4 × 1.6 mm
Half-Fourier acquisition single-shot turbo spin echo (HASTE) multislice imaging in a transverse orientation	TR 700, TE 42, slice thickness 6 mm, matrix 2.3 × 1.3 mm
Steady-state free precession (SSFP) multislice imaging in the transverse, coronal and sagittal oblique orientations	TR 292.2, TE 1.22, slice thickness 6 mm, matrix 2.0 × 1.3 mm
SSFP cine imaging	TR 40.2, TE 1.13, slice thickness 7 mm, matrix 1.7 × 1.7 mm, temporal resolution 25 frames
Phase contrast flow and velocity quantification: in-plane and through plane flow	In-plane: TR 61, TE 3.09, slice thickness 6 mm, matrix 2.5 × 1.3 mm, temporal resolution 20 frames
	Through plane: TR 60, TE 2.32, slice thickness 10 mm, matrix 2.5 × 1.3 mm, temporal resolution 20 frames
Turbo spin echo (TSE) imaging	TR 700, TE 29, slice thickness 6 mm, matrix 2.2 × 1.3 mm
Contrast enhanced magnetic resonance angiography (MRA)	TR 2.85, TE 1.19, slice thickness 1.3 mm, matrix 1.1 × 0.9 × 1.3 mm
3D whole heart balanced steady-state precession with fat suppression (3D whole heart)	TR 275.81, TE 1.63, slice thickness 1.5 mm, matrix 1.5 × 1.0 × 1.0 mm

disease such as asthma. The aorta is not easily visualised in its entirety and especially in an adult. Detailed examination of aneurysms or stenosis in the arch or proximal descending aorta and arch vessel anomalies cannot be done easily on echo, but excellent imaging of these regions can be achieved using CMR. Echocardiography is limited also in its ability to assess aortic dissection and rupture. Similarly, the pulmonary artery and its branches are best assessed by CMR. Transesophageal echocardiography can provide more detailed examination compared to transthoracic echocardiography, but is semi-invasive and require at least partial sedation.

12.2.2 Indications and Goals for CMR Imaging

CMR is indicated for diagnosis, planning management strategies, serial follow up for progression of disease or the development of complications, and reassessment after intervention. Imaging has to demonstrate the anatomy and functional significance of the anomaly, and be precise in the alignment of the imaging planes so that measurements of aortic dimensions including aneurysms and stenosis may be as accurate as possible and reproducible in subsequent repeated studies for follow up. Assessment for associated anomalies and cardiac function must also be performed.

12.2.3 CMR Assessment of the Aorta

A suggested protocol (to be altered accordingly to suit the particular condition under assessment) is tabulated on Table 12.1

12.2.3.1 Anatomical Imaging
- The aorta may be examined using any or all of the sequences in the suggested protocol. The entire aorta is imaged, from the left ventricular outflow tract to the descending aorta at

diaphragm level. A cross sectional plane through the aortic valve for valve morphology is also recommended. The 'hockeystick' or 'candycane' image of the aorta (Fig. 12.1a) gives an overview of the aorta but may not necessarily be completely aligned in all the segments of the aorta as the aorta is rarely in one plane. Therefore, separate specifically aligned images to the aortic segments (ascending aorta, arch and descending aorta) may be necessary for accurate assessment and measurement.

- Careful alignment of the imaging plane is crucial. The aorta is usually circular in the cross sectional plane, and the most accurate measurement of aortic diameters is at its widest point, that is, through the middle of the vessel. Several cross cuts of the area of interest may be required to obtain the most accurately aligned imaging plane. This is particularly important for repeated studies over years, for patients with conditions such as CoA and aortic aneurysms with regular follow up studies for disease progression. It is difficult to attribute differences in measurement as true changes in dimensions if the imaging planes are not exactly the same. This is particularly relevant and important to clinical management decisions with regard to reintervention or not as a result of the CMR study. It is recommended that previous studies should be available at the time of the present study and comparative images acquired.

- Aortic root: A diastolic cross sectional plane through the widest diameter of the aortic sinus is recommended for the measurement of aortic root dimension [8] (Fig. 12.2a). To account for through plane movement that may cause inaccuracies in measuring the diameters, it is recommended that two consecutive slices without an interslice gap are acquired.

- Dark blood sequences using half-Fourier acquisition single-shot turbo spin echo (HASTE) and T1 weighted turbo spin echo (TSE) sequences are useful for vessel wall inspection, for example in aortic dissection.

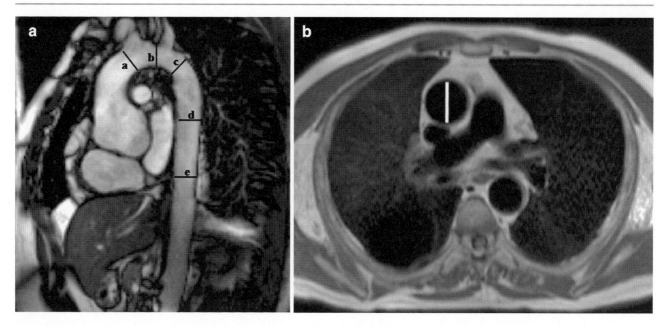

Fig. 12.1 (**a**) Sites of aortic measurement from the arch to the descending aorta: *a*=proximal arch just before the origin of the right brachiocephalic artery; *b*=mid aortic arch, between the origins of the left common carotid and subclavian arteries; *c*=distal arch; *d*=mid descending thoracic aorta, between *c* and *e*; *e*=descending aorta at the diaphragm. (**b**) Site of measurement of the ascending aorta, performed at the level of the right pulmonary artery in the transaxial orientation

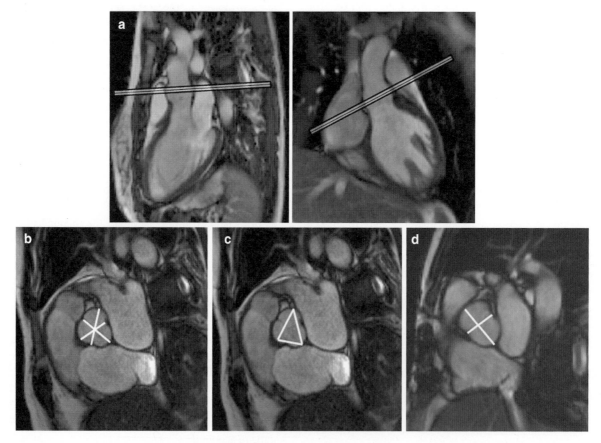

Fig. 12.2 (**a**) Two slice imaging without a gap transecting the aortic sinus at its widest dimension, in the sagittal and oblique coronal orientations to obtain the image in (**b–d**). (**b**) Diastolic cusp-commissure measurements of the aortic root in its cross sectional orientation. (**c**) Diastolic cusp-cusp measurements of the aortic root in its cross sectional orientation. (**d**) Diastolic cusp-cusp and cusp-commissure measurements of the aortic root of a bicuspid aortic valve in its cross sectional orientation

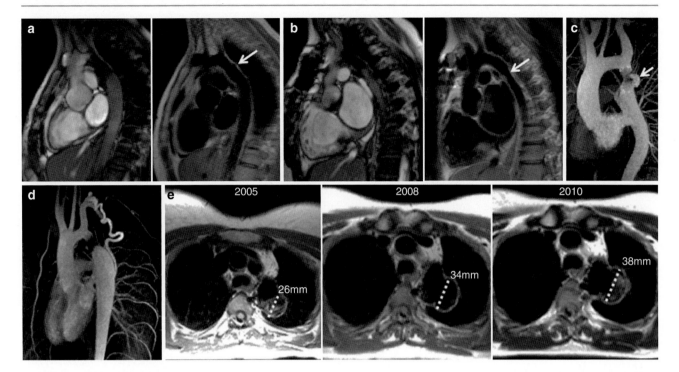

Fig. 12.3 Imaging after stent implantation in CoA. (**a**, **b**) SSFP images on the left and TSE images on the right. Metallic artefact precludes detailed examination on SSFP, but the aortic lumen is well visualised in TSE. A small aneurysm (*arrowed*) in the proximal stent is seen on TSE but not on SSFP in (**a**), and narrowing of the descending aorta distal to the stent (*arrowed*) is visualised on TSE but not easily on SSFP in (**b**). (**c**) An aneurysm seen in the stent (*arrowed*) on MRA. (**d**) Collateral on MRA supporting the suspicion of stenosis within the stent. (**e**) Serial CMR studies 2005–2010 to assess progression of an aneurysm at the site of a stent. TSE imaging in similar planes show increasing dimensions

- Metallic artefacts (due to stents for example) preclude detailed examination of the aorta on steady-state free precession (SSFP) cine and multislice imaging (Fig. 12.3). Dark blood and fast low angle shot imaging (FLASH) sequences can be used in this circumstance, although FLASH is also susceptible to metallic artefact. A stent cannot be seen on dark blood images, but the lumen of the vessel is visible, and therefore some assessment of the diameter of the lumen can be made. Complications such as an in-stent aneurysm which cannot be seen on cine imaging, but may be visualised on TSE or HASTE imaging (Fig. 12.3a, e).
- Contrast or non-contrast enhanced magnetic resonance angiography (MRA) is useful for its 3-dimensional assessment, particularly for planning of intervention

12.2.3.2 Function
- Judgement on the severity of the lesions such as stenosis or the relationship of the vessel to and its impact on its surrounding structures may be made using cine imaging, phase contrast flow and velocity mapping.
- Again, careful alignment of the imaging plane to the jet whether in the long axis or transacted planes, is crucial for accurate assessment.
- MRA is useful for the detection of collateral vessels for example, in the severe CoA.

12.2.4 Reporting a CMR Study

Important features to include are:
- Detailed description of the aortic abnormality: Anatomical detail and dimensions, location, severity of and impact of the anomaly on its surrounding structures (for example trachea compression from a vascular sling) should be reported.
- Aortic dimensions: Measurements may be made on images acquired using any of the sequences described previously. For consistency and repeatability, measurements should be made on the same type of sequence on subsequent follow up studies. Documentation of where the measurements were made and on which sequence especially in the presence of a stent should ideally be made in the report. Previous documentation is useful for repeated studies over years for accurate assessment of progression of stenosis or increasing aneurysm size. If previous record is not available, then it is recommended that measurements of the previous study at similar locations to the current study are performed by the same reporter (Fig. 12.3e). Maximum extra-luminal dimensions perpendicular to the aortic wall are recommended [8]. The intra-luminal diameter does not always reflect the external aortic diameter when there is intraluminal throm-

bus, wall inflammation or dissection. Both diameters, external and internal, are useful in these circumstances. Cine SSFP and dark blood spin echo images such as HASTE or TSE are recommended for these measurements. Figure 12.1a illustrates the recommended sites of measurement from the ascending aorta to the descending aorta at the diaphragm. The ascending aorta is best measured in its cross sectional plane at the level of the RPA (Fig. 12.1b). Measurement of the aortic root at the sinus level is recommended from the cross sectional image described above using the diastolic cusp-commissure diameters (Fig. 12.2b) as they correspond closer with respect to age and body surface area compared to other measurements using diastolic cusp-cusp or systolic cusp-commissure or the widest diameters measured from the left ventricular outflow tract images in the coronal and sagittal oblique orientations [9]. Diastolic cusp-cusp diameters may also be measured for an overall assessment of aortic root dimensions (Fig. 12.2c). In bicuspid aortic valve, the aortic sinus may be measured using the diastolic cusp-cusp and commissure-commissure diameters (Fig. 12.2d). Normal values for aortic root dimensions in males and females by CMR have been reported previously and can be used as a reference [9].

- Associated anomalies: Coexisting congenital defects such as ventricular septal defect or bicuspid aortic valve and/or consequences of the disease such as aortic valve regurgitation or left ventricular hypertrophy.
- Cardiac function: Dimensions, ejection fraction and hypertrophy of the right and left ventricles must be reported.

12.3 Coarctation of the Aorta

Coarctation of the aorta (CoA) is a narrowing in the aortic lumen (Movie 12.1). It is usually discrete, commonly located distal to the left subclavian artery and opposite the ligamentum arteriosum, but may also be found in the aortic arch, descending thoracic or abdominal aorta, or as complete interruption of the aorta [10]. More diffuse narrowing may be present, and usually in association with other congenital anomalies such as a bicuspid aortic valve, ventricular septal defect, Shone's syndrome (subvalvular, valvular and supravalvular aortic stenosis, and mitral valve abnormality) or complex congenital heart disease for example, transposition of the great arteries. CoA is present in about 7 % of congenital heart disease with a male preponderance of 1.5:1 [4]. The region of coarctation is related to posterior infolding of the aorta, seen as a ridge that protrudes into the lumen. It is likely that CoA represents a more diffuse arteriopathy, as cystic medial necrosis is present not only at the site of coarctation, but also in the aorta proximal and distal to coarctation [11].

These aortic wall abnormalities may account for aneurysmal dilatation in the descending aorta distal to the site of coarctation, and aneurysms found around the site of previous repair. Other associated abnormalities are aneurysms of the circle of Willis (in 10 %) and Turners syndrome.

The mode of presentation depends on the severity of the lesion. In the more severe cases, patients present soon after birth commonly with heart failure, or in the less severe, with hypertension, claudication in the lower limbs during exercise, or non-specific symptoms of headache or epistaxis. After CoA repair, patients with recurrent or residual stenosis may present with hypertension or lower limb claudication. Aneurysms that develop after intervention are usually silent, unless there is dissection or rupture of the aneurysm.

Management is usually surgical repair for young children. Percutaneous balloon angioplasty and stent implantation (Fig. 12.3) may be an option for adults or older children and have the advantages of a smaller procedure without the use of cardiopulmonary bypass. There are various options for surgical repair: resection and end to end anastomosis (Fig. 12.4a), subclavian flap repair (Fig. 12.4b, c), patch repair using artificial material such as Dacron (Fig. 12.4d, e), interposition graft repair (Fig. 12.4f) and bypass graft repair (Fig. 12.4g, h). The most common complications after repair are stenosis (residual or recurrent or at suture lines, Fig. 12.4a–b, d) or/and aneurysm formation (Fig. 12.4c, e, f, h). In subclavian flap repair, residual stenosis is probably due to inadequate resection of the periductal tissue, and may be seen on CMR as a indenting ridge at the site of previous repair (Fig. 12.4b) [10]. Aneurysms may form at the site of previous repair (Figs. 12.3a, c, e and 12.4c, e), or may occur at or/and around suture lines (Fig. 12.4f and 12.4h). Dacron patch repair for example, is predisposed to aneurysm formation [11] in the aortic wall around the patch (Fig. 12.4e). Discrete aneurysms may form as a result of percutaneous balloon angioplasty, or at the suture lines after interposition graft repair (Fig. 12.4f).

12.3.1 CMR of CoA

The protocol may be followed as described previously, but with additional attention to:

- Site of coarctation, native or post repair: Precise alignment through the region of coarctation is crucial and should be done in at least two planes perpendicular to each other, and aligned through the centre of the aortic lumen. Any aneurysm formation should be interrogated, taking cross sectional planes through the aneurysm at its widest points. Consider high temporal resolution imaging for small aneurysms.
- The aortic root and remaining thoracic aorta as described previously.

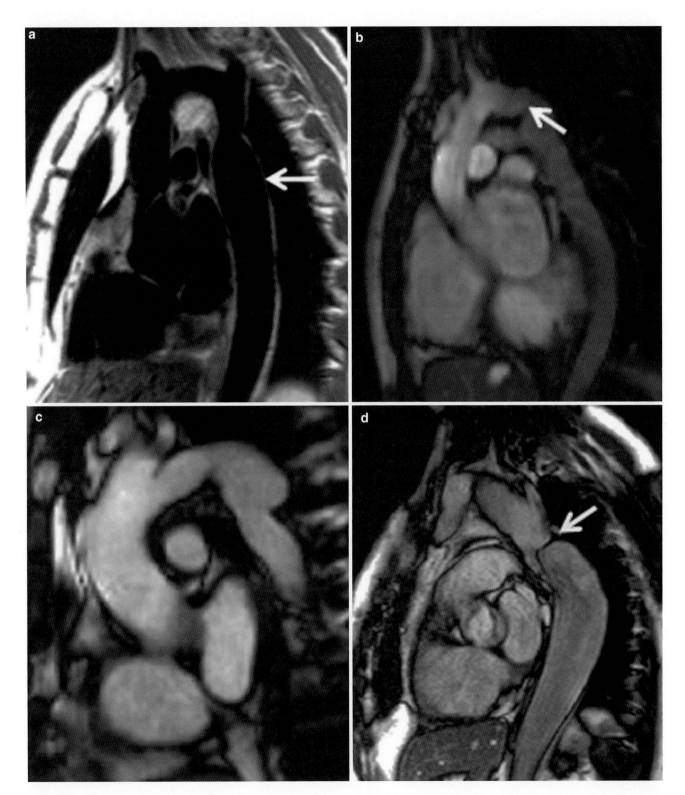

Fig. 12.4 (**a**) Resection and end to end repair with post stenotic dilatation (*arrowed*). (**b**, **c**) Subclavian flap repair showing a residual infolding ridge (**b**, *arrowed*), and aneurysm formation (**c**). (**d**, **e**) Patch repair with stenosis and jet formation, (**d**, *arrowed*) and aneurysm formation (**e**). (**f**) Interpositional graft repair with discrete aneurysms at the proximal and distal suture lines (*arrowed*). (**g**, **h**) Two bypass graft repairs. In (**g**), the bypass is connected to the ascending aorta and the descending aorta at the diaphragm. In (**h**), the bypass is located just distal to the origin of the left subclavian artery and connected to the mid descending thoracic aorta. There is a discrete aneurysm at the distal suture line (*arrowed*)

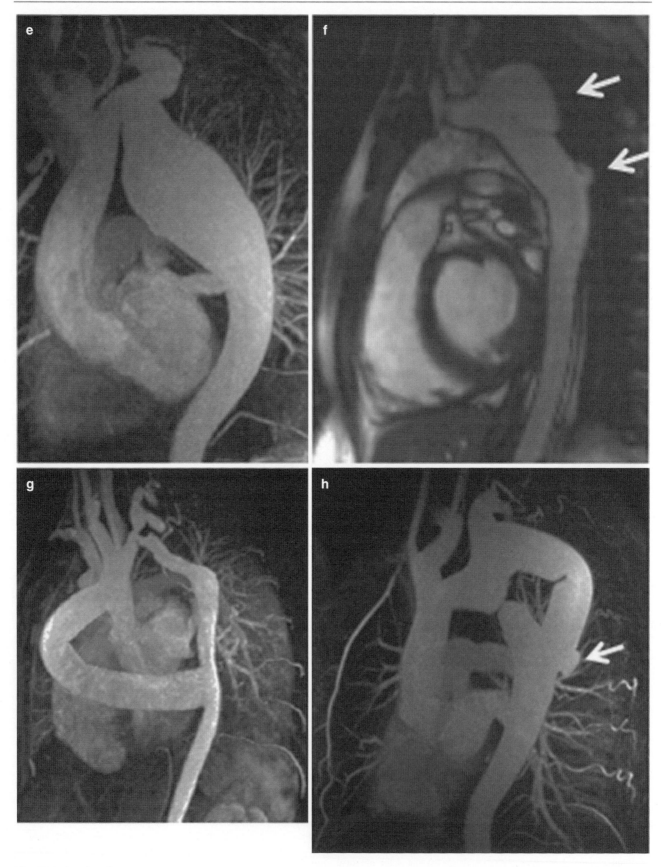

Fig. 12.4 (continued)

- Through-plane flow: most commonly, done at the level just distal to the site of coarctation at the point of highest velocity as seen on the in-plane flow. This allows peak velocity measurement, and also quantification of flow through the site of coarctation. Through-plane aortic flows at the level of coarctation and at the diaphragm can also be performed for comparative flow quantification at these sites [12].
- MRA: Important for detailed anatomical information on dimensions, anatomy and assessment for collaterals (which are not so easily assessed on cine imaging alone).
- Stent: Metallic artefact may be problematic in imaging. As described previously, dark blood and FLASH sequences may be used. Instent aneurysm or stenosis in or near the stent for instance, may be better visualised (Fig. 12.3a, b) on dark blood imaging. In addition, MRA may be useful for closer examination and measurement of an aneurysm at the site of the stent (Fig. 12.3c). MRA may also provide evidence of instent stenosis by demonstrating collateral flow (Fig. 12.3d). SSFP cine imaging is still useful, as in the case of aneurysms, it may demonstrate flow into the aneurysm (Movie 12.2).

12.3.2 Analysis of CoA

The following should be reported:
- Site of coarctation, native: Dimensions of the stenosis and its location. Intra-luminal dimensions are recommended. The anatomy is also crucial, for example, angulation or tortuosity of the site can have important implications on the type of intervention needed. The dimension of the stenosis, presence or absence of collaterals, and peak recorded velocity through the stenosis (normal <1.5 m/s) can and should be used to assess severity of the stenosis. A diastolic tail, or forward flow persisting into diastole is also indicative of severity, but is not always easy to see on through plane flow mapping done distal to the site of CoA. Flow curves may be helpful in demonstrating a diastolic tail on the flow curve. The presence of collaterals can also be demonstrated by higher aortic flow at the level of the diaphragm compared to flow at the coarctation [12]. Associated aneurysm formation or anomalous neck vessels such as an anomalous origin of the right subclavian artery from the proximal descending aorta close to the coarctation, must also be reported as they must also be considered in planning management strategies.
- The aortic root and the remaining aorta: Measurement of the diameters of the aortic root and ascending aorta must be made as one or both segments of the aorta may be dilated, particularly in the presence of a bicuspid aortic valve. It is not uncommon to find dilatation of the descending aorta distal to the site of CoA even after successful repair (Figs. 12.3d and 12.4a). This is commonly referred to as 'post-stenotic' dilatation.
- Left ventricle: Left ventricular hypertrophy indicates systemic hypertension, and is another sign of severity of stenosis. Hypertension may also occur in the absence of stenosis and is a recognised complication of CoA.
- Associated anomalies: bicuspid aortic valve, ventricular septal defect, left ventricular outflow obstruction from supra or/and subaortic valve stenosis, mitral valve abnormalities, other anomalies.

Assessment after repair: As described above, but with special attention to:
- Site of coarctation: Detailed assessment of the repair site for restenosis and aneurysm formation (anatomy, dimensions and severity). Serial CMR studies may be done to assess progression of an aneurysm, and it is therefore crucial that there is consistency in measurements. Stents may be difficult to assess because of metallic artefact. Dark blood sequences should be used to assess for intra-stent aneurysm. Stent waisting may not be seen. Stenosis proximal or distal to the stent may not be visualised adequately on SSFP cine imaging, but may be seen on dark blood imaging (Fig. 12.3b). MRA is useful to assess for any aneurysm formation as measurements and detailed assessment of its anatomy can be made. Evidence for stenosis may be indicated on MRA by the presence of collaterals (Fig. 12.3d).

12.4 Aortic Aneurysms

Aortic aneurysms secondary to congenital defects affect predominantly, the aortic root and ascending aorta. Marfan syndrome is the most common genetic cause of aortic aneurysm, and its estimated prevalence is between 1 in 5,000 and 1 in 10,000 [2]. Intrinsic wall architecture abnormality from mutations in the fibrillin 1 gene cause aneurysmal dilatation of the aorta, predominantly in the aortic root. A bicuspid aortic valve also predisposes to aortic aneurysms, previously reported to be about 60 % in the ascending aorta, and 40 % in the aortic root by echocardiography study [13] and appear to be due to multiple mechanisms. Cystic medial degeneration, fibrillin 1 gene defect that is also found in the main pulmonary artery of these patients, and 'post-stenotic' dilatation of the ascending aorta due to jet flow from a stenotic aortic valve and other causes have all been proposed [2, 3, 14].

Aneurysm of the sinus of Valsalva differs from aortic root dilatation as it is enlargement of one aortic sinus (Fig. 12.5a–d), between the aortic annulus and the sinotubular junction, and accounts for 0.14–0.23 % of Western surgical series, and 0.46–3.5 % of Asian surgical series [15]. It is due to a weakness in the aortic wall from congenital absence of elastic lamellae causing disruption of the aortic

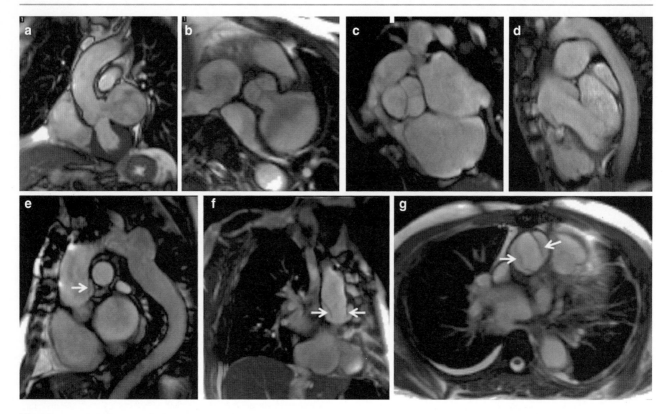

Fig. 12.5 (**a–d**) Left sinus of valsalva aneurysm without rupture in (**a**, **b**). Right sinus of valsalva aneurysm with compression into and rupture into the RVOT in (**c–d**). (**e–g**) Bicuspid aortic valve with patch aneu- rysm after CoA patch repair and dissection in the ascending aorta (**e**). (**f**) Is a slice from a coronal stack through the area of dissection, and (**g**) from a transaxial stack, the dissection flaps are arrowed in images e-g.

media in the sinus and the media adjacent to the aortic annulus [16]. The most common aortic sinus involved is the right sinus (65–85 %) and less commonly, the non-coronary sinus accounting for 10–30 % and the left sinus in less than 5 % of cases [17].

Arch and descending aortic aneurysms in the context of congenital heart disease are rarer, and mostly due to complications of previous repair. CoA is the main cause, and aneurysms (Figs. 12.3 and 12.4) can be found at the site of previous repair, or as a 'post-stenotic' dilatation in the descending aorta and is thought to be due to flow disturbance from the stenosis (native or recurrent). CoA is described in more detail earlier in this chapter.

12.4.1 Associated Cardiac Defects

1. Marfan syndrome: mitral regurgitation due to either mitral valve prolapse or annular dilatation.
2. Bicuspid aortic valve: aortic stenosis or/and regurgitation, CoA (Fig. 12.5e).
3. Aneurysm of the sinus of Valsalva: most commonly, a ventricular septal defect (30–60 %), aortic regurgitation (up to 30 %), bicuspid aortic valve, CoA, pulmonary stenosis and atrial septal defect [15]. Coronary artery anomalies may rarely coexist.

4. Coarctation of the aorta: bicuspid aortic valve in up to 85 % of patients and associated aortic stenosis or/and regurgitation, ventricular septal defect. CoA may occur as part of complex congenital heart disease, in which other defects such as transposition of the great arteries may be present.

12.4.2 Complications

The main complications of aortic aneurysms are aortic regurgitation due to annular dilatation from an aortic root aneurysm, and aortic dissection or rupture. Clinical presentation in the acute setting of dissection and rupture is usually with chest pain radiating to the back, or more dramatically, with haemodynamic compromise with or without heart failure. Dissection may also present more insidiously, with chronic back pain, or incidentally found on follow-up imaging. Aortic regurgitation presents either with a murmur found on clinical examination, or in the more severe cases, with heart failure. Other complications are more specific to the underlying condition. In aneurysm of the sinus of Valsalva, obstruction to the right ventricular outflow tract (RVOT) (Fig. 12.5c), coronary artery ostium or rarely the left ventricular outflow tract, may occur, and depends on the particular sinus involved. A right sinus aneurysm usually ruptures into the RVOT

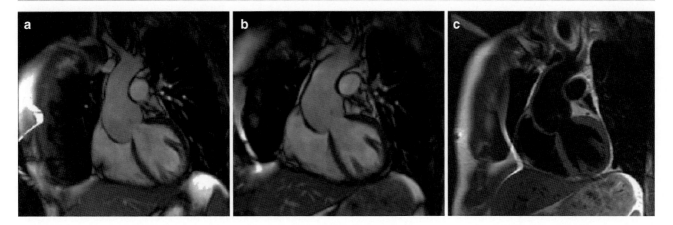

Fig. 12.6 (**a**) Marfan syndrome with dilated aortic root, unrepaired. (**b, c**) Same patient as (**a**), post EARS insertion. The device is seen as a thickened layer of aortic wall, seen in the SSFP image (**b**), and better seen on TSE imaging in (**c**)

(Fig. 12.5d) or more rarely the pulmonary artery, the noncoronary sinus into the right atrium and the left sinus into the left ventricular outflow tract. Coronary artery tear or dissection, and thrombus formation may also present following rupture of a sinus of Valsalva aneurysm.

12.4.3 Management

Surgical repair with or without aortic valve replacement (for concurrent aortic valve disease) is the treatment of choice for aortic aneurysms. For smaller aneurysms of the aortic root and ascending aorta that do not need surgical repair, medical therapy may be instituted [14]. A more recent innovation for Marfan syndrome is the bespoke external aortic root support (EARS), a support structure that is wrapped around the external surface of the aorta from the level of the annulus to just beyond the right brachiocephalic artery [18] (Fig. 12.6). The support structure is fashioned after a computer derived model adjusted specifically to the patient's aortic measurements made from preliminary CMR images acquired according to a dedicated protocol. Initial results have shown reduction in the aortic root dimensions at 1 year follow-up [18].

12.4.4 CMR of Aortic Aneurysms

Early detection and intervention of aortic aneurysms result in more successful management and better prognosis [8]. Baseline imaging should be performed at the time of diagnosis of the underlying condition, and then repeated imaging at a time frequency appropriate for the condition, for example, annual imaging for Marfan syndrome [8]. More frequent imaging should be done if the aneurysm is increasing in size. CMR is the modality of choice for patients with hemodynamically stable chronic aortic dissection who require regular follow-up imaging for surveillance. A patient with acute aortic dissection and unstable hemodynamic should not undergo

CMR as the study is longer in duration than that of cardiac CT or transesophageal echocardiography. Furthermore, monitoring of and quick access to the patient should there be any deterioration in haemodynamics is difficult within the confines of a CMR scanner. Although access to the patient in a CT scanner may also be similarly difficult, a CT scan is much quicker to perform in comparison to a CMR study.

In addition to that already described for imaging of the aorta, particular attention should also be given to:

- Dissection or rupture: A stack of transaxial slices from the aortic arch to the aortic root or in another orientation aligned with the area of interest is useful (Fig. 12.5f and g) to assess the extent of dissection.
- Localised aneurysm: This may occur after repair of CoA, for example as a discrete aneurysm (usually a pseudoaneurysm) at the suture line of an interpositional graft (Fig. 12.4). Images carefully aligned to the widest points of the aneurysm is useful for measurements. High spatial and temporal resolution SSFP may be helpful if the aneurysm is small.
- Aortic valve: For functional assessment particularly of aortic regurgitation in aortic root aneurysm.
- Flow mapping: May be helpful in rupture to visualise leakage better or to visually assess the amount of leakage.
- Dissection flap: May be assessed using either SSFP cine imaging, TSE or MRA.
- Thrombus in dissection: May be seen on SSFP, TSE, MRA or alternatively, in the early phase after contrast injection
- Imaging for complications such as RVOT obstruction from a right sinus of Valsalva aneurysm.

12.4.5 Analysis of Aortic Aneurysms

The following should be reported:

- Dimensions of the aorta: It is useful to record the location of the measurements as a reference for repeated studies in the future. Either the external or internal aortic dimensions can be used, but the key is consistency especially as most of these patients will have repeated studies for follow-up. If there is intramural thrombus, the internal and external diameters will be quite different. TSE imaging is useful in this instance for measurement of the internal diameter.

- Aneurysm: The shape of the aneurysm should be described (for example, asymmetrical, fusiform or saccular). Measurements will depend on its form. The widest and the longest (for aneurysms apart from aortic root aneurysm) dimensions are recommended. Discrete aneurysms should also be similarly measured and described.
- Dissection and rupture: The extent of the dissection including branch artery involvement, intramural haematoma, relative widths of the false and true lumen, and leakage from rupture should be described. The chamber or region that the aneurysm has ruptured into, if it is contained or not, persistent leakage from the aorta and the impact on the surrounding structures should also be reported.
- Aortic valve structure and function. Severity of stenosis and/or regurgitation should be reported.

Assessment after repair:

- The site of repair and the aorta: report on dimensions, presence of further or new dissection, intramural haematoma and any new aneurysm formation.
- Assessment of aortic valve replacement if that has also been done at the time of aortic aneurysm repair.

12.5   Truncus Arteriosus

Truncus arteriosus is a single arterial trunk arising from the heart that divides into the pulmonary, systemic and coronary artery circulations and results from failed septation of the aortopulmonary septum [1] and accounts for <1 % of all congenital heart anomalies. The truncal valve is tricuspid in 70 % of patients, bicuspid in 21 % and quadricuspid in 9 % (Fig. 12.7a). A subarterial ventricular septal defect is invariably present, and is usually large and non-restrictive. Other associated anomalies are right aortic arch (30 %), interrupted aortic arch (10 %) in association with a patent ductus arteriosus (PDA) (Fig. 12.7b), coronary artery abnormalities and the Di George syndrome.

Classification according to Collette and Edwards [19] is commonly used (Fig. 12.8). In type 1 (48–68 %), the main pulmonary artery arises from the common arterial trunk and

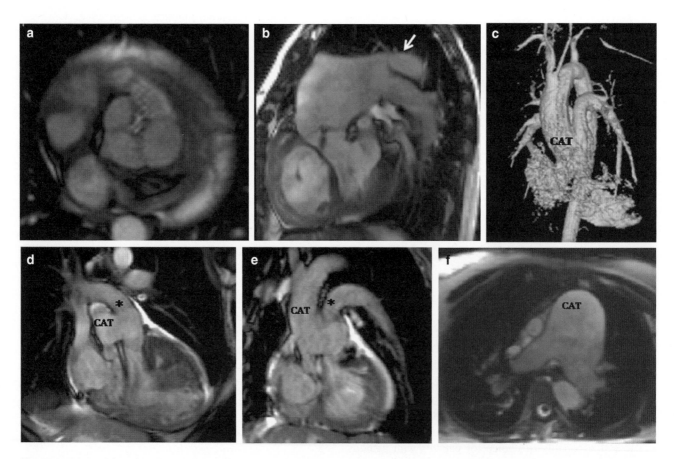

Fig. 12.7 (a) Quadricuspid truncal leaflet. (b) Truncus arteriosus type 2 with interrupted arch and PDA (*arrowed*). (c–e) Surface rendered 3D reconstruction after contrast enhanced MRA of truncus arteriosus type 1 in (c). There is a short main pulmonary arising from the common trunk (labelled *CAT*) and then dividing into the right pulmonary artery (labelled * in d) and left pulmonary artery (labelled * in e). (f) Truncus arteriosus type 2 with the pulmonary arteries arising separately from the posterior aspect of the common truncus (labelled *CAT*)

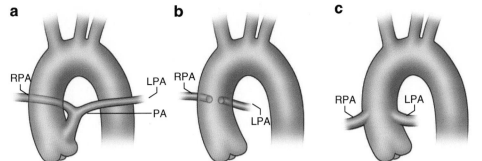
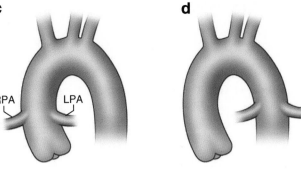

Fig. 12.8 Classification of Truncus Arteriosus. Type 1 (**a**) the main pulmonary artery arises from the common arterial trunk. Type 2 (**b**) separate but close origins of the left and right pulmonary arteries from the common arterial trunk. Type 3 (**c**) separate but distant origins of the left and right pulmonary arteries from the common arterial trunk. Type 4 (**d**) absence of the pulmonary arteries with aorto-pulmonary collaterals supplying blood flow to the lungs. *RPA* right pulmonary artery, *LPA* left pulmonary artery, *PA* pulmonary artery

branches into the right and left pulmonary arteries (Movie 12.3 and Fig. 12.7c–e); in type 2 (29–48 %), the main pulmonary artery is absent, and the right and left pulmonary arteries arises separately but close to each other on the posterior aspect of the common arterial trunk (Fig. 12.7f); in type 3 (6–10 %), the branch pulmonary arteries arise separately and further away from each other. There is complete absence of the pulmonary arteries in type 4. The lungs are perfused by aorto-pulmonary collaterals, and type 4 is no longer considered as part of the spectrum of truncus arteriosus, but instead, a variant of pulmonary atresia.

Patients present early in infancy with cyanosis or heart failure. Rarely, survival without repair may occur and is mainly due to the development of pulmonary hypertension. However, it is uncommon to survive beyond the third decade without intervention.

Surgical repair involves detachment of the pulmonary arteries from the arterial trunk, closure of the ventricular septal defect, connection of the pulmonary arteries to the right ventricle using a valved or valveless conduit, and repair of the truncal valve if regurgitatant.

12.5.1 CMR of Truncus Arteriosus

In addition to the previously described suggested protocol, imaging of:

- Common arterial trunk and pulmonary arteries, prior to repair: Two planes perpendicular to each other aligned to the left ventricular outflow tract for assessment of the outflow tract and truncal valve function. A cross-section through the truncal valve to define valve morphology should be done. Planes aligned to the pulmonary arteries for anatomical assessment of the pulmonary arteries and through flow mapping is useful if there is pulmonary stenosis to evaluate the severity of stenosis.

- MRA: May be helpful to further delineate pulmonary artery anatomy and if present, CoA.
- Ventricular septal defect.
- Associated aortic interruption and PDA with phase contrast flow mapping for shunt direction and quantification.
- After repair: Interrogation of the RVOT to assess pulmonary homograft valve function and homograft conduit stenosis. Careful assessment of the pulmonary arteries and flow mapping should be done if there is pulmonary arterial stenosis. The function of the truncal valve or the replaced valve, and the truncal root dimension should all be assessed.

12.5.2 Analysis of Truncus Arteriosus

The following should be reported:
- Definition of the type of truncus arteriosus
- Pulmonary artery: Morphology and function. If there is stenosis, report on its location and severity.
- Dimensions of the common arterial trunk.
- Truncal valve morphology and function.
- Ventricular septal defect: Report on the size, location, shunt direction and quantification.
  Assessment after repair:
- Pulmonary homograft valve and conduit: Report on the competency of the valve, and if there is any stenosis in the conduit.
- Pulmonary arteries: Location and severity of pulmonary arterial stenosis should be reported.
- Truncal valve: Assessment of the function of the native or replaced valve.
- Arterial trunk: Report on its dimensions.
- Residual ventricular septal defect and other anomalies such as CoA or a patent ductus arteriosus.

12.6   Aortopulmonary Window

An aortopulmonary window is a rare congenital anomaly and result from a defect in the aorticopulmonary septum [1]. The pulmonary artery and aorta have separate pulmonary and aortic valves. The defect is usually located midway between the level of the aortic and pulmonary valves and the pulmonary bifurcation (Fig. 12.9), and may be circular or helical in shape. This defect may occur in isolation, or in association with CoA, aortic interruption, tetralogy of Fallot and anomalous origin of one branch pulmonary artery, usually the right, from the ascending aorta [20].

Aortopulmonary window causes a left to right shunt. Large defects present early in childhood with heart failure. Late presentation with pulmonary hypertension and cardiac failure is rarer. Repair is usually with a direct suture or patch closure. There are reports of a limited number of small defects that have been closed using a percutaneous device.

12.6.1 CMR of Aortopulmonary Window

In addition to the protocol already described:
- Aortopulmonary window: A large defect should be easily seen on the initial multislice images and followed by appropriately aligned SSFP cine and phase contrast flow mapping for shunt direction and quantification. If the defect is small and not easily seen on the multislice images, then a stack of thin sliced (5 mm thick) SSFP cine images in a transverse orientation taken from the level of the pulmonary bifurcation down to the level of the aortic and pulmonary valve should be done. If the defect cannot be seen on those images, a stack in the sagittal oblique orientation, aligned parallel to the wall of the ascending aorta may be helpful.

12.6.2 Analysis of an Aortopulmonary Window

The following should be reported:
- Aortopulmonary window: The size and location of the defect including shunt size and direction and any associated anomalies should be reported.
- Evidence of pulmonary hypertension: Dilated branch pulmonary arteries with limited expansion, right ventricular hypertrophy, and septal flattening in systole.
- After repair: Report on any residual defect and shunt size.

12.7   Patent Ductus Arteriosus

A PDA is a vascular connection between the proximal descending aorta and the pulmonary artery, usually near the origin of the left pulmonary artery. It forms from the left 6th aortic arch [1], and in fetal life, functions as a conduit for the portion of blood flow that passes between the right ventricle and the descending aorta. The duct normally closes after birth, but may persist in preterm babies because of immaturity, or in term babies due to a combination of structural, genetic and environmental factors [21]. The incidence of PDA in term babies is about 5–10 % of all congenital heart disease. It may occur as an isolated finding, or as part of a group of other congenital anomalies. A PDA is usually on the left, but occasionally, a right sided PDA can occur particularly if the aortic arch is also right sided.

Presentation of a PDA depends on the size of the duct and the shunt. A duct may be silent and only discovered as an incidental finding for example, on transthoracic echocardiography performed for other reasons. A continuous murmur is heard on clinical examination. Infective endarteritis can complicate a small PDA and in those with more significant shunts, heart failure, arrhythmia and pulmonary hypertension (Fig. 12.10) may present later in life [20, 21]. In the most severe cases, there is differential cyanosis of the lower limbs.

Other intra-cardiac shunts such as an atrial or ventricular septal defect may coexist with a PDA. A PDA may also occur in the context of complex congenital heart disease such as pulmonary atresia or hypoplastic left heart syndrome.

Treatment for a PDA is either surgical ligation or clip, or percutaneous device closure using coils or an Amplatzer (or other similar) device.

12.7.1 CMR of PDA

The transaxial, coronal and sagittal SSFP multislice localizer stacks should be used to locate the PDA prior to SSFP cine imaging. It should be possible to see it on one or more of these stacks, but may be difficult if it is small in size. If it is not obvious on the initial stacks, look also for a hint of it on the coronal SSFP stack, as a bright spot in the main pulmonary artery as it passes below the aortic arch.

Once a PDA is visualised on the initial stacks, cine imaging should be performed first to delineate the structure of the PDA and its relation to its surrounding structures.
- PDA: Ideally, at least two images in different orientations should be acquired. An in-plane flow map to demonstrate the direction of the shunt is useful, however, a through plane flow map through the PDA is not essential. Shunt quantification is done by through plane ascending aortic to main pulmonary artery flow ratio.
- If a PDA cannot be easily seen on the initial transaxial, coronal and sagittal stacks, it is probably small and may be difficult to find on CMR. In this instance, a stack of SSFP cine imaging in the transaxial orientation from the aortic arch to the main pulmonary artery, done using thin slices of 5 mm without gaps, can be very useful to pick up

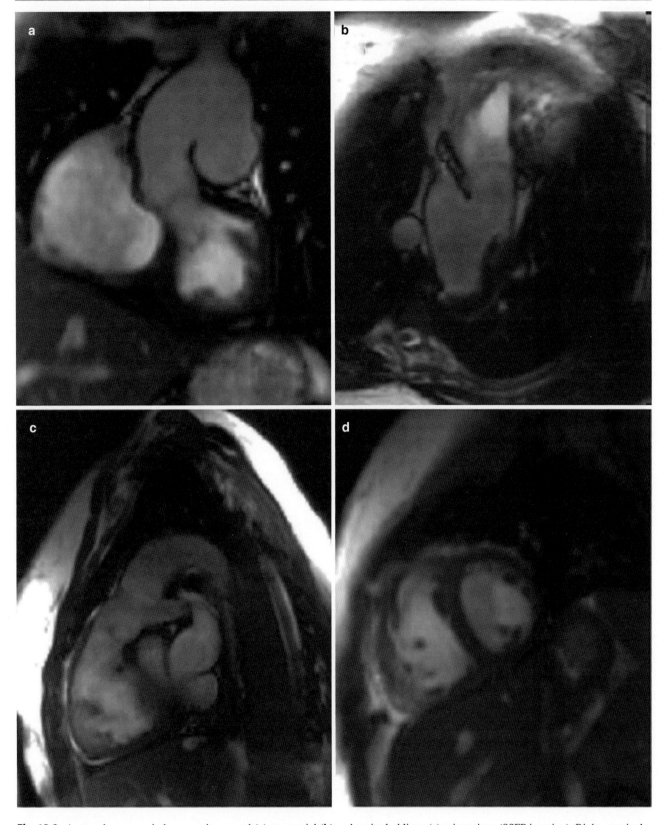

Fig. 12.9 Aortopulmonary window seen in coronal (**a**), transaxial (**b**) and sagittal oblique (**c**) orientations (SSFP imaging). Right ventricular hypertrophy on short-axis SSFP (**d**) imaging, suggestive of pulmonary hypertension

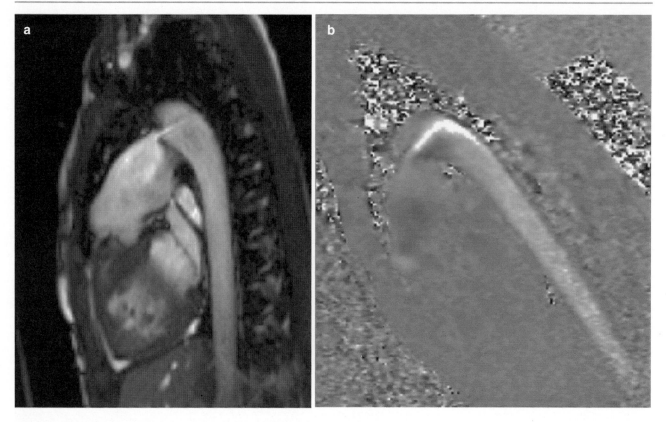

Fig. 12.10 Patent ductus arteriosus with Eisenmenger physiology. There is reversed flow into the descending aorta on SSFP (**a**) and flow mapping (**b**), and RV hypertrophy

a small PDA. If this stack fails to show a PDA, then a similar stack but in a sagittal oblique orientation, aligned perpendicular to the descending aorta and the left pulmonary artery as seen in the transaxial orientation can be used. If a PDA cannot be seen on these images, then ensure that the aortic and pulmonary artery through plane flows for shunt quantification is done to confirm the presence (in this case then, a small PDA) or absence of a PDA.

- Repaired PDA: Metallic artifact from the clip or device may preclude detailed examination of the site of repair. FLASH imaging may be used to try and overcome the problem with the artifacts. Shunt quantification should be done to assess for a residual defect.

12.7.2 Analysis of a PDA

The following should be reported:
- PDA: Size, structure and dimensions of the PDA. These are useful in clinical decisions on management and the type of intervention.
- Shunt direction and quantification.
- Evidence for pulmonary hypertension: dilated branch pulmonary arteries with limited expansion, right ventricular hypertrophy, and septal flattening in systole.

- Biventricular volumes and function: Overloading of the left ventricle may be present and indicates a more significant shunt.
  Assessment after repair:
- Assess for a residual PDA and improvement in ventricular function if there was pre-surgical impairment.

12.8 Vascular Rings and Sling

The aortic arch, its branches, and the pulmonary arteries are the result of the embryologic development or regression of the six paired aortic arches that are connected to the ventral and dorsal aortas. Of these arches, the 3rd, 4th and 6th pairs normally develop into the carotid arteries, the aortic arch, and the proximal right pulmonary artery, left pulmonary artery and ductus arteriosus respectively [1]. Abnormalities in the pattern of regression or persistence of these arches result in vascular rings and sling.

Vascular rings are rare with a prevalence of <1 % of all congenital heart defects. It forms a ring around the oesophagus and trachea and causes respiratory and feeding difficulties by compression. It may be complete or partial, depending on whether the oesophagus and trachea are fully surrounded by the ring or not [22].

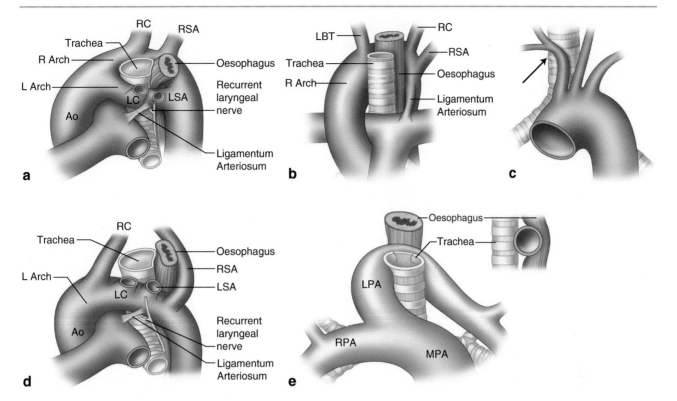

Fig. 12.11 Complete and partial vascular rings. (**a**) Double aortic arch. (**b**) Right aortic arch and a persistent ligamentum arteriosus. (**c**) Compression of the trachea by a more leftward origin of the right brachiocephalic artery (*arrowed*). (**d**) Anomalous origin of the right subclavian artery from the proximal descending aorta with a retroesophageal and tracheal course. (**e**) Left pulmonary artery arising from a right pulmonary artery. *RC* right carotid artery, *LC* left carotid artery, *RSA* right subclavian artery, *LSA* left subclavian artery, *LBT* left brachiocephalic trunk, *Ao* ascending aorta, *LPA* left pulmonary artery, *RPA* right pulmonary artery, *MPA* main pulmonary artery

Complete vascular ring (Fig. 12.11a, b): A double aortic arch (Movie 12.4) is the most common complete vascular ring (40 %) and results from persistence of the right aortic arch. Both arches with their respective arch branches fuse dorsally to form the descending aorta. The second most common complete ring is a right aortic arch with a persistent left ligamentum arteriosum. The ring is formed by the ascending aorta anteriorly, the arch on the right, an aberrant left subclavian artery that arises as the fourth arch vessel and passes posterior to the oesophagus and trachea, and on the left, is a persistent ligamentum arteriosus between the descending aorta and the left pulmonary artery.

Partial vascular rings (Fig. 12.11c–d) include an aberrant origin of the right brachiocephalic artery from a more leftward position on the arch and causes compression as it passes anteriorly towards the right, and anomalous origin of the right subclavian artery as the fourth neck vessel on a left sided aortic arch and passing posterior to the oesophagus (or anomalous left subclavian artery origin from a right sided aortic arch, Movie 12.5 and Fig. 12.12a).

A vascular sling is an anomalous left pulmonary artery origin from the right pulmonary artery, and causes compression as it passes between the trachea and the oesophagus during its course to the left lung (Fig. 12.12b).

Symptoms and clinical presentation depend on the severity of trachea and oesophageal compression, and are mainly replated to respiratory compromise. Dysphagia is less common. Associated anomalies are tetralogy of Fallot, transposition of the great arteries, CoA and ventricular septal defects.

Surgery is not commonly indicated. If needed, division can be done of the smaller of the arches in double aortic arch or the ligamentum arteriosum for a right aortic arch ring, and for a vascular sling, division and reimplantation of the left pulmonary artery.

12.8.1 CMR of a Vascular Ring or Sling

Diagnosis is possible using CMR, but most rings are diagnosed on clinical symptoms and by barium esophagography. CMR is extremely useful in examining the relationship between the vascular ring and the surrounding structures.

- SSFP cine imaging: unless the anomaly can be visualised in a single plane (and often it is not as vessels may be tortuous and traverse more than one plane), a stack of images is recommended (Fig. 12.12c). Orientation may be in the transaxial or coronal (or both) whichever follows the course of the vessel best. Thin slices of 5 mm without

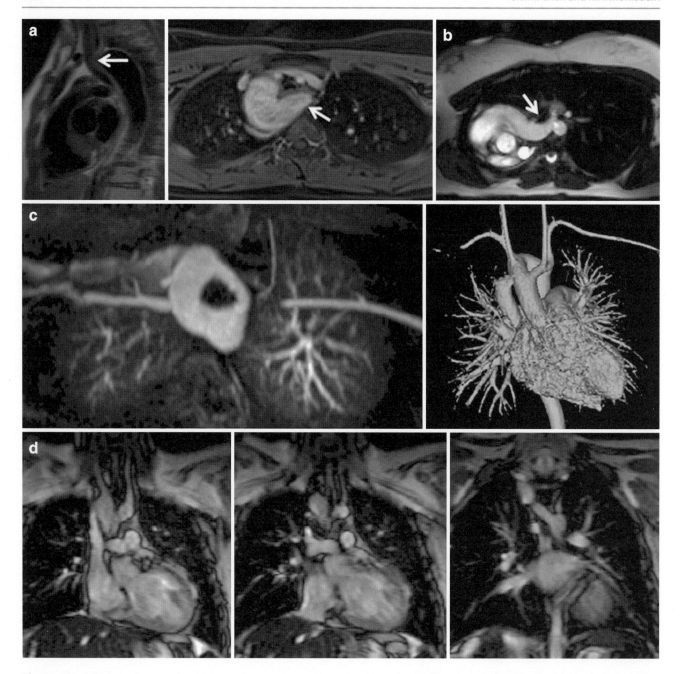

Fig. 12.12 (**a**) Right aortic arch with a Kommerell diverticulum at the origin of an anomalous left subclavian artery. The left subclavian artery courses behind the oesophagus and trachea (*arrowed*), causing compression (HASTE and SSFP multislice imaging). (**b**) Unusual left pulmonary artery sling causing oesophageal and tracheal compression (*arrowed*). (**c**) Double aortic arch. Contrast enhanced (near transaxial orientation) image showing a complete vascular ring on the left, and a surface rendered 3D reconstruction after contrast enhanced MRA on the right. (**d**) SSFP multislice imaging showing a double aortic arch

gaps are recommended as vessels may be small in diameter. Cine imaging may be advantageous over a 3D whole heart or SSFP multislice imaging as assessment may also be made (to a degree) of the effect of systolic expansion of the anomalous vessels on the trachea and oesophagus.

- 3D whole heart: This method may be useful, and may be used as an adjunct to cine imaging.
- MRA: this is not essential, but may be useful if there is concurrent stenosis in the vessels of interest.

12.8.2 Analysis of a Vascular Ring or Sling

The following should be reported:
- The morphology and course of the vascular ring or sling.
- The relationship of the vascular ring or sling to its surrounding structures, and the degree of compression.
- After repair: report on any evidence of residual compression.

12.9 Limitations and Common Pitfalls

CMR is somewhat limited by the image degrading effect of metallic artefacts, but this can be overcome to a degree as described earlier in the chapter. Tortuous aortas and branch vessels may be difficult to image on SSFP cine imaging, but MRA largely compensates. The most common pitfall is inaccurate measurements due to malalignment of the imaging planes, and reproducibility in measurements of studies done over time may be difficult. Again, by careful planning of the planes prior to imaging and using previous studies as a guide, reproducibility and accuracy of measurements and therefore assessment may be improved.

Conclusion

Aortic anomalies comprise a heterogenous group of defects and can be assessed in detail using CMR for diagnosis and in planning management strategies, surveillance and follow up for residual or progressive and/or recurrent abnormalities. Its ability to image the aorta in all orientations and projections is an advantage as detailed and accurate assessment of can be made. In addition, phase contrast and velocity mapping allow measurement of blood flow, useful in quantification of severity of the lesions. CMR is a versatile imaging modality for the evaluation of the aorta with the added advantages of its non-invasive nature, and the lack of radiation and use of iodinated contrast agents.

References

1. Moore KL, Persaud TVN. The developing human, clinically orientated embryology. 7th ed. Philadelphia: Saunders; 2003. p. 329–80.
2. Pearson GD, Devereux R, Loeys B, Maslen C, milewicz D, Pyeritz R, Ramirez F, Rifkin D, Sakai L, Svensson L, Wessels A, Van Eyk J, Dietz HC. Report of the National Heart, Lung and Blood Institute and National Marfan Foundation Working Group on research in Marfan syndrome and related disorders. Circulation. 2008;118:785–91.
3. Fedak PW, de Sa MP, Verma S, Nili N, Kazemian P, Butany J, Strauss BH, Weisel RD, David TE. Vascular matrix remodelling in patients with bicuspid aortic valve malformations: implications for aortic dilatation. J Thorac Cardiovasc Surg. 2003;126:797–806.
4. Aboulhosn J, Child JS. Left ventricular outflow obstruction: subaortic stenosis, bicuspid aortic vavle, supravalvar aortic stenosis, and coarctation of the aorta. Circulation. 2006;114:2412–22.
5. Warnes CA, Williams RG, Bashore TM, Child JS, Connolly HM, Dearani JA, del Nido P, Fasules JW, Graham Jr TP, Hijazi AM, Hunt SA, King ME, Landzberg MJ, Miner PD, Radford MJ, Walsh EP, Webb GD. ACC/AHA 2008 guidelines for the management of adults with congenital heart disease: a report of the American College of Cardiology/American Heart Association Task Force on practice guideline (writing committee to develop guidelines on the management of adults with congenital heart disease): developed in collaboration with the American Society of Echocardiography, Heart Rhythm Society, International Society for Adult Congenital Heart Disease, Society for Cardiovascular Angiography and Interventions, and Society of Thoracic Surgeons. Circulation. 2008; 118:e714–833.
6. Morgan-Hughes GJ, Marshall AJ, Roobottom C. Morphologic assessment of patent ductus arteriosus in adults using retrospectively ECG-gated multidetector CT. AJR Am J Roentgenol. 2003;181:749–54.
7. Hoey ETD, Kanagasingam A, Sivananthan MU. Sinus of valsalva aneurysms: assessment with cardiovascular MRI. AJR Am J Roentgenol. 2010;194:W494–504.
8. ACCF/AHA/AATS/ACR/ASA/SCA/SCAI/SIR/STS/SVM guidelines for the diagnosis and management of patients with Thoracic Aortic Disease: a report of the American College of Cardiology Foundation/American Heart Association Task Force on Practice Guidelines, American Association for Thoracic Surgery, American College of Radiology, American Stroke Association, Society of Cardiovascular Anesthesiologists, Society for Cardiovascular Angiography and Interventions, Society of Interventional Radiology, Society of Thoracic Surgeons, and Society for Vascular Medicine. Hiratzka LF, Bakris GL, Beckman JA, Bersin RM, Carr VF, Casey DE Jr, Eagle KA, Hermann LK, Isselbacher EM, Kazerooni EA, Kouchoukos NT, Lytle BW, Milewicz DM, Reich DL, Sen S, Shinn JA, Svensson LG, Williams DM; American College of Cardiology Foundation/American Heart Association Task Force on Practice Guidelines; American Association for Thoracic Surgery; American College of Radiology; American Stroke Association; Society of Cardiovascular Anesthesiologists; Society for Cardiovascular Angiography and Interventions; Society of Interventional Radiology; Society of Thoracic Surgeons; Society for Vascular Medicine. Circulation. 2010 Apr 6;121(13):e266-369
9. Burman ED, Keegan J, Kilner PJ. Aortic root measurement by cardiovascular magnetic resonance: specification of planes and lines of measurement and corresponding normal values. Circ Cardiovasc Imaging. 2008;1:104–13.
10. Rocchini AP. Coarctation of the aorta and interrupted aortic arch. In: Moller JH, Hoffman IE, editors. Pediatric cardiovascular medicine. Philadelphia: Churchill Livingstone; 2000. p. 567–93.
11. Isner JM, Donaldson RF, Fulton D, Bhan I, Payne DD, Cleveland RJ. Cystic medial necrosis in coarctation of the aorta: a potential factor contributing to adverse consequences observed after percutaneous balloon angioplasty of coarctation sites. Circulation. 1987;75:689–95.
12. Steffens JC, Bourne MW, Sakuma H, O'Sullivan M, Higgins CB. Quantification of collateral blood flow in coarctation of the aorta by velocity encoded cine magnetic resonance imaging. Circulation. 1994;90:937–43.
13. Nistri S, Sorbo MD, Palisi M, Scognamiglio R, Thiene G. Aortic root dilatation in young men with normally functioning bicuspid aortic valves. Heart. 1999;82:19–22.
14. Isselbacher EM. Thoracic and abdominal aortic aneurysms. Circulation. 2005;111:816–28.
15. Ring WS. Congenital heart surgery nomenclature and database project: aortic aneurysm, sinus of valsalva aneurysm, and aortic dissection. Ann Thorac Surg. 2000;69:S147–63.
16. Edwards JE, Burchell HB. The pathological anatomy of deficiencies between the aortic root and the heart, including aortic sinus aneurysms. Thorax. 1957;12:125–39.
17. Swan L. Sinus of valsalva aneurysms. In: Gatzoulis MA, Webb GD, Daubeney PEF, editors. Diagnosis and management of adult congenital heart disease. London: Churchill Livingston; 2003. p. 239–44.
18. Pepper J, Golesworthy T, Utley M, Chan J, Ganeshalingam S, Lamperth M, Mohiaddin R, Treasure T. Manufacturing and placing a bespoke support for the Marfan aortic root: description of the method and technical results and status at one year for the first ten patients. Interact Cardiovasc Thorac Surg. 2010;10:360–5.

19. Collett RW, Edwards JE. Persistent truncus arteriosus; a classification according to anatomic types. Surg Clin North Am. 1949;29:1245–70.

20. Gersony WM, Apfel HD. Patent ductus arteriosus and other aortopulmonary anomalies. In: Moller JH, Hoffman IE, editors. Pediatric cardiovascular medicine. Philadelphia: Churchill Livingstone; 2000. p. 323–34.

21. Schneider DJ, Moore JW. Patent ductus arteriosus. Circulation. 2006;114:1873–82.

22. Park MK. Paediatric cardiology for practitioners. 4th ed. Philadelphia: Mosby; 1984. p. 241–6.

Inherited Cardiomyopathies

13

Rory O'Hanlon and Raad H. Mohiaddin

13.1 Introduction

In order to plan optimal management and treatment strategies in patients with a suspected cardiomyopathy, the key initial factor is to establish the diagnosis and underlying etiology at an early stage. While many patients will present with symptoms and demonstrable ventricular dysfunction on echocardiography, often the underlying cause is not apparent, thus necessitating many "routine" invasive and noninvasive investigation such as angiography, echocardiography, holter monitoring, treadmill testing, and nuclear studies. There has been considerable progress in recent years in the development of imaging technologies which are now able to characterize a much wider number of cardiomyopathic processes than ever before in a non-invasive manner. The advent of gadolinium enhanced cardiac magnetic resonance imaging (CMR) has dramatically changed the non-invasive workup of patients with a suspected cardiomyopathy. In a single scan setting it is now possible to provide a comprehensive assessment of both ischemic and non-ischemic cardiomyopathies providing detailed information on cardiac anatomy, function, tissue characterization, assessment of epicardial and microvascular perfusion, valvular flows, and coronary and peripheral angiography (Fig. 13.1). This comprehensive examination can be completed in a short period of time, typically 30–45 min, without the need for prolonged breath holds (5–10 s) or ionizing radiation. Establishing definitive diagnoses with the greatest degree of clarity, helps guide and

monitor therapeutic response, and assists in optimal risk stratification. Gadolinium based contrast agents are remarkably safe and the incidence of adverse reactions or nephrogenic systemic sclerosis (NSF) is exceedingly low. Follow up imaging to monitor progression and response to interventions can be performed safely and without any concern regarding cumulative radiation exposure.

In this chapter we will primarily focus on the inherited/congenital cardiomyopathies with a defined genetic basis. There will be significant scope for the discussion of non-inherited cardiomyopathies as there is often a phenotypic overlap since patients typically do not present with a known genetic diagnosis; rather they present with symptoms or are incidentally found to have an abnormal clinical exam or screening test and are subsequently found to have a hypertrophied or dilated heart warranting further workup.

13.2 CMR Techniques

In the CMR workup of a suspected cardiomyopathy a wide range of sequences are acquired following dedicated protocols as outlines by the Society of Cardiovascular Magnetic Resonance [1]. Initial dark blood single shot images are acquired in transaxial, coronal, and saggital imaging planes using Half-Fourier Acquisition Single-Shot Turbo Spin-Echo (HASTE) imaging to readily identify important congenital anomalies and obvious shunts. Following this, dynamic cine images of the heart are acquired along its long and short-axis using gradient-echo steady state free precession (TrueFISP; SSFP) cine imaging. Cine images can be acquired in any given imaging plane without the limitation of acoustic windows as seen with echocardiography. CMR is validated as the gold standard imaging tool to quantify biventricular volumes and function using short axis cine images of

R. O'Hanlon, M.D., MRCPI
Department of Cardiology, St. Vincent's University Hospital, Dublin, Ireland

Centre for Cardiovascular Magnetic Resonance, Blackrock Clinic, Rock Road, Dublin, Ireland
e-mail: r.ohanlon9@btinternet.com

R.H. Mohiaddin, M.D., Ph.D., FRCR, FESC, FRCP, FACC (✉)
Cardiovascular Magnetic Resonance Unit, Royal Brompton Hospital and National Heart and Lung Institute, Imperial College London, Sydney Street, London, SW3 6NP, UK
e-mail: r.mohiaddin@imperial.ac.uk

Electronic supplementary material The online version of this chapter (doi:10.1007/978-1-4471-4267-6_13) contains supplementary material, which is available to authorized users.

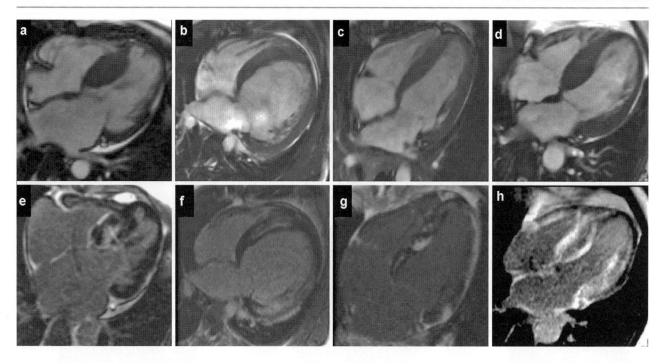

Fig. 13.4 Four chamber SSSP images of different patterns of left ventricular hypertrophy (**a–d**) and corresponding late gadolinium enhancement images (LGE) (**e–h**). Hypertrophic cardiomyopathy (**a+e**) typically shows patchy mid wall LGE in the regions of maximal hypertrophy. Fabry's (**b+f**) shows mid wall LGE in the basal lateral wall and septum. Sarcoidosis (**c+g**) typically shows focal LGE scarring which is typically patchy and involving the basal and lateral segments. Cardiac amyloidosis (**d+f**) showing diffuse subendocardial LGE with "sparing" of the epicardium and septum characteristically referred to as a "zebra" pattern

HCM patients, inappropriate ICD discharge events occurred in 25 % of the studied population, at a rate of approximately 7 % per year. A more recent study has suggested that a single risk factor for SCD in HCM patients may warrant ICD implantation [19].This has led to a search for better predictors of risk and CMR may prove useful in this regard.

CMR has a unique ability to determine myocardial tissue characteristics in-vivo using the late gadolinium enhancement technique (LGE). The presence of fibrosis is an important marker of risk and those patients with greater number of risk factors for SCD typically have more fibrosis, which is consistent with post-mortem data (Fig. 13.5) [20, 21].The presence of fibrosis contributes to the disruption of the electrical synchrony that exists between myocytes and hence increases arrhythmia potential [22, 23]. Several recent studies have demonstrated risk of ventricular tachyarrhythmias and atrial fibrillation to be associated with LGE [24, 25]. It also promotes increased myocardial stiffness with LV adverse remodeling leading to cavity dilatation and eventually systolic dysfunction, and is detected in 85 % of patients with end stage dilated HCM, and importantly may be a progressive process over time, hence potentially representing a potential therapeutic target [26] (Fig. 13.6). The main mechanism driving the formation of fibrosis is thought to be myocardial ischemia due to abnormal microvasculature and/or a mismatch between the greatly increased LV mass and coronary flow [27, 28]. Abnormal perfusion in HCM patients despite normal coronary angiography has been linked to SCD and has been traditionally difficult to assess in HCM patients being principally performed using PET, which to date remains the gold standard tool to evaluate myocardial ischemia. CMR stress perfusion can now be performed in the same setting as the LGE study and has been validated against PET perfusion studies [29, 30]. The addition of adenosine perfusion imaging and LGE in the evaluation of HCM vastly enhances our ability to define very different phenotypic sarcomeric HCM than can be appreciated using cine imaging alone (Fig. 13.7). A recent paper by Petersen et al. demonstrated that severity of myocardial perfusion defects correlate with areas of maximal wall thickness and the presence of fibrosis in patients with HCM [31]. A further hypothesis is that microvascular abnormalities may precede and predispose to the development of myocardial fibrosis and if present may represent an earlier risk marker and possible therapeutic target [32].

An as yet unappreciated potential marker of risk is the total left ventricular (LV) mass and LV mass index. In vivo assessment of LV mass by echocardiography is unreliable due to assumptions based on the due to the asymmetric distribution of hypertrophy. In a recent study by Olivotto et al., the authors demonstrated that LVMI was a

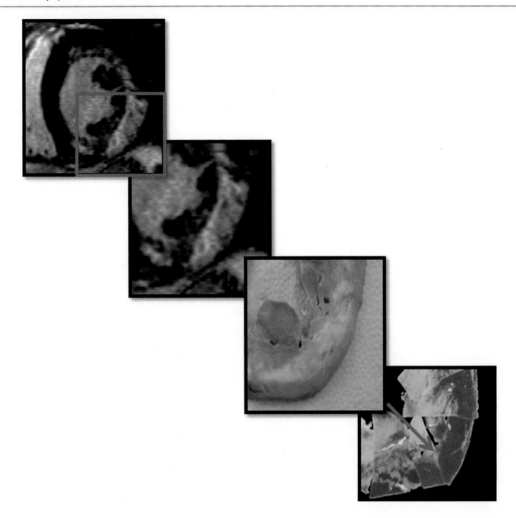

Fig. 13.5 Comparison of in vivo late gadolinium enhancement (LGE) images (**a+b**) matching macroscopic assessment from autopsy (**c**), and confirmed as myocardial replacement fibrosis on histology sections stained with Picrosirius red (**d**)

more sensitive indicator of risk of death than peak wall thickness [33]. Other potential prognostic markers evaluated by CMR could be the presence of right ventricular hypertrophy or even the presence of myocardial edema [34, 35].

Two recent papers have prospectively studied the independent prognostic role of LGE in predicting adverse events in HCM. In a study by O' Hanlon et al., 217 patients with HCM scanned with CMR were followed for a mean of 3.1 years for a combined primary end point of cardiovascular death, unplanned cardiovascular-related hospital admission, sustained ventricular tachycardia or ventricular fibrillation, or appropriate ICD discharge [36]. During follow-up, 9 cardiovascular- related deaths occurred, of which eight (89 %) were in patients with fibrosis seen by CMR. The primary end point was reached in 40 patients (18.4 %), of whom 34 had fibrosis seen by CMR (HR 3.4, 95 % CI 1.4–8.1, P=0.006). On multivariate analysis, the presence and extent of fibrosis remained an independent predictor of outcome (Fig. 13.9). A secondary end point was focused on heart failure, and included unplanned hospital stay owing to heart failure, progression to a NYHA functional class III or IV, or death related to heart failure. This end point was reached in 41 patients (19 %), of whom 33 had fibrosis seen by CMR (HR 2.51, 95 % CI 1.1–5.5, P=0.021). The presence and extent of fibrosis remained a significant predictor of this secondary outcome (Fig. 13.8). Another secondary end point was focused on arrhythmias (including sustained ventricular tachycardia or ventricular fibrillation, appropriate ICD discharge, and SCD). This end point was reached in 12 patients (5.5 %), with 10 patients in the fibrosis group (Hr 3.15, 95 % CI 0.69–14.4, P=0.138). Although the presence and extent of fibrosis was predictive of this end point in the univariate analysis, this association was not significant in the multivariate analysis, which was possibly due to the low event rates observed. A second study by Bruder et al. prospectively enrolled 220 patients with HCM and followed them for 3 years. The primary end points of the study were all-cause mortality and SCD [37]. Importantly, 75 % of patients had no risk factors for SCD. Over 65 % had fibrosis as seen by contrast-enhanced CMR. The patients with fibrosis were not different from those without fibrosis in terms of clinical characteristics, except that patients with fibrosis had a higher burden of hypertrophy and more often had a history of arrhythmias. During follow-up, 20 patients (9 %) died and 2 (0.9 %) had ICD shocks. Importantly, 91 % of the patients who died had no previous symptoms and 8 of 11 patients (73 %) who experienced SCD had no risk factors. The presence of fibrosis, as detected by CMR, was significantly associated with all-cause mortality (OR 5.47, 95 % CI 1.24–24.08, $P=0.01$) and cardiac-related mortality (OR 8.01, 95 % CI 1.04–61.9, $P < 0.05$); its association with SCD did not however quite reach statistical significance. In a multivariable analysis fibrosis seen on CMR was the only predictor of all-cause mortality and cardiac death.

In summary, CMR provides a robust single imaging modality to diagnose HCM, outrule phenocopies, and add significantly to risk stratification for major adverse cardiac events including HF and possibly SCD.

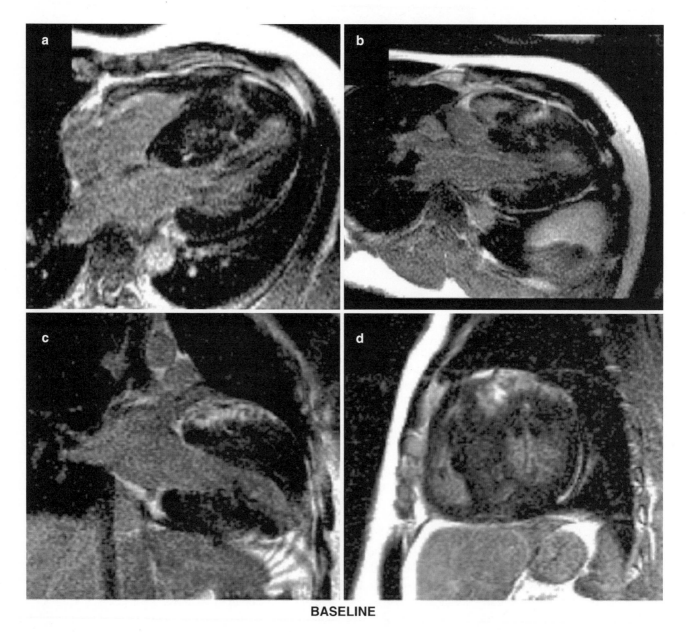

BASELINE

Fig. 13.6 LGE images in a patient with HCM in 4-chamber, 3-chamber, 2-chamber, and short axis views (**a–d**) at the time of the baseline scan. Follow up scanning 4 years later shows marked increase in the severity of LGE in the anterior, septal, and inferior walls (**e–h**)

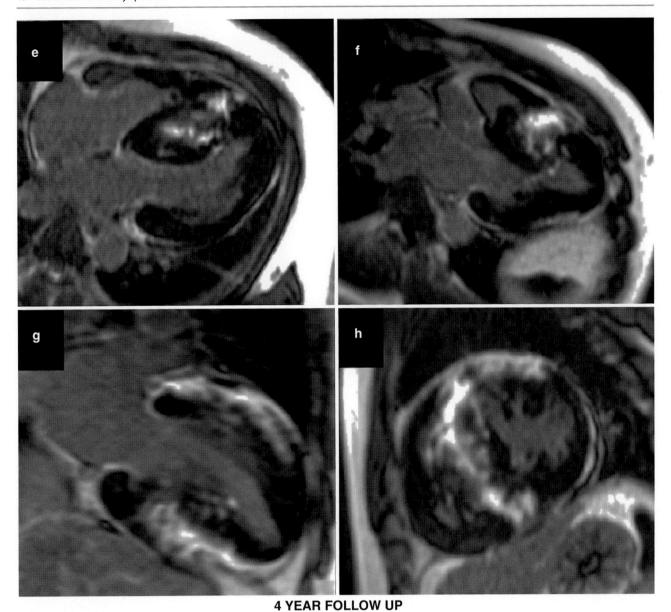

4 YEAR FOLLOW UP

Fig. 13.6 (continued)

13.4 Dilated Cardiomyopathy

Dilated cardiomyopathy (DCM) is the most common cardiomyopathy worldwide and has many causes. In this disorder, dilation and impaired contraction of the left or both ventricles develops (Movies 13.9 and 13.10). It can be primary (genetic, mixed or predominantly familial non-genetic, or acquired) or secondary (e.g., infiltrative or autoimmune). It is characterized mainly by left ventricular systolic dysfunction with an associated increase in mass and volume. In some cases, left ventricular diastolic abnormal findings are present. Right ventricular dilation and dysfunction can also develop but are not needed for diagnosis. Prevalence in the general population remains undefined. This disorder develops at any age, in either sex, and in people of any ethnic origin. In many cases, the disease is inherited, and is called familial dilated cardiomyopathy. The familial type might account for 20–48 % of all cases [38].

13.4.1 CMR and Diagnosis

The most pressing clinical question in a patient presenting with a dilated heart with systolic reduction is whether or not it is due to underlying ischemic heart disease. This differentiation carries important therapeutic implications

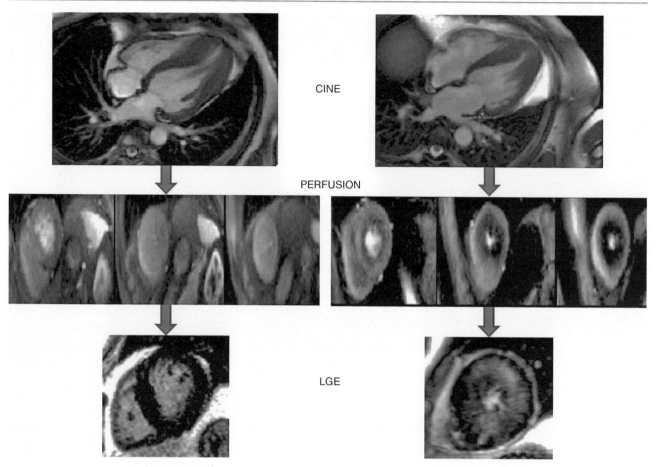

CINE

PERFUSION

LGE

Fig. 13.7 Two cases of mid to apical HCM (**a**+**b**) appearing phenotypically similar on cine imaging. By performed adenosine stress perfusion followed by *LGE* imaging, two very different phenotypes emerge. Patient A demonstrates preserved microvascular perfusion at basal, mid and apical ventricular levels without evidence of myocardial fibrosis on *LGE* imaging. Patient B shows a similar pattern of hypertrophy but with marked circumferential microvascular perfusion abnormalities (*dark regions*) at basal, mid and apical ventricular levels, and evidence of diffuse fibrosis in the regions of maximal hypertrophy

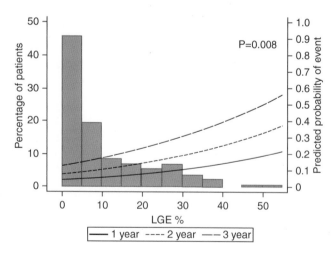

Fig. 13.8 The prognostic impact of myocardial fibrosis in HCM. The predicted probability of cardiovascular death, unplanned cardiovascular hospital admission, sustained ventricular tachycardia or ventricular fibrillation, or appropriate implantable cardioverter-defibrillator (ICD) at 1, 2, and 3 years on the basis of the overall percentage of fibrosis (*broken and unbroken lines*), plotted against the x-axis on the right. The *bar charts* represent the overall percentage of patients with this amount of fibrosis, plotted on the x-axis on the left (Modified from O' Hanlon et al. [36])

since recovery of function and reverse LV remodeling may occur if the CAD is appropriately revascularized. To this end, in many centers coronary angiography is routinely performed in the workup of patients presenting with left ventricular dysfunction [39]. Identifying DCM carries equal importance since contributory causes such as alcohol excess or post viral cardiomyopathies should be considered. The diagnosis of DCM may also have importance familial implications. There are many studies using the LGE technique as a novel non-invasive test to determine if LV dysfunction has an ischemic cause. In the absence of LGE in those with a dilated cardiomyopathy, an ischemic etiology is extremely unlikely (97 % negative predictive value), and in the presence of an ischemic etiology, the amount of LGE correlates with the degree of severity of underlying CAD (Fig. 13.9) [40, 41]. By contrast, patients with normal coronaries by angiography and LV dysfunction may still have an ischemic etiology for LV dysfunction (up to 13 % of individuals), and may have been inappropriately diagnosed as having a non-ischemic cardiomyopathy leading potentially to important therapeutic implications. The results of this technique as a

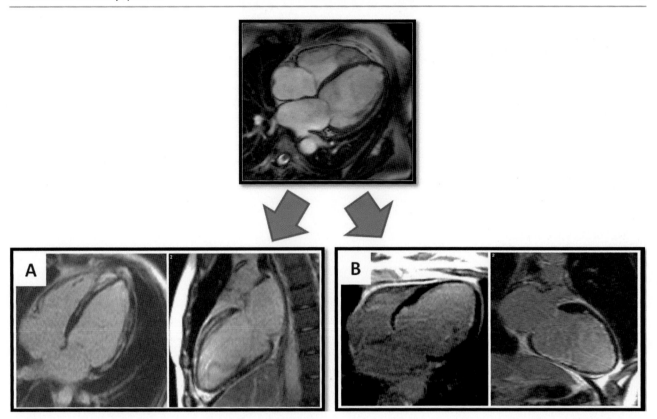

Fig. 13.9 Dilated cardiomyopathy appearing "phenotypically" one disease on cine imaging (*Top row*). Late gadolinium enhanced images (*Bottom row*) demonstrating two different disease processes leading to similar phenotype. Mid wall fibrosis is seen in example (**a**) consistent with DCM, whereas extensive subendocardial fibrosis is seen in example (**b**), consistent with prior myocardial infarction, and diagnostic of an ischemic etiology

non-invasive method of differentiating ischemic and non-ischemic cardiomyopathy are superior to other techniques because the myocardial substrate can be interrogated with such high resolution. Additionally, CMR is superior to nuclear scintigraphic techniques to distinguish non-ischemic from ischemic etiologies since CMR is not limited by attenuation artifacts, leading to false positive results [42]. Comparative studies between SPECT and CMR perfusion imaging have demonstrated that CMR can identify regional reductions in myocardial perfusion over a wider range than current nuclear techniques. These techniques provide sensitivity and specificity values ranging between 83 and 95 % and 53 and 95 % respectively [43].

While the absence of LGE does not completely out rule an ischemic etiology in the potential rare setting of true myocardial hibernation in the absence of infarction, stress and rest first pass perfusion imaging can be performed with gadolinium to assess transmural myocardial blood flow to the microvascular level.

13.4.2 CMR and Prognosis

Risk stratification for DCM has tended to focus on traditional markers such as ejection fraction to predict SCD risk.

Histologically, DCM is characterized by progressive interstitial fibrosis and degeneration of myocytes. Replacement fibrosis is also often seen and unlike in CAD, there is mid-wall rather than subendocardial fibrosis due to involvement of the circumferential fiber layer. This pattern of mid wall fibrosis is seen in 30 % of patients with DCM (Figs. 13.9 and 13.10). This finding carries important prognostic implications and has been found to represent an important substrate for inducible ventricular arrhythmias independent of ejection fraction [44]. There have to date been a number of prospective studies evaluating the independent prognostic value of myocardial fibrosis in DCM [45, 46]. The first of these studies was published by Assomul et al. in 2006. The authors followed 101 consecutive patients with DCM for a mean of 658 ± 355 days. Mid wall fibrosis (seen in 35 % of patients) was an independent predictor of major adverse cardiac events, including all-cause death and hospitalization for a cardiovascular event (HR 3.4; p=0.01). Multivariate analysis showed midwall fibrosis as the sole significant predictor of death or hospitalization. Midwall fibrosis also predicted secondary outcome measures of sudden cardiac death (SCD) or ventricular tachycardia (HR 5.2, p=0.01). Midwall fibrosis remained predictive of SCD/VT after correction for baseline differences in left ventricular ejection fraction between those with and without fibrosis. In the work by Wu et al. in 2008,

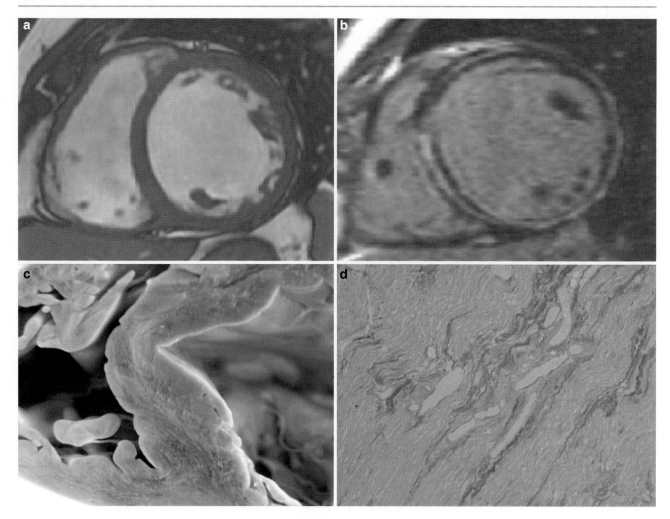

Fig. 13.10 Dilated cardiomyopathy. Cine image (**a**) showing dilated LV with wall thinning and mild increase in lateral wall trabeculation. Late gadolinium images (**b**) show typical mid wall enhancement, confirmed macroscopically (**c**) and microscopically as myocardial fibrosis (**d**)

65 prospective patients with non-ischemic cardiomyopathy undergoing ICD implantation were followed for a median of 17 months. Forty two percent of this cohort had myocardial fibrosis, the presence of which was associated with an eight fold increased risk of the primary endpoint (cardiac death, appropriate ICD discharge, and heart failure hospitalization). Recently Cho and colleagues have shown that myocardial fibrosis in DCM is predicative of recovery of function over time as well as rehospitalizations (n=79; 11 rehospitalizations in LGE+ group vs. 1 in LGE – group; HR 8.06, p > 0.05) [47].

13.5 Arrhythmogenic Right Ventricular Cardiomyopathy (ARVC)

Arrhythmogenic right ventricular cardiomyopathy/dysplasia (ARVC/D) is a primary heart muscle disorder presenting clinically with ventricular arrhythmias, sudden death, or heart failure and characterized pathologically by progressive myocardial loss with fibrous or fibrofatty replacement mostly of the right ventricle caused by abnormal cell connections through the desmosome and generally affects young males [48, 49]. The estimated prevalence of ARVC/D in the general population ranges from 1 in 2,000 to 1 in 5,000, and men are more frequently affected than women, with an approximate ratio of 3:1. The condition is a major cause for SCD in the young and athletes. To date, 12 genes have been identified which are linked to ARVC/D, encoding several components of the cardiac desmosome. Dysfunctional desmosomes resulting in defective cell adhesion proteins, such as plakoglobin (JUP), desmoplakin (DSP), plakophilin-2 (PKP-2), and desmoglein-2 (DSG-2) consequently cause loss of electrical coupling between cardiac myocytes, leading to myocyte cell death, fibrofatty replacement and arrhythmias. RV dilatation and functional impairment often result leading to regional wall motion abnormalities and regional aneurysmal dilatation (Movies 13.11 and 13.12). Structural changes may be absent in the early stage of the disease and therefore can be difficult to diagnose. Subtle early changes are typically confined to the inflow tract, outflow tract, or apex of the RV, the so called 'triangle of dysplasia' [50]. Progression to more diffuse RV disease leading to left ventricular involvement, typically affecting the posterior lateral wall, is common. Histological findings suggest the RV changes occur as a result of repair of injury. LV involvement is typically a late manifestation. In the early 'concealed phase', individuals are often asymptomatic but may nonetheless be at risk of sudden cardiac death, notably during exertion [51]. In the 'electrical phase', individuals present with symptomatic arrhythmias, and RV morphological abnormalities are readily discernible by conventional imaging. Later, diffuse disease may result in biventricular heart failure, and ventricular arrhythmias may or may not be present. In the very advanced stage of disease, it can be difficult to differentiate from DCM [52].

Echocardiography remains the most extensively used imaging tool to evaluate the heart including the right ventricle. The RV however is difficult to completely evaluate with echocardiography owing to near field signal dropout and its crescent shape. CMR is considered the gold standard method to image the RV and has attracted much interest over the years as a method to diagnose ARVC owing to the ability to image the heart in any given imaging plane acquiring unparalleled images of the RV structure and function. While localized and diffuse RV wall abnormalities are easily visualized (chamber dilatation, wall thinning, diastolic bulging, and localized aneurysmal dilatation) the positive predictive value is uncertain owing to concerns regarding interobserver variability, lack of experience with the modality at most imaging centers, insufficient resolution for detection of wall thinning, over interpretation of RWMA, and difficulties in differentiating normal epicardial fat from true myocardial adipose replacement [53]. The ability of fast-spin echo sequences to differentiate fat from normal myocardium aroused considerable interest in assisting ARVC diagnosis. CMR studies that focused on imaging fat in the RV as a diagnostic criterion for ARVC suffered from a low sensitivity and many false positives since fatty deposits in the RV can occur in a wide variety of conditions and small focal fatty deposits are not easy to visualize [54]. LGE permits myocardial tissue characterization in the LV but can be difficult to be certain of LGE in the thin walled RV and due to possible confusion with fat [55, 56]. A recent study has shown however that subtle RV abnormalities detected by CMR and missed by echocardiography may in fact be identifying an early form of ARVC [57]. In this study CMR criteria to diagnose ARVC in a genotyped population achieved a sensitivity of 96 % and specificity of 78 %. These impressive figures were achieved by acquiring high temporal resolution cine images which improved assessment of RWMA, plus the majority of patients received gadolinium contrast. DCE is found to variable degrees and locations in ARVC. In a study of 200 affected patients, over 80 % had CMR evidence of LV LGE.

The inferolateral wall was most commonly affected (85 %) in subepicardial and mid wall locations. Other locations include the inferoseptal junction, anterolateral wall, and anterior wall (Fig. 13.11) [58].

In 2010, ARVC Task force criteria were modified to make allowance for the advances in genetics and diagnostic modalities [59]. High resolution RV volumetric analysis has led to regional CMR defined RV akinesia, dyskinesia, or aneurysmal dilatation *and* one of the following: indexed RV volumes (RVEDV/BSA >110 for males and >100 for females) or an RVEF < 40 % to be incorporated into the major criteria (sensitivity 76 % (males) and 68 % (females) and specificity 90 % (males) and 98 % (females)). The accuracy of these revised task force criteria were recently studied in a paper by Protanorious et al. [60]. The authors studied 103 consecutive carriers of pathogenic desmosome mutations and 102 mutation positive relatives belonging to 22 families with dominant and 14 families with recessive ARVC using the original 1994 task force criteria and the 2010 criteria. They found that the revised Task force criteria improved sensitivity from 92 to 99 %. Importantly fat visualization on CMR is not and cannot be included in the revised criteria, because it has not been found to be specific for ARVC and has a poor inter-reader agreement.

The accuracy and reproducibility for CMR diagnosis of ARVC is strongly operator dependent and challenges exist, especially regarding subjective interpretation of RV wall motion abnormalities and thus it is recommended that evaluation should be performed in dedicated centers and interpreted by individuals with both a clinical background in the condition and extensive CMR experience [61]. Currently, fat or fibrosis imaging using CMR is not a validated tool to diagnose ARVC or risk stratify patients with the disease. On the other hand, CMR is preferable to RV angiography, CT, or echocardiography for serial assessment of index cases and prospective evaluation of asymptomatic relatives, and further allows simultaneous examination of both ventricles and without the need for ionizing radiation making the technique more suitable for periodic reassessment and familial screening.

13.6 Left Ventricular Non-compaction

Left ventricular non-compaction (LVNC) is a rare form of cardiomyopathy believed to be a result of impaired/arrested compaction of the developing myocardium [62]. There are a variety of gross patterns of non-compaction, including anastomosing broad trabeculae, coarse trabeculae resembling multiple papillary muscles, and interlacing smaller muscle bundles resembling a sponge (Movies 13.13, 13.14, and 13.15). Occasionally, the entity can be somewhat subtle viewed on gross features only although the absence of well-formed

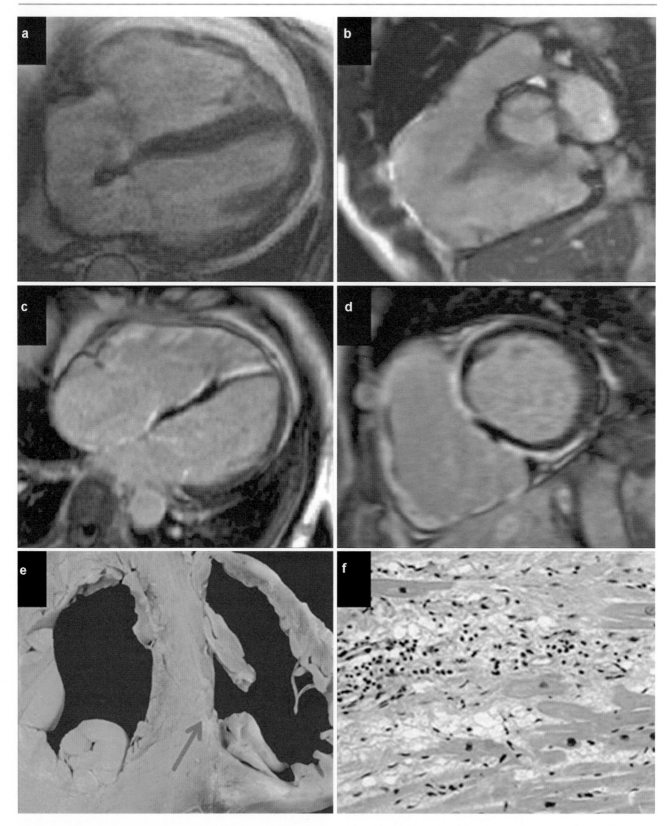

Fig. 13.11 Arrhythmogenic right ventricular cardiomyopathy. Four-chamber and RVOT view cine images show a markedly dilated RV (**a**) with local aneurysmal in the RVOT (**b**). Corresponding LGE imaging shows extensive fibrosis in the RV walls and in the septum, preferentially in the RV septal wall extending to the LV inferior and anterior epicardial regions (**c**+**d**). A representative post mortem heart showing RV septal fibrosis (*red arrow*) confirmed as ARVC on microscopy showing typical fibrofatty replacement

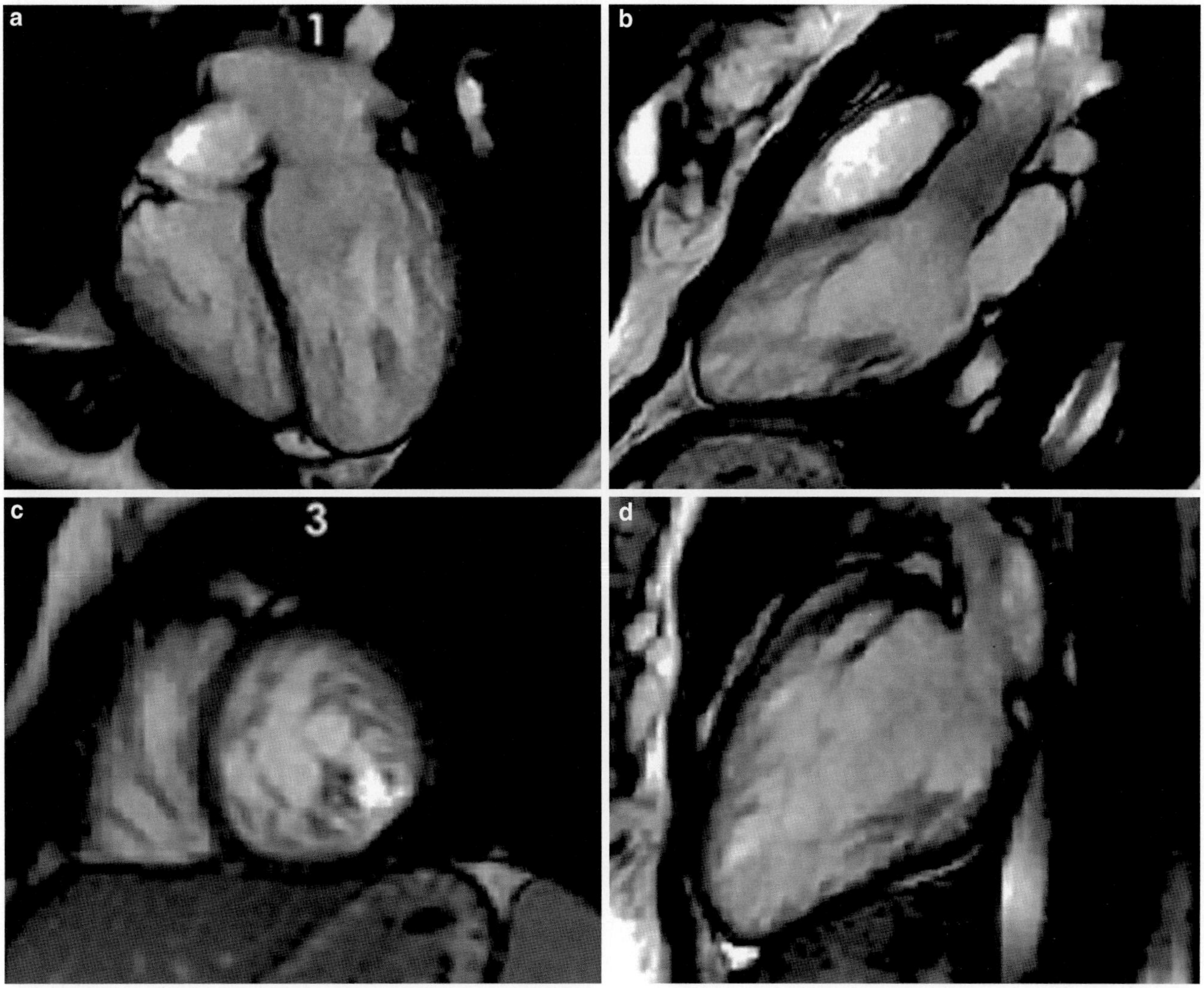

Fig. 13.12 Left ventricular non compaction (LVNC). Representative cine images in 4-chamber, 3-chamber, 2-chamber, and short axis imaging planes (**a–d**) demonstrating marked increase in trabecular meshwork, with a non-compact trabecular to compact trabecular ratio >2.3:1 at end diastole. The apical regions are easily visualized using CMR

papillary muscles is a clue to the diagnosis, even when the recesses are microscopic [63]. The RV can be involved in 30–50 % of cases. Persistence of non-compacted myocardium may be associated with structural heart defects or may be isolated [64]. Associated conditions include coronary artery anomalies, coronary to ventricular fistulae, TGA, and pulmonary and tricuspid valve abnormalities. The disease can present throughout life with progressive LV systolic dysfunction and may be associated with an increased incidence of thrombo-embolism and ventricular arrhythmia [65].

There is an increasing interest in this condition as well as a marked increase in publications in the past 12 months, possibly reflecting the ability of higher resolution imaging modalities to delineate the morphological appearance of the myocardium. This has however raised the question that "standard" diagnostic criteria may be too sensitive and the use of higher resolution imaging may lead to over diagnosis of LVNC [66]. The pattern of most marked non-compaction typically affects the apical and lateral walls (Figs. 13.12 and 13.13). Three principle publications have detailed various echocardiographic criteria for LVNC. Chin et al. proposed echocardiographic diagnostic criteria quantifies the ratio between the depth of penetration of the intertrabecular recesses relative to the posterior wall thickness at end-diastole [67]. The criteria by Jenni et al. focus n the ratio of non-compact endocardial layer to compact epicardium at end-systole [68]. A third set of criteria set out by Stollberger focuses on the number of trabeculae and perfusion in the intertrabecular recesses [69]. The sensitivity and specificity to diagnose the condition is still being established, principally owing to the lack of standardized definitions as to what represents LVNC, with less than a third of patients fulfilling all three established

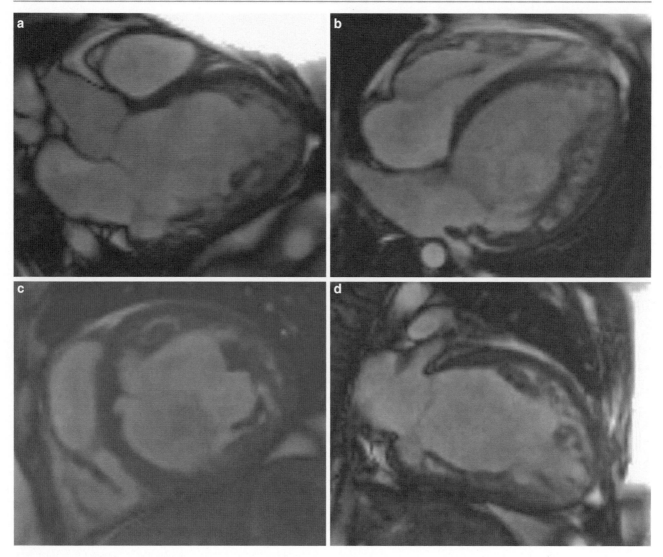

Fig. 13.13 Left ventricular non compaction (LVNC). Representative cine images in 3-chamber, 4-chamber, 2-chamber, and short axis imaging planes (**a–d**). This example demonstrates the more "traditionally" described trabecular pattern in LVNC with predominant non-compact trabeculations seen in the lateral and apical walls

echocardiography criteria in one study and up to 10 % of normal subjects fulfill one or more LVNC criteria based on the above studies [70].

Due to near signal dropout, the apex can be difficult to image with echocardiography. CMR is ideally placed to comprehensively image the condition owing to the wide field of view, and the ability to image the right heart structures and assess for associated congenital abnormalities in a single examination. In the work by Petersen et al., the accuracy of CMR to distinguish pathological LVNC from lesser degrees of trabecular layering seen in those with normal hearts, and in those with LV hypertrophy and cardiomyopathies was tested [71]. Areas of non-compaction were common and occurred more frequently in all groups studied in the apical and lateral, rather than in basal and septal segments as reported in echocardiographic studies. A non-compacted

to compacted ratio of 2.3 in diastole distinguished pathological non- compaction with values for sensitivity and specificity, and positive and negative predictions of 86, 99, 75, and 99 %, respectively. A subsequent study by Jacquier et al. proposed different CMR criteria to diagnose LVNC by measuring the total left ventricular mass and total trabeculated mass in patients with various cardiomyopathies (HCM, DCM, LVNC, and normals) and found that the percentage trabeculated mass in LVNC was 3 times higher than in other subjects. Of key importance, however, was that the compacted mass was not different in normal subjects, DCM and LVNC [72].

A recent paper compared echocardiography and CMR in the evaluation of LVNC, with CMR shown to be superior to echocardiography in the assessment of non-compact myocardium [73].

Fibrosis is seen at post mortem and histologically and may be imaged by CMR using LGE imaging. Recent papers have demonstrated LGE to correlate with disease severity and EF [74]. LGE is seen in 55 % of LVNC subjects averaging approximately 5 % if LV mass, and typically located in the mid wall and RV-LV insertion points.

Conclusion

CMR allows for a comprehensive and single imaging modality to diagnose congenital cardiomyopathies; to differentiate phenotypes, and to provide key prognostic information utilizing high resolution cine imaging, T1 and T2 images, adenosine stress perfusion, and late gadolinium imaging to image and quantify fibrosis. The use and requests for CMR imaging is increasing at a phenomenal rate internationally. Unique insights into disease manifestation and progression are being acquired and in time, CMR should hopefully provide more data on genotype-phenotype correlations beyond what standard imaging currently provides.

13.7 Practical Pearls

- In a single scan setting, CMR can acquire high resolution cine cardiac images with a wide field of view, can tissue characterize to define fat, edema, infarction, fibrosis, and infiltration, and assess epicardial and microvascular blood flow using adenosine perfusion imaging.
- CMR is increasingly appreciated as the gold standard imaging modality of choice in the assessment and risk stratification in inherited cardiomyopathies.
- CMR accurately in a single scan setting diagnoses HCM, outrules HCM phenocopies, and provides novel risk stratification information including the presence and amount of myocardial fibrosis.
- Adenosine perfusion imaging may provide a novel tool to risk stratify inherited cardiomyopathies
- The presence of mid wall fibrosis is an important independent marker of risk in patients with DCM
- CMR imaging has now been incorporated into the new Task force criteria for ARVC, highlighting the important role CMR plays in the assessment of the right ventricle.

References

1. CMR image acquisition protocols. www.scmr.org.
2. Maceira AM, Prasad SK, Khan M, Pennell DJ. Normalized left ventricular systolic and diastolic function by steady state free precession cardiovascular magnetic resonance. J Cardiovasc Magn Reson. 2006;8:417–26.
3. Maceira AM, Prasad SK, Khan M, Pennell DJ. Reference right ventricular systolic and diastolic function normalized to age, gender and body surface area from steady-state free precession cardiovascular magnetic resonance. Eur Heart J. 2006;27:2879–88.
4. Anderson LJ, Holden S, Davis B, et al. Cardiovascular T2-star (*) magnetic resonance for the early diagnosis of myocardial iron overload. Eur Heart J. 2001;21:2171–9.
5. Caruthers SD, Lin SJ, Brown P, et al. Practical value of cardiac magnetic resonance imaging for clinical quantification of aortic valve stenosis. Comparison with echocardiography. Circulation. 2003;108:2236–43.
6. Rademakers FE, Bogaert J. Cardiac dysfunction in heart failure with normal ejection fraction: MRI measurements. Prog Cardiovasc Dis. 2006;49:215–27.
7. Maron BJ, Gardin JM, Flack JM, et al. Prevalence of hypertrophic cardiomyopathy in a general population of young adults: echocardiographic analysis of 4111 subjects in a CARDIA study. Circulation. 1995;92:785–9.
8. Maron BJ, McKenna WJ, Danielson GK, et al. American College of Cardiology/European Society of Cardiology Clinical Expert consensus document on hypertrophic cardiomyopathy. A report of the American College of Cardiology Task Force on clinical expert consensus documents and the European Society of Cardiology Committee for practice guidelines committee to develop an expert consensus document on hypertrophic cardiomyopathy. J Am Coll Cardiol. 2003;42:1687–713.
9. Elliott P, Andersson B, Arbustini E, et al. Classification of the cardiomyopathies: a position statement from the European society of cardiology working group on myocardial and pericardial diseases. Eur Heart J. 2009;29:270–6.
10. Klues HG, Schiffers A, Maron BJ. Phenotypic spectrum and patterns of left ventricular hypertrophy in hypertrophic cardiomyopathy: morphologic observations and significance as assessed by two-dimensional echocardiography in 600 patients. J Am Coll Cardiol. 1995;26:1699–708.
11. Sipola P, Magga J, Husso M, et al. Cardiac MRI assessed left ventricular hypertrophy in differentiating hypertensive heart disease from hypertrophic cardiomyopathy attributable to a sarcomeric gene mutation. Eur Radiol. 2011;21(7):1383–9.
12. Basavarajaiah S, Boraita A, Whyte G, et al. Ethnic differences in left ventricular remodeling in highly-trained athletes relevance to differentiating physiologic left ventricular hypertrophy from hypertrophic cardiomyopathy. J Am Coll Cardiol. 2008;51:2256–62.
13. Rickers C, Wilke NM, Jerosch-Herold M, et al. Utility of cardiac magnetic resonance imaging in the diagnosis of hypertrophic cardiomyopathy. Circulation. 2005;112:855–61.
14. Moon JCC, Fisher NG, McKenna WJ, et al. Detection of apical hypertrophic cardiomyopathy by cardiovascular magnetic resonance in patients with nondiagnostic echocardiography. Heart. 2004;90:645–9.
15. Pennell DJ, Sechtem UP, Higgins CB, et al. Society for cardiovascular magnetic resonance; Working Group on Cardiovascular Magnetic Resonance of the European Society of Cardiology. Clinical indications for cardiovascular magnetic resonance (CMR): consensus panel report. Eur Heart J. 2004;25:1940–65.
16. Smedema JP, van Kroonenburgh JPG, Snoep G, et al. Cardiac sarcoidosis in a patient with hypertrophic cardiomyopathy demonstrated by magnetic resonance imaging and single photon-emission computed tomography dual-isotope scintigraphy. Circulation. 2004;110:e529–31.
17. Elliott PM, Poloniecki J, Dickie S, et al. Sudden death in hypertrophic cardiomyopathy: identification of high risk patients. J Am Coll Cardiol. 2000;36:2212–8.
18. Maron BJ, Shen WK, Link MS, et al. Efficacy of implantable cardioverter-defibrillators for the prevention of sudden death in patients with hypertrophic cardiomyopathy. N Engl J Med. 2000;342:365–73.

19. Maron BJ, Spirito P, Shen W-K, et al. Implantable cardioverter-defibrillators and prevention of sudden cardiac death in hypertrophic cardiomyopathy. JAMA. 2007;298:405–12.

20. Moon JC, McKenna WJ, McCrohan JA, et al. Toward clinical risk assessment in hypertrophic cardiomyopathy with gadolinium cardiovascular magnetic resonance. J Am Coll Cardiol. 2003;41:1561–7.

21. Varnava AM, Elliott PM, Sharma S, et al. Hypertrophic cardiomyopathy: the interrelation of disarray, fibrosis, and small vessel disease. Heart. 2000;84:476–82.

22. Kuribayashi T, Roberts WC. Myocardial disarray at junction of ventricular septum and left and right ventricular free walls in hypertrophic cardiomyopathy. Am J Cardiol. 1992;70:1333–40.

23. Kawara T, Derksen R, de Groot JR, et al. Activation delay after premature stimulation in chronically diseased human myocardium relates to the architecture of interstitial fibrosis. Circulation. 2001;104:3069–75.

24. Adabag AS, Maron BJ, Applebaum E, et al. Occurrence and frequency of arrhythmias in hypertrophic cardiomyopathy in relation to delayed enhancement on cardiovascular magnetic resonance. J Am Coll Cardiol. 2008;51:1369–74.

25. Dimitrow PP, Klimeczek P, Vliegenthart R, et al. Late hyperenhancement in gadolinium-enhanced magnetic resonance imaging: comparison of hypertrophic cardiomyopathy with and without sustained ventricular tachycardia. Int J Cardiovasc Imaging. 2008;24:77–83.

26. Harris KM, Spirito P, Maron MS, et al. Prevalence, clinical profile, and significance of left ventricular remodeling in the end-stage phase of hypertrophic cardiomyopathy. Circulation. 2006;114:216–25.

27. Cecchi F, Olivotto I, Gistri R, et al. Coronary microvascular dysfunction and prognosis in hypertrophic cardiomyopathy. N Engl J Med. 2003;349:1027–35.

28. Olivotto I, Cecci F, Gistri R, et al. Relevance of coronary microvascular flow impairment to long-term remodelling and systolic dysfunction in hypertrophic cardiomyopathy. J Am Coll Cardiol. 2006;47:1043–8.

29. Sipola P, Lauerma K, Husso-Saastamoinen M, et al. First-pass MR imaging in the assessment of perfusion impairment in patients with hypertrophic cardiomyopathy and the Asp175Asn mutation of the alpha-tropomyosin gene. Radiology. 2002;226:129–37.

30. Knaapen P, van Dockum WG, Gotte MJW, et al. Regional heterogeneity of resting perfusion in hypertrophic cardiomyopathy is related to delayed contrast enhancement but not to systolic function: a PET and MRI study. J Nucl Cardiol. 2006;13:660–7.

31. Petersen SE, Jerosch-Herold M, Hudsmith L, et al. Evidence for microvascular dysfunction in hypertrophic cardiomyopathy: new insights from multiparametric magnetic resonance imaging. Circulation. 2007;115:2418–25.

32. Sotgia B, Sciagra R, Olivotto I, et al. Spatial relationship between coronary microvascular dysfunction and delayed contrast enhancement in patients with hypertrophic cardiomyopathy. J Nucl Med. 2008;49:1090–6.

33. Olivotto I, Maron MS, Autore C, et al. Assessment and significance of left ventricular mass by cardiovascular magnetic resonance in hypertrophic cardiomyopathy. J Am Coll Cardiol. 2008;52:559–66.

34. Maron MS, Hauser TH, Dubrow E, et al. Right ventricular involvement in hypertrophic cardiomyopathy. Am J Cardiol. 2007;100:1293–8.

35. Abdel-Aty H, Cocker M, Strohm O, et al. Abnormalities in T2-weighted cardiovascular magnetic resonance images of hypertrophic cardiomyopathy: regional distribution and relation to late gadolinium enhancement and severity of hypertrophy. J Magn Reson Imaging. 2008;28:242–5.

36. O' Hanlon R, Grasso AE, Roughton M, et al. Prognostic significance of myocardial fibrosis in hypertrophic cardiomyopathy. J Am Coll Cardiol. 2010;56(11):867–74.

37. Bruder O, Wagner A, Jensen CJ, et al. Myocardial scar visualized by cardiovascular magnetic resonance imaging predicts major adverse events in patients with hypertrophic cardiomyopathy. J Am Coll Cardiol. 2010;56(11):875–87.

38. Taylor MR, Carniel E, Mestroni L. Cardiomyopathy, familial dilated. Orphanet J Rare Dis. 2006;1:27.

39. Bart BA, Shaw LK, McCants Jr CB, et al. Clinical determinants of mortality in patients with angiographically diagnosed ischemic or nonischemic cardiomyopathy. J Am Coll Cardiol. 1997;30:1002–8.

40. Casolo G, Minneci S, Manta R, et al. Identification of the ischaemic etiology of heart failure by cardiovascular magnetic resonance imaging: diagnostic accuracy of late gadolinium enhancement. Am Heart J. 2006;151:101–8.

41. McCrohon JA, Moon JC, Prasad SK, et al. Differentiation of heart failure related to dilated cardiomyopathy and coronary artery disease using gadolinium-enhanced cardiovascular magnetic resonance. Circulation. 2003;108:54–9.

42. Bulkley BH, Hutchins GM, Baileyy I, et al. Thallium 201 imaging and gated cardiac blood pool scans in patients with ischemic and idiopathic congestive cardiomyopathy: a clinical and pathological study. Circulation. 1977;55:753–60.

43. Barkhausen J, Hunold P, Jochims M, et al. Imaging of myocardial perfusion with magnetic resonance. J Magn Reson Imaging. 2004;19:750–7.

44. Nazarian S, Bluemke DA, Lardo AC, et al. Magnetic resonance assessment of the substrate for inducible ventricular tachycardia in non-ischaemic cardiomyopathy. Circulation. 2005;112:2821–5.

45. Assomull RG, Prasad SK, Lyne J, et al. Cardiovascular magnetic resonance, fibrosis, and prognosis in dilated cardiomyopathy. J Am Coll Cardiol. 2006;48:1977–85.

46. Wu KC, Weiss RG, Thiemann DR, et al. Late gadolinium enhancement by cardiovascular magnetic resonance heralds and adverse prognosis in nonischemic cardiomyopathy. J Am Coll Cardiol. 2008;51:2414–21.

47. Cho JR, Park S, Choi BW, et al. Delayed enhancement magnetic resonance imaging is a significant prognostic factor in patients with non-ischemic cardiomyopathy. Circ J. 2010;74:476–83.

48. Thiene G, Nava A, Corrado D, Rossi L, Pennelli N. Right ventricular cardiomyopathy and sudden death in young people. N Engl J Med. 1988;318:129–33.

49. McKenna WJ, Thiene G, Nava A, et al. Diagnosis of arrhythmogenic right ventricular dysplasia/cardiomyopathy. Task force of the Working Group Myocardial and Pericardial Disease of the European Society of Cardiology and of the Scientific Council on Cardiomyopathies of the International Society and Federation of Cardiology. Br Heart J. 1994;71:215–8.

50. Corrado D, Basso C, Thiene G, et al. Spectrum of clinicopathologic manifestation of arrhythmogenic right ventricular cardiomyopathy/dysplasia: a multicenter study. J Am Coll Cardiol. 1997;6:1512–20.

51. Thiene G, Nava A, Corrado D, et al. Right ventricular cardiomyopathy and sudden death in young people. N Engl J Med. 1988;318:129–33.

52. Casolo G, Di Cesare E, Molinari G, et al. Diagnostic work up of arrhythmogenic right ventricular cardiomyopathy by cardiovascular magnetic resonance (CMR). Consensus statement. Radiol Med (Torino). 2004;108:39–55.

53. Hamid MS, Norman M, Quraishi A, et al. Prospective evaluation of relatives for arrhythmogenic right ventricular cardiomyopathy/dysplasia reveals a need to broaden diagnostic criteria. J Am Coll Cardiol. 2002;40:1445–50.

54. Burke A, Farb A, Tashko G, et al. Arrhythmogenic right ventricular cardiomyopathy and fatty replacement of the right ventricular myocardium: are they different diseases? Circulation. 1998;97:1571–80.

55. Bomma C, Rutberg J, Tandri H, et al. Misdiagnosis of arrhythmogenic right ventricular dysplasia/cardiomyopathy. J Cardiovasc Electrophysiol. 2004;15:300–6.

56. Tandri H, Saranathan M, Rodriguez R, et al. Noninvasive detection of myocardial fibrosis in arrhythmogenic right ventricular cardio-

myopathy using delayed-enhancement magnetic resonance imaging. J Am Coll Cardiol. 2005;45:98–103.

57. Sen-Chowdry S, Prasad SK, Syrris P, et al. Cardiovascular magnetic resonance in arrhythmogenic right ventricular cardiomyopathy revisited: comparison with task force criteria and genotype. J Am Coll Cardiol. 2006;48:2132–40.

58. Sen-Chowdry S, Syrris P, Ward D, et al. Clinical and genetic characterisation of families with arrhythmogenic right ventricular dysplasia/cardiomyopathy provides novel insights into patterns of disease expression. Circulation. 2007;115:1710–20.

59. Marcus FI, McKenna WJ, Sherill D, et al. Diagnosis of arrhythmogenic right ventricular cardiomyopathy/dysplasia. Proposed modification of the task force criteria. Eur Heart J. 2010;31:806–13.

60. Protonotarios N, Anastasakis A, Antoniades L, et al. Arrhythmogenic right ventricular cardiomyopathy/dysplasia on the basis of the revised diagnostic criteria in affected families with desmosomal mutations. Eur Heart J. 2011;32(9):1097–104.

61. Bluemke DA, Krupinski EA, Ovitt T, et al. MRI imaging of arrhythmogenic right ventricular cardiomyopathy: morphological findings and intraobserver reliability. Cardiology. 2003;99:153–62.

62. Jenni R, Wyss CA, Oechslin EN, et al. Isolated ventricular noncompaction is associated with coronary microcirculatory dysfunction. J Am Coll Cardiol. 2002;39(3):450–4.

63. Burke A, Mont E, Kutys MS, et al. Left ventricular noncompaction: a pathological study of 14 cases. Hum Pathol. 2005;36:408–11.

64. Jenni R, Rojas J, Oechslin E. Isolated noncompaction of the myocardium. N Engl J Med. 1999;340:966–7.

65. Oechslin EN, Attenhofer Jost CH, Rojas JR, et al. Long-term follow-up of 34 adults with isolated left ventricular noncompaction: a distinct cardiomyopathy with poor prognosis. J Am Coll Cardiol. 2000;36:493–500.

66. Lewin M. Left ventricular noncompaction: travelling the road from diagnosis to outcomes. J Am Soc Echocardiogr. 2010;23:54–7.

67. Chin TK, Perloff JK, Williams RG, et al. Isolated noncompaction of left ventricular myocardium. A study of eight cases. Circulation. 1990;82:507–13.

68. Jenni R, Oechslin E, Schneider J, et al. Echocardiographic and pathoanatomical characteristics of isolated left ventricular noncompaction: a step towards classification as a distinct cardiomyopathy. Heart. 2001;86:666–71.

69. Stollberger C, Finsterer J, Blazek G. Left ventricular hypertrabeculation/noncompaction and association with additional cardiac abnormalities and neuromuscular disorders. Am J Cardiol. 2002;90:899–902.

70. Kohli SK, Pantazis AA, Shah JS, et al. Diagnosis of left-ventricular non-compaction in patients with left-ventricular systolic dysfunction: time for a reappraisal of diagnostic criteria? Eur Heart J. 2007;29:89–95.

71. Petersen SE, Selvanayagam JB, Wiesmann F, et al. Left ventricular non-compaction: insights from cardiovascular magnetic resonance imaging. J Am Coll Cardiol. 2005;46:101–5.

72. Jacquier A, Thuny F, Jop B, et al. Measurement of trabeculated left ventricular mass using cardiac magnetic resonance imaging in the diagnosis of left ventricular noncompaction. Eur Heart J. 2010;31:1098–104.

73. Thunt F, Jacquier A, Jop B, et al. Assessment of left ventricular non-compaction in adults: side-by-side comparison of cardiac magnetic resonance imaging with echocardiography. Arch Cardiovasc Dis. 2010;103:150–9.

74. Nucifora G, Aquaro GD, Pingitore A, et al. Myocardial fibrosis in isolated left ventricular non-compaction and its relation to disease severity. Eur Heart J. 2011;13:170–6.

Coronary Artery Anomalies

Andrew M. Crean

14.1 Introduction

Anomalies of the coronary arteries are paradoxically amongst the simplest and most difficult of subjects to get to grips with in congenital heart disease. Disconcertingly, even the definition of what constitutes an 'anomalous' vessel has been disputed in the past. Prevalence data for coronary anomalies vary widely between published reports, undoubtedly reflecting institutional bias and degree of enthusiasm for the topic.

Whilst the identification of one of the many published anomalies is rarely difficult with modern imaging methods, the clinical relevance of the uncovered abnormality is often unclear, forcing patients and their physicians to live with an unsettling degree of uncertainty at times [1–3].

The purpose of this chapter is first to establish what is meant by normal and anomalous coronary anatomy, then to describe the principal subtypes of anomaly and finally to review the strengths and weaknesses of potentially applicable CMR imaging protocols.

14.2 Definition

Recognition of 'abnormal' assumes knowledge of 'normal' – a statement which appears facile but reflects the debate that has occurred on this topic. Leonardo da Vinci (1452–1519) was perhaps amongst the first to publish a description of normal coronary anatomy in which he described not only separate right and left coronary ostia but also pointed out that the normal coronary tree diminishes progressively in size from base of the heart to apex [4].

Works by other authors from a similar period in history, however, elaborated on cases with single coronary arteries

and it would not be for another 200 years before Morgagni would clearly establish the normality of a dual coronary system in the human [5]. A further leap forward occurred in the 60s with the advent of selective invasive coronary angiography and subsequent publications on coronary variants and anomalies in large cohorts.

Finally, the era of multi-detector row computed tomography (MDCT) has opened Pandora's box with significant numbers of coronary artery anomalies (CAAs) being uncovered for the first time in adult patients with widely varying degrees of symptomatology (and in some cases, no symptoms at all).

Angelini et al. suggested over 20 years ago that recognition of CAAs must stem from an appreciation of normal coronary anatomy and proposed a number of guiding principles for the definition of this [6]. These remain valid today:

(a) A coronary artery is defined as any artery or arterial branch that carries blood to the cardiac parenchyma.

(b) The name and nature of a coronary artery or branch is defined by that vessel's distal vascularization territory, not by its origin.

(c) The sinuses of Valsalva are identified not by the coronary arteries but rather by their own topographic location.

(d) 'Normal' should mean 'what is commonly observed'

(e) 'Abnormal' or 'anomalous' should be employed for any form observed in less than 1 % of the general (human) population. Thus, an abnormality which occurs in a population with an observed frequency of greater than 1 % is better described as a (normal) variant than an anomaly.

(f) Classification schemes are helpful for cataloguing CAAs but not for clinical prognostication.

(g) Normally (i.e. in >1 %) the human coronary arteries have 2 or 3 coronary ostia.

(h) The proximal segment of a coronary artery arises at a nearly orthogonal angle from the aortic wall.

A.M. Crean, M.D., B.Sc., BM, MRCP, M.Sc., FRCR, M.Phil. (✉)
Departments of Medicine (Cardiology) & Medical Imaging,
Peter Munk Cardiac Center, Toronto General Hospital,
585 University Avenue, Toronto, ON M5G 2C4, Canada
e-mail: crean67@hotmail.com

Electronic supplementary material The online version of this chapter (doi:10.1007/978-1-4471-4267-6_14) contains supplementary material, which is available to authorized users.

(i) The coronary ostia are typically equal to, or larger in size, than the proximal segment of the related coronary artery.

(j) The course of the coronary arteries is mostly epicardial.

(k) The coronary arteries normally terminate in the capillary network.

(l) All myocardial segments should have a congenitally adequate arterial circulation with respect to basal and exercise requirements.

14.3 Morphology

Many complex classification schemes bedevil this topic – a nice summary was recently published by Jacobs et al. [7]. A simplified structure for the classification of anomalies is best provided by a simple three part framework – (1) anomalies of origin, (2) anomalies of course and (3) anomalies of termination. Although this scheme provides anatomic neatness it has little bearing on the clinical importance of selected anomalies as will be discussed below. Nonetheless it is an appropriate starting point.

14.4 Associated Anomalies

Coronary artery anomalies may occur alone or in conjunction with other cardiac abnormalities and malformations. Most commonly an incidental recognition of an anomaly in an otherwise well individual is usually an isolated finding. Several important anomalies occur reliably in association with major congenital malformations. These range from the clockwise rotation of the aortic root common to most cases of tetralogy of Fallot to the varied coronary patterns (including single coronary artery) associated with transposition of the great arteries as well as the coronary-cameral fistulas seen in children with pulmonary atresia with intact interventricular septum (PA-IVS) [8].

Not surprisingly there is a moderate association with aortic valve disease in up to 20 % of cases of coronary anomaly in angiographic series [9] and it is possible that this represents an underestimate of the true incidence of associated valvular pathology. Prospective registries with newer cross-sectional imaging techniques will be ideally placed to resolve this [10].

Coronary abnormalities may also be seen in heart muscle disease, principally hypertrophic cardiomyopathy (HCM) in which an excessive degree of myocardial bridging is not infrequently seen. This is more correctly regarded as a variant than an anomaly since it occurs with a frequency well in excess of 1 %. Bridging has been claimed to result in demonstrable myocardial ischemia in the absence of atherosclerotic disease [11]. Although coronary 'milking' is a systolic phenomenon there is evidence to suggest impact on diastolic coronary flow also [12]. On occasion this may be sufficiently severe as to warrant surgery.

Sometimes overlooked, also, are the *acquired* coronary anomalies, including aneurysms, that may develop as a result of systemic illness particularly Behcet's and Kawasaki's diseases. Although not congenital (except perhaps by virtue of genetic predisposition), they are likely to be encountered by most CMR imagers and are included here for completeness.

14.5 Clinical Presentation

The frequency of CAAs is debated and it seems likely that many individuals with coronary anomalies never present during their lifetime. The literature is biased with series of either otherwise healthy individuals who experienced sudden cardiac death or those with symptoms of myocardial ischemia. The diagnosis is established in some cases by invasive angiography and in others by autopsy alone. Extreme populations are often over represented (for example military recruits or athletes who undergo extreme levels of conditioning and physical exertion) making it difficult to know whether outcomes in these groups are truly representative of those in the general (more sedentary) population with the same or similar anomaly [13–15]. The one consistent finding, however, has been that there is a higher incidence of coronary anomalies in victims of sudden death than is seen in *routine* autopsy series [16, 17]. It is this fact that generates the most angst for physicians attempting to counsel these patients.

One retrospective surgical series of 36 patients documented preoperative symptoms of angina, shortness of breath or syncope in 81 % but importantly, abnormalities of perfusion were only identifiable in 43 % [18]. In contrast another small series demonstrated inducible perfusion defects by nuclear perfusion imaging in 80 % of subjects with an interarterial vessel [19]. However, it is the lack of reproducible ischemia in survivors of sudden cardiac death with known coronary anomalies that has led to some arguing in favor of surgical repair upon identification, regardless of stress test results. This is held to be particularly true for anomalous left coronary artery from the opposite sinus (ALCAOS) which appears to have a much stronger association with sudden death than its counterpart anomalous right coronary artery from the opposite sinus (ARCAOS) [2]. There is generally a lower threshold for operating on asymptomatic children than there is in adults unless myocardial ischemia can be demonstrated.

At the Texas Heart Institute almost 2,000 angiograms were reviewed for evidence of CAA. In this study approximately 5 % of men and 8 % of women had an identifiable anomaly [9]. The commonest anomalies were as shown in Table 14.1.

Thus a total of 5.6 % of the sample had an identifiable CAA – a much higher figure than the 1.3 % detected in the large angiographic series from the Cleveland Clinic [20]. Furthermore, in a recent paper from the Netherlands looking at a little under 2,000 patients examined by dual source CT,

Table 14.1 Frequency of coronary anomalies in the Texas Heart Institute angiographic series [9]

Anomaly	Percentage
Ectopic RCA from left cusp	0.92
Fistulas	0.87
Absent left main coronary artery	0.67
Circumflex arising from the right cusp	0.67
Left coronary artery from the right cusp	0.15
Low origin of the RCA	0.1
Other anomalies	0.27

the incidence of anomalies was identical to the Cleveland angiographic series at 1.3 % [21]. Thus the true incidence of coronary anomalies remains uncertain and is a question likely to be answered by large CT registries in the future.

14.6 How Good is CMR for the Detection of Anomalous Coronary Vessels?

14.6.1 Anomalies of Origin

These are generally simple to identify by CMR since the vessels are usually of a reasonable size and the number of options for their origin is relatively limited. By far the commonest abnormality is origin of one coronary from the opposite sinus. Careful imaging of the aortic root with thin slice cine, black blood or angiographic images usually uncovers the abnormality in a matter of minutes. Slightly more challenging are rarer coronary origins such as that of the left or right coronary artery from the pulmonary artery. The first clue to the presence of this condition is the unusually dilated nature of most

of the coronary arterial branches – enlarged because of increased volume flow as blood passes down a pressure gradient from the coronary with an aortic origin to that connecting to the pulmonary artery. Multiple small fistulous branches anastomose between left and right coronary systems including septal branches, giving the appearances of twinkling lights or 'Christmas tree septum' on Doppler echocardiography. Once recognized, the search for the coronary origin from the pulmonary artery is then straightforward.

The other very rare anomalies of origin cannot be dealt with here. Suffice it to say that most CMR practitioners may never encounter one in an entire career. However the best way of ensuring that a rare anomaly (coronary or otherwise) is not missed is to ensure that every CMR protocol includes full thoracic coverage in either axial, sagittal or coronal planes (or all three) with thin slice overlapping SSFP single shot single phase acquisitions. These can be run in quiet respiration and are a very rapid method of acquiring a comprehensive overview of the heart and great vessels.

14.6.2 Anomalies of Course

At this point it is appropriate to consider what precisely is meant by an 'anomalous' coronary course. When a coronary artery arises anomalously it may travel along four principal courses and these are not all of equal clinical importance. The vessel may pass:

(a) inter-arterially between the aorta and pulmonary trunk (Fig. 14.1);
(b) retro-aortic (Fig. 14.2);
(c) trans-septal (Fig. 14.3) i.e. the proximal portion is tunneled through the septal myocardium (below the level of the pulmonary valve) or

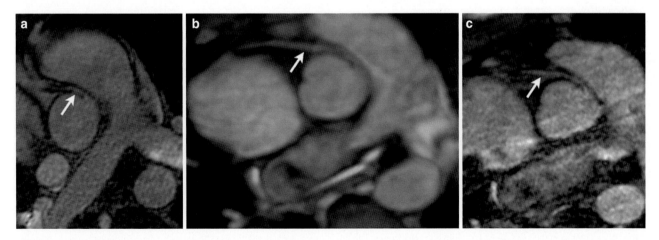

Fig. 14.1 Inter-arterial course of the right coronary artery. The right coronary artery (*arrow*, all three panels) can be identified originating from the contra-lateral sinus. SSFP cine imaging (**a**) alone is often adequate for identification of inappropriate sinus origin – performed here with a voxel size of 1.0 × 1.0 × 3 mm. Whole heart coronary MRA (**b**) demonstrates the same finding in this patient with clarity achieved by a 1.5 × 1.5 × 1.5 mm voxel size. The relationship of the proximal vessel to the aortic wall (intramural course – see text) is however more clearly defined with higher resolution MRA images (**c**) acquired at an isotropic 1.0 mm resolution

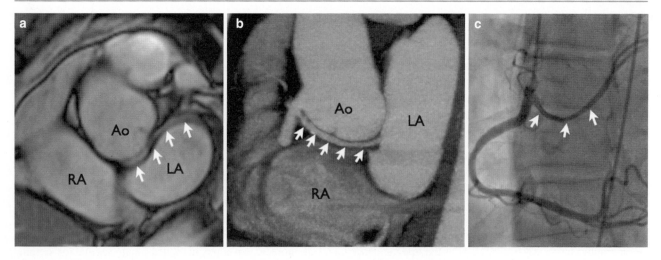

Fig. 14.2 Retro-aortic course of the circumflex artery (arrows a–c). A vessel (*arrows*) can be seen to take an unusual course infero-posterior to the aortic root on the freeze frame from a short axis SSFP cine stack (**a**). Cardiac-gated tomography (**b**) in the same patient clearly shows its origin from the right coronary artery. Although this anomalous vessel is readily identified by catheter angiography (**c**) its 3 dimensional course in space is much more clearly understood by a cross sectional technique. *Ao* aorta; *LA* left atrium; *RA* right atrium

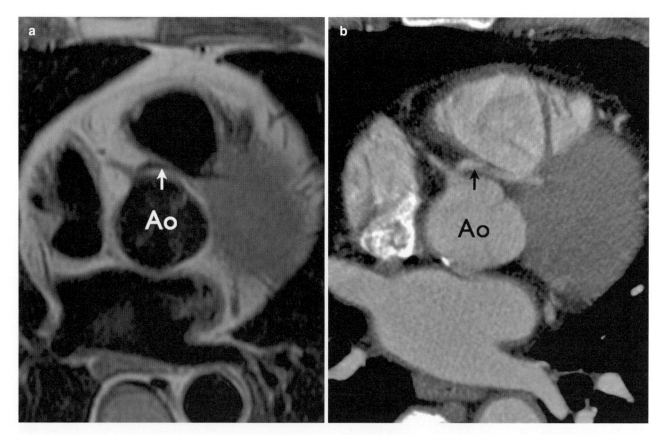

Fig. 14.3 Trans-septal course of the left main coronary artery. The left main coronary vessel (*arrow*) arises from a common ostium with the right coronary artery. Note however that it is clearly extramural in relation to the aortic root. It passes anterior to the aorta below the level of the pulmonary valve and dives into septal myocardium prior to gaining a normal position in the anterior interventricular groove. A simple double inversion black blood technique (**a**) demonstrates the abnormality every bit as clearly as the companion slice from a cardiac-gated CT scan (**b**). Ao=aorta

position for the subsequent whole heart acquisition. The navigator pulse takes approximately 40 ms to run.

14.10.3 Fat Saturation Pulse

The coronary arteries are surrounded by epicardial fat which is usually high signal on many cMRA pulse sequences. In order to reduce this signal a fat suppression pre-pulse is commonly applied prior to data acquisition. There is a spectral shift of approximately 3.5 ppm between lipid and water and this can be exploited to either saturate the lipid signal or instead selectively excite the water molecules to emphasize the signal within the coronary arteries. It should be noted that the distal coronary tree which is less often surrounded by fat benefits more from T2 preparation than from fat saturation per se.

14.10.4 Data Acquisition Window

The requirement to 'freeze' coronary motion during image acquisition necessitates identification of that portion of the cardiac cycle when the coronary arteries appear relatively static. Since the RCA typically exhibits a wider arc of motion than the left coronary system, this vessel is usually employed as a marker to identify the coronary rest period.

A 4 chamber cine SSFP image of the heart can be used which, when 'stepped through' frame by frame, allows recognition of the first time point at which RCA motion stops and the duration (in ms) until it begins moving again Movie (14.3). This determines the period of time during each end-expiratory cardiac cycle that the operator will set for data acquisition during the whole heart MRA itself. The data acquisition window can in theory equal the coronary rest period, which at slow heart rates may be as long as 150 ms. In practice, and at the more typical higher patient heart rates, an acquisition window of 50–60 ms usually produces excellent results. An incorrect selection of window starting point or duration will of course introduce coronary motion during data acquisition with predictable and uninterpretable results.

For fine tuning of the window at higher heart rates it may be necessary to use a 4 chamber scout with a higher than normal temporal resolution. For example reducing the temporal resolution of the cine image to 10 ms frames and reconstructing 80 phases rather than the more typical 35–50 ms reconstructed at 25 phases, permits very accurate delineation of the coronary rest period which would otherwise be difficult to achieve Movie (14.4). (However, achieving this kind of temporal resolution with adequate spatial resolution in a single breath hold requires the use of 3–4 times acceleration with parallel imaging).

Finally it should be remembered that diastolic length is a function of heart rate. As heart rate increases systole remains unchanged in duration but diastole shrinks. Above 80 bpm there may be little or no available diastolic rest period in which to image. In this case we have learned from our contemporaries in the cardiac CT world that – with a sufficiently short acquisition window of around 50 ms – good images may be acquired in late systole when there is also a brief period of coronary rest. Although it is seldom done in clinical practice, the use of betablockers and sublingual nitrate is as pertinent to coronary MRA as it is to CTA.

With close attention to the foregoing details, the results from whole heart MRA are sometimes gratifyingly good (Fig. 14.9). Unlike other methods of visualizing the coronary arteries, whole heart MRA also has the advantage that the data set is an isotropic volume which can therefore be displayed in a number of ways, like cardiac CT, including multiplanar reformats, curved reformats and center line extractions (Fig. 14.10).

14.11 Stress CMR for Coronary Anomalies

Since the relevant clinical endpoint for patients with coronary anomalies is sudden cardiac death, and since the mechanism is assumed to be ischemia-induced ventricular arrhythmia or infarction it appears logical to extend the role of CMR beyond the simple identification of a coronary anomaly and seek to uncover the underlying ischemic pathophysiology as well. Despite the logic of this approach there has been surprisingly little published in this area using CMR as the primary tool.

CMR, nonetheless, is ideally suited to the task. Both dobutamine and vasodilator stress CMR have been validated in the setting of adult coronary disease and neither poses a significant technical challenge in congenital heart disease. The unobstructed field of view and lack of ionizing radiation are both major benefits of a CMR-led approach to ischemia detection in this relatively young population who have – at times – complex and confusing anatomy.

The only paper in the literature to deal specifically with stress MRI and coronary anomaly relates to coronary surveillance for asymptomatic children and young adults following arterial switch surgery for transposition of the great arteries, a situation in which there has been concern regarding asymptomatic but significant post-operative distortion of the proximal coronary vessels. The authors reported high technical success rates with no detectable ischemia under adenosine stress [25]. We have had a similar experience at the Toronto General Hospital where we also make routine efforts to image the proximal coronary tree by either whole heart MRA or targeted thin slice cine imaging.

Similarly, there is almost no published experience with dobutamine stress MR for coronary anomalies although it has been applied to other questions in the congenital field. One paper in

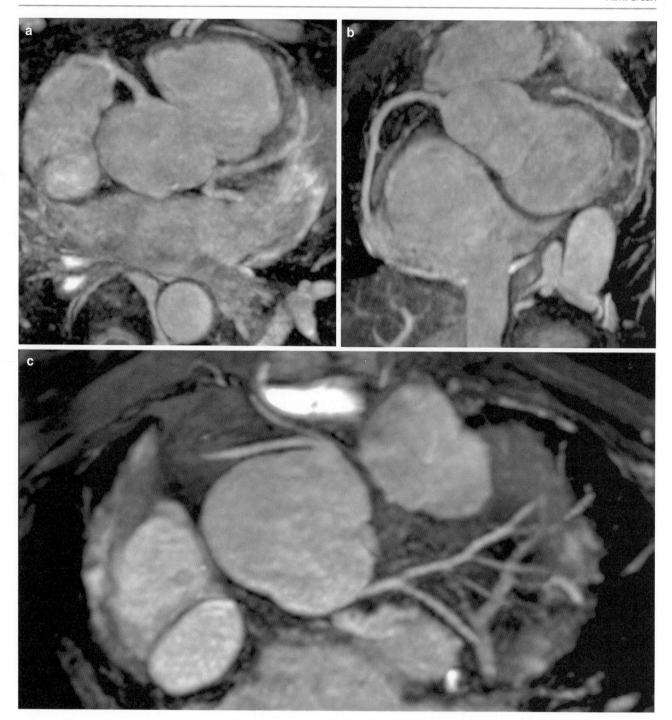

Fig. 14.9 Examples of successful whole heart coronary MRA. Three separate examples (**a–c**) of good coronary definition achieved with use of a whole heart technique. Note that although the presence of gadolinium contrast agent is not required for the SSFP-based whole heart sequence used at 1.5 T, where present in the blood pool it tends to produce slightly better image quality and our practice is therefore to run this sequence after the usual late gadolinium enhancement images have been acquired

the last few years reported high technical success rates with an aggressive protocol that involved graded infusion of dobutamine up to 40 mcg/kg/min plus atropine as done in standard stress echocardiography [26]. However a new wall motion abnormality was identified in only 1 out of 32 studies in a relatively heterogeneous congenital patient cohort. It is worth noting that two

thirds of the studies were performed under general anesthesia. In the author's experience, high dose dobutamine stress is often less well tolerated by patients than vasodilator stress and is more complicated to perform in the magnet environment.

Finally the technique of late gadolinium enhancement which is now accepted as the reference standard for the

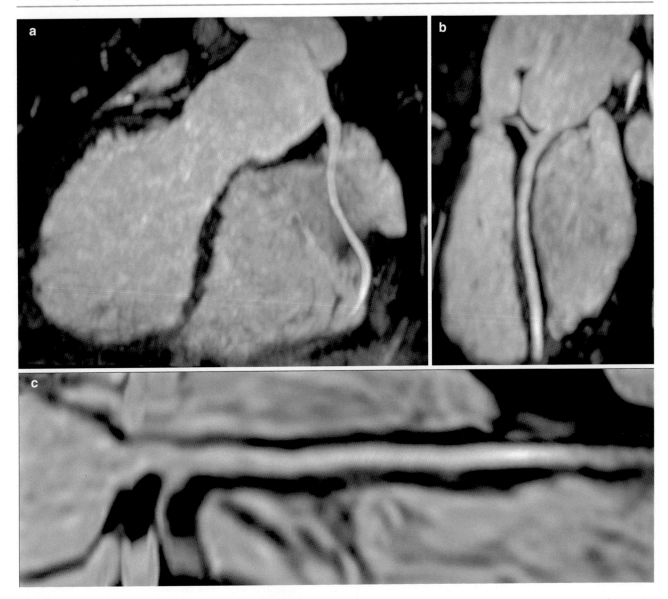

Fig. 14.10 Post-processing of the volumetric data set. Since whole heart acquisitions are usually 3D isotropic volume acquisitions they may be post-processed in just the same way that thin slice CT data sets can be. This includes production of multiplanar coronary reformats (**a**, **b**) as well as straightened center line extractions (**c**)

identification of myocardial viability clearly merits incorporation into a standard CMR protocol for coronary assessment since infarction is assumed to be one of the modes of morbidity and patient attrition.

14.12 The Comprehensive CMR Examination in Suspected Coronary Anomalies

In general there are three main categories of coronary anomaly patient; those in whom an anomaly is suspected; those in whom an anomaly has been surgically repaired; and those in whom the discovery of an anomaly is incidental during a study performed for another purpose. The aim of the

examination must therefore be tailored to some extent to the background history and the current clinical question under consideration.

In general, a minimum CMR exam should include assessment of the coronary origin and proximal course adequate to categorize the anomaly as either high risk (interarterial, ALCAPA, ARCAPA) or a lower risk group (prepulmonic, retroaortic, intraseptal etc.). Coronary aneurysms should be excluded in patients with childhood Kawasaki disease – a situation where CMR has been proved to be as accurate as catheter angiography [27] – or adult Behcet's disease (Figs. 14.11 and 14.12). Coronary narrowing may be ostial as a result of re-implantation following the arterial switch procedure, Ross operation or Bentall procedure or may occur due to

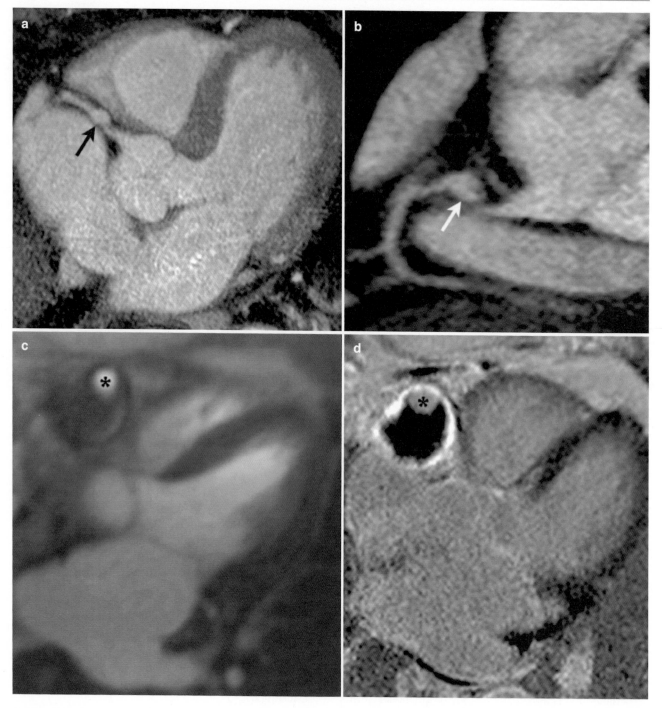

Fig. 14.11 CMR in Kawasaki Disease. Patient 1 has a small proximal right coronary artery aneurysm (*arrows*, **a**, **b**) that is well delineated by coronary MRA. Patient 2 has a much larger aneurysm lying in the right atrioventricular groove (**c**, **d**). Dynamic perfusion CMR (**c**) demonstrates an enlarged but centrally patent portion of the aneurysm (*aster-* *isk*) which represents the ectatic right coronary artery. Late gadolinium enhancement images (**d**) reveal low signal thrombus posterior to the lumen. Note also the circumferential enhancement surrounding the aneurysm (**d**) which hints at the inflammatory etiology of the lesion

enlargement of adjacent vascular structures – this latter situation is sometimes encountered in the tetralogy variant with absent pulmonary valve when gross pulmonary arterial enlargement is the norm and can result in left main or left anterior descending coronary compression (Fig. 14.13 and Movie 14.5).

Since myocardial infarction is a recognized complication both of many anomalies as well as a possible iatrogenic sequela of surgery, assessment of ventricular function and myocardial scar can also be considered mandatory Movie (14.6, Fig. 14.14).

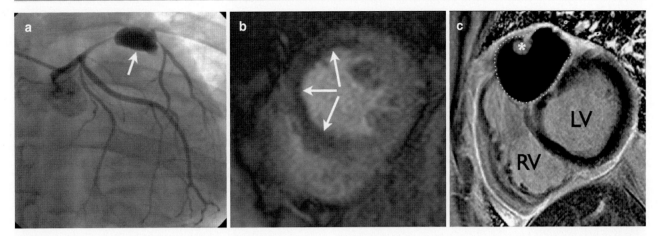

Fig. 14.12 CMR in Behcet Disease. Coronary angiography (**a**) shows a large aneurysm involving the mid portion of the left anterior descending coronary artery in this patient with confirmed Behcet disease. The vessel appears to taper both on its entrance into and exit from the aneurysm. The physiological significance of this is confirmed by adenosine stress perfusion cardiac MRI (**b**) in which a substantial perfusion defect is visible in the antero-septum (*white arrows*). Late enhancement imaging (**c**) reveals a large portion of the aneurysm to contain low signal thrombus with a central patent core (*asterisk*) representing the native vessel. *LV* left ventricle; *RV* right ventricle

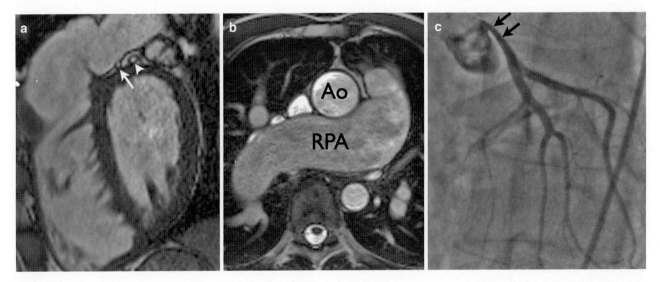

Fig. 14.13 Compression of the left main coronary artery. This rare complication was seen in a patient with the tetralogy-absent pulmonary valve complex. In this condition life long absence of the pulmonary valve results in severe pulmonary arterial enlargement. This 55 year old manual worker presented with typical angina and subsequently had a strongly positive treadmill exercise test. Cine SSFP demonstrates his left main coronary artery (*arrow*, **a**) to be compressed between the undersurface of the main and right pulmonary artery (**b**) and the heart. The left anterior descending portion (**a**, *arrowhead*) appears spared. Catheter angiography confirms significant extrinsic compression of the left main (*arrows*, **c**). Left main osteoplasty and pulmonary arterial plication was performed at open heart surgery with subsequent full relief of symptoms. *Ao* aorta; *RPA* right pulmonary artery

In some instances there may be a more specific clinical question relating to known pre-existing anatomy and planned percutaneous intervention. In patients with tetralogy of Fallot and significant pulmonary insufficiency, for example, an increasingly important role for CMR is to establish the relationship between the site of 'touchdown' for a percutaneous pulmonary valve in the main pulmonary artery and any adjacent coronary artery which might be at risk of compression by stent placement (Fig. 14.15).

14.13 Unoperated CAA

Unoperated patients may be particularly challenging since the question usually concerns not only the course of the anomalous artery but its physiological consequences in the form of myocardial ischemia or volume loading of a ventricle due to shunt flow. Standard anomalies of origin or course will not cause shunting (since termination is normal), although may cause ischemia. As discussed there is little practical experience

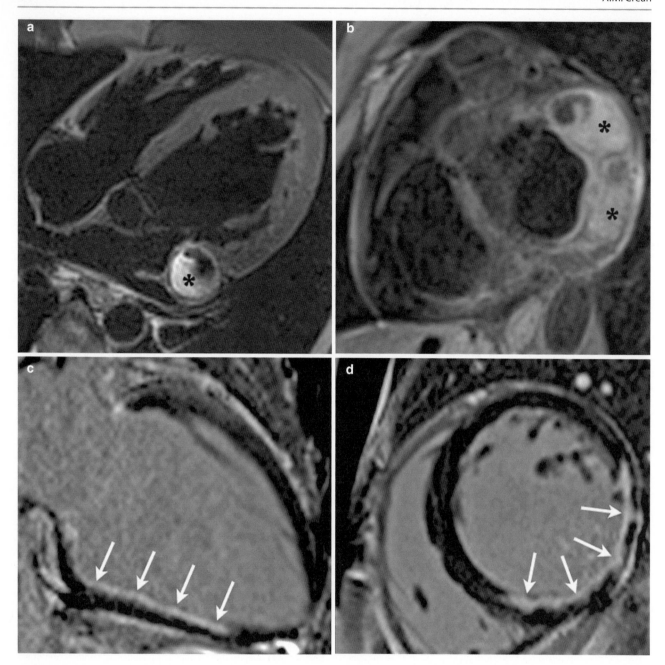

Fig. 14.14 Example of myocardial scar secondary to Kawasaki's disease. Several large aneurysms are evident in the left atrio-ventricular groove (**a**, **b**, *asterisks*). These inflammatory aneurysms contain thrombus which has the potential to embolize distally. This has occurred in this patient whose late enhancement (LGE) imaging depicts a subendo-cardial area of infarction in the inferolateral wall (**c**, **d**, *arrows*). This was unknown prior to the CMR exam and highlights the importance of including LGE imaging as part of the CMR protocol in congenital or inflammatory coronary disease

and no consensus on whether CMR is adequate for the detection of ischemia using any method in these cases. The three most common lesions leading to shunting as well as possible ischemia are the RCA to coronary sinus fistula, the ALCAPA and the ARCAPA anomalies. The ALCAPA lesion is only rarely encountered de novo in an adult patient [28–31].

However its 'sister' lesion – ARCAPA – is less often life threatening and occasionally presents for the first time in adult life. Either lesion results in a bulk steal of blood from the contrary coronary artery down a diastolic pressure gradient from the aortic root to the pulmonary artery. The coronary arteries generally become severely dilated as a consequence of significantly increased flow and increased size and tortuosity of coronary vessels is a sign that a coronary shunt lesion should be expected Movie (14.6). Since multiple collateral pathways exist in this type of lesion it is

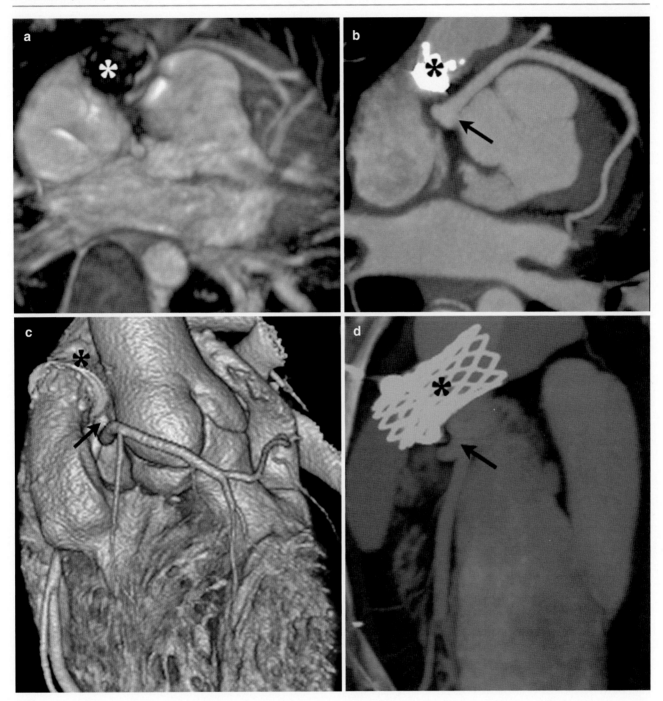

Fig. 14.15 Suboptimal coronary visualization at CMR due to metal stent. This patient required re-stenting of an RV conduit which had previously been stented. One of the concerns of conduit stenting is any possible compression effect on adjacent coronary arteries. The origin of the anomalous left coronary artery (*arrow*) shown in (**a**) was obscured by susceptibility artifact from the adjacent pre-existing stent (*asterisk*). This is one situation in which switching to cardiac CT is required – the relationship of the vessel to the conduit pre re-stenting (**b**) and post re-stenting (**c**, **d**) is clearly appreciated

also common for the smaller intramyocardial vessels to be dilated and this is usually most obvious in the interventricular septum (Fig. 14.16). Again there is little experience with stress CMR in these clinical conditions and in our experience with vasodilator stress the result is generally negative, although this has not been the universal experience.

14.14 Operated CAA

Surgical repair of coronary anomalies depends on the nature of the anomaly itself [32]. Interarterial left main or LAD lesions are generally treated with coronary artery bypass for which follow up is conventional and generally beyond the

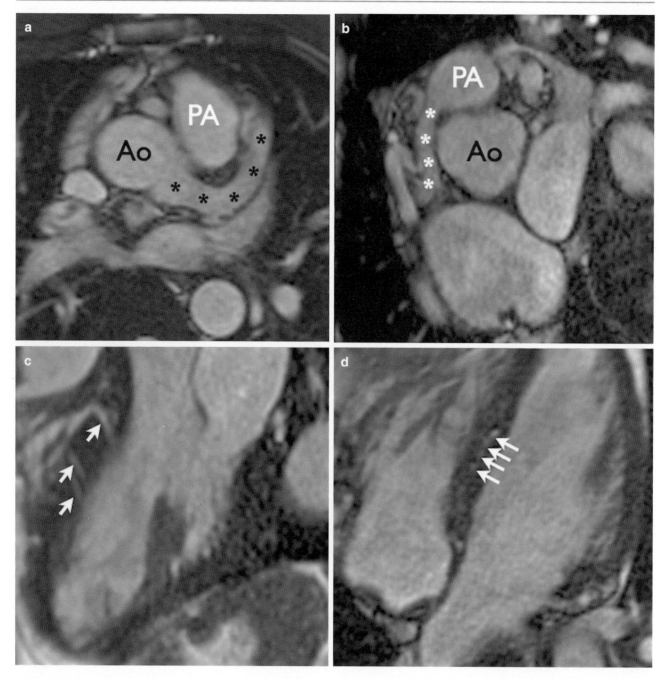

Fig. 14.16 Anomalous right coronary artery from the pulmonary artery. The left main and left anterior descending coronary arteries (**a**, *asterisks*) are severely dilated. This is often a clue that there is a high pressure to low pressure shunt with high volume flow occurring down a pressure gradient. This is seen to be true on the short axis SSFP image (**b**) where the right coronary artery (*asterisks*) is observed to drain into the pulmonary artery (*PA*) rather than arise from the aorta (*Ao*). Multiple dilated collateral networks connect the left and right coronary systems, most often visible in the interventricular septum (**c**, **d**, *arrows*)

scope of CMR except perhaps for assessment of LV function and myocardial perfusion. Only a true enthusiast would endeavour to image the bypassed coronary circulation by MRI instead of CT or conventional angiography although the potential for this has been demonstrated by several groups [33–35].

Repaired ARCAPA/ALCAPA or coronary artery to coronary sinus fistula lesions are, however, eminently suitable for follow up by CMR. The chief focus of interest is the anastomotic site of the re-implanted anomalous artery into the aortic root since in some cases there may be asymptomatic post-surgical distortion or even atresia of the proximal vessel with demonstrable ischemia and/or scar (Fig. 14.17).

14.15 When the Going Gets Tough

Although the preference at our institution is to perform whole heart MRA for most coronary anomalies, simple cine SSFP or black blood imaging is acceptable where the principal question relates to the proximal course of the artery. At times,

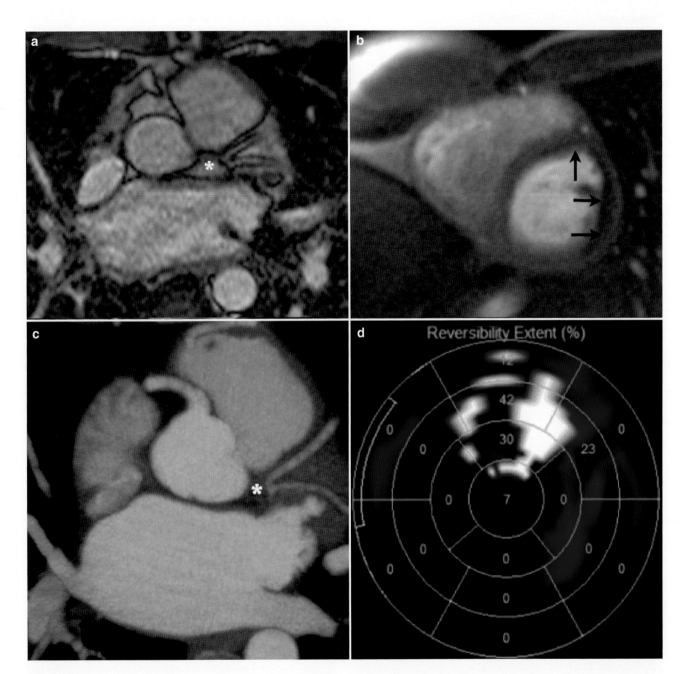

Fig. 14.17 Post operative chronic ischemia following ALCAPA repair. Routine imaging in this young adult following infantile repair of anomalous left coronary artery from the pulmonary artery (ALCAPA) demonstrated unexpected absence of the left main coronary segment (**a**, *asterisk*). Cardiac CT (**c**) was equally unable to visualize the re-implanted left main segment at the aortic origin (*asterisk*). Stress perfusion CMR (**b**) and technetium MIBI (**d**) both confirmed the presence of a large area of reversible ischemia (arrows in (**b**)). The patient has been offered surgical revascularization

Table 14.3 Relative merits of imaging modalities in the assessment of coronary anomalies

	CMR	Cardiac CT	Echo	Invasive angiography
Spatial resolution	Good	Excellent	Excellent	Excellent
Temporal resolution	Good	Fair	Excellent	Excellent
Potential morbidity	Low	Low	None[a]	High
Coronary visibility	Good	Excellent	Poor (except children)	Excellent
Coronary course	Good to Excellent	Excellent	Poor	Fair/Difficult
Coronary origins	Excellent	Excellent	Fair (except children)	Excellent
Demonstration of small fistulae	Fair	Good	Fair	Excellent
Demonstration of large fistulae	Excellent	Excellent	Fair	Fair (often incomplete opacification)
Wall motion abnormalities	Excellent	Fair	Excellent	Good
Scar demonstration	Excellent	Poor	Poor	Poor
Perfusion abnormality	Excellent	Not established	Good	Fair
Radiation exposure	None	Low to moderate[b]	None	Moderate
Dependence on patient window for image quality	None	Low (noise if obese)	High	Low
Suitability for sick patients or those unable to breath hold	Poor	Good	Excellent	Good to excellent
Identification of coronary thrombus	Excellent	Excellent	Poor	Poor
Claustrophobia	Can be problematic	Rarely problematic	Not problematic	Not problematic
Presence of metal	Can be problematic	Rarely problematic	Not problematic	Not problematic

[a]Unless intravenous contrast given
[b]Low if a prospective trigger technique is used, moderate if retrospective gating applied

however, it can be difficult to comment on ostial narrowing or fully comprehend the course of complex tortuous fistulas even with good quality coronary MRA and cine imaging – and in those instances prompt transfer of the patient to the cardiac CT scanner is a wise action rather than a nihilistic expression of defeat [36]!

14.16 Limitations of CMR and Considerations for Imaging Coronary Anomalies

As Mark Twain is reported (without evidence) to have said: "to a man with a hammer everything looks like a nail". However, no handyman relies upon a single tool and the same should apply to the cardiac imager. CMR may not always be the modality of choice to assess all cases of coronary anomaly and the multiple multi-modality figures provided in this chapter speak for themselves in this regard.

Selection between CMR, CT, catheter angiography, echo etc. depends partly on the age of the patient, partly on the question being asked and partly also on the physical condition of the patient. For example young children are considered highly radiosensitive such that echo or CMR would usually be the preferred methods of investigation.

In contrast a sick patient or claustrophobic patient, or one immediately post-operative in whom a surgical complication is suspected, may not tolerate the prolonged examination times common to CMR. In this situation cardiac CT may be quicker and kinder as well as less susceptible to breathing artifacts. On the other hand if an assessment of myocardial perfusion or scar is required nuclear medicine or CMR are the modalities of choice.

Finally the presence of metallic coils, calcified conduits or stents within the thorax may limit the visibility of the coronary arteries by CMR and cardiac CT is usually an excellent alternative in this situation (Fig. 14.15).

Points to consider in selection of the most appropriate technique for depiction of a coronary anomaly and its potential consequences are given in Table 14.3.

Conclusion

Coronary anomalies may appear to be one of the more arcane topics for the CMR practitioner but they appear surprisingly often in any busy cardiac practice and a working knowledge of the principal types of anomaly is essential. Most anomalies are straightforward to image without great technical prowess or advanced imaging techniques. Ventricular function, myocardial perfusion and scar are often intrinsic parts of the patient assessment since it is these aspects that in many cases will dictate subsequent management.

14.17 Practical Pearls

Standard imaging sequences will likely be adequate for the demonstration of a coronary anomaly in more than 90 % of patients but if you do perform coronary MRA then consider:

1. Coronary MRA requires a high degree of physician involvement at the scanner. If you delegate the study acquisition to an unsupervised technologist then expect poor quality images unless you have extremely experienced CMR technologists.
2. A whole heart approach is often easier for the novice than a targeted approach
3. A high temporal resolution cine scout for identifying the coronary rest period more than repays the small time investment required to perform it.
4. Select a relatively narrow data acquisition window – no more than 70 ms at heart rates of 65 bpm or less and <50 ms at heart rates higher than this
5. Tighten the respiratory belt until the patient feels mildly uncomfortable when breathing in – this has the effect of limiting diaphragmatic excursion somewhat and in our experience (and that of others [37]) tends to increase navigator acceptance by 10–15 %.
6. Consider giving sublingual nitrate and oral beta blockers prior to acquisition
7. Don't forget that it's not just the vessel origin and course, but also the consequences of the anomaly that should be sought (perfusion, LGE etc.)
8. CMR may not be the imaging modality of choice in some circumstances
9. It is a sign of wisdom – not failure – to terminate the CMR study early and send the patient to the CT scanner occasionally!

References

1. Brothers J, Gaynor JW, Paridon S, Lorber R, Jacobs M. Anomalous aortic origin of a coronary artery with an interarterial course: understanding current management strategies in children and young adults. Pediatr Cardiol. 2009;30(7):911–21.
2. Cheitlin MD, De Castro CM, McAllister HA. Sudden death as a complication of anomalous left coronary origin from the anterior sinus of valsalva, a not-so-minor congenital anomaly. Circulation. 1974;50(4):780–7.
3. Cheitlin MD. Finding asymptomatic people with a coronary artery arising from the wrong sinus of valsalva: consequences arising from knowing the anomaly to be familial. J Am Coll Cardiol. 2008; 51(21):2065–7.
4. Boon B. Leonardo da Vinci on atherosclerosis and the function of the sinuses of valsalva. Neth Heart J. 2009;17(12):496–9.
5. Morgagni G. The seats and causes of diseases investigated by anatomy; in five books,: Containing A great variety of dissections, with remarks. to which are added very accurate and copious indexes of the principal things and names therein contained. translated from the latin of john baptist morgagni, chief professor of anatomy, and president of the university at padua, by benjamin alexander, M. D. in three volumes. …. London: Printed for A. Millar; and T. Cadell.
6. Angelini P. Normal and anomalous coronary arteries: definitions and classification. Am Heart J. 1989;117(2):418–34.
7. Jacobs ML, Mavroudis C. Anomalies of the coronary arteries: nomenclature and classification. Cardiol Young. 2010;20 Suppl 3:15–9.
8. Anderson RH, Spicer D. Fistulous communications with the coronary arteries in the setting of hypoplastic ventricles. Cardiol Young. 2010;20 Suppl 3:86–91.
9. Angelini P, Fairchild VD, editors. Coronary artery anomalies: a comprehensive approach. Philadelphia: Lippincott Williams & Wilkins; 1999.
10. Brothers JA, Gaynor JW, Jacobs JP, Caldarone C, Jegatheeswaran A, Jacobs ML, et al. The registry of anomalous aortic origin of the coronary artery of the congenital heart surgeons' society. Cardiol Young. 2010;20 Suppl 3:50–8.
11. Gawor R, Kusmierek J, Plachcinska A, Bienkiewicz M, Drozdz J, Piotrowski G, et al. Myocardial perfusion GSPECT imaging in patients with myocardial bridging. J Nucl Cardiol. 2011;18(6): 1059–65.
12. Hakeem A, Cilingiroglu M, Leesar MA. Hemodynamic and intravascular ultrasound assessment of myocardial bridging: fractional flow reserve paradox with dobutamine versus adenosine. Catheter Cardiovasc Interv. 2010;75(2):229–36.
13. Thiene G, Carturan E, Corrado D, Basso C. Prevention of sudden cardiac death in the young and in athletes: dream or reality? Cardiovasc Pathol. 2010;19(4):207–17.
14. Maron BJ, Doerer JJ, Haas TS, Tierney DM, Mueller FO. Sudden deaths in young competitive athletes: analysis of 1866 deaths in the United States, 1980–2006. Circulation. 2009;119(8):1085–92.
15. Eckart RE, Scoville SL, Campbell CL, Shry EA, Stajduhar KC, Potter RN, et al. Sudden death in young adults: a 25-year review of autopsies in military recruits. Ann Intern Med. 2004;141(11):829–34.
16. Hill SF, Sheppard MN. Non-atherosclerotic coronary artery disease associated with sudden cardiac death. Heart. 2010;96(14): 1119–25.
17. Baroldi G, Scomazzoni G. Coronary circulation in the normal and the pathologic heart. Washington, D.C.: Armed Forces Institute of Pathology, 1967.
18. Davies JE, Burkhart HM, Dearani JA, Suri RM, Phillips SD, Warnes CA, et al. Surgical management of anomalous aortic origin of a coronary artery. Ann Thorac Surg. 2009;88(3):844–7. discussion 847–8.
19. De Luca L, Bovenzi F, Rubini D, Niccoli-Asabella A, Rubini G, De Luca I. Stress-rest myocardial perfusion SPECT for functional assessment of coronary arteries with anomalous origin or course. J Nucl Med. 2004;45(4):532–6.
20. Yamanaka O, Hobbs RE. Coronary artery anomalies in 126,595 patients undergoing coronary arteriography. Cathet Cardiovasc Diagn. 1990;21(1):28–40.
21. Zhang LJ, Yang GF, Huang W, Zhou CS, Chen P, Lu GM. Incidence of anomalous origin of coronary artery in 1879 Chinese adults on dual-source CT angiography. Neth Heart J. 2010;18(10):466–70.
22. Angelini P, Flamm SD. Newer concepts for imaging anomalous aortic origin of the coronary arteries in adults. Catheter Cardiovasc Interv. 2007;69(7):942–54.
23. Crean AM, Kilcullen N, Younger JF. Arrhythmic acute coronary syndrome and anomalous left main stem artery: culprit or innocent bystander. Acute Card Care. 2008;10(1):60–1.
24. Gui D, Tsekos NV. Dynamic imaging of contrast – enhanced coronary vessels with a magnetization prepared rotated stripe keyhole acquisition. J Magn Reson Imaging. 2007;25(1):222–30.
25. Manso B, Castellote A, Dos L, Casaldaliga J. Myocardial perfusion magnetic resonance imaging for detecting coronary function anomalies in asymptomatic paediatric patients with a previous arterial switch operation for the transposition of great arteries. Cardiol Young. 2010;20(4):410–7.

26. Strigl S, Beroukhim R, Valente AM, Annese D, Harrington JS, Geva T, et al. Feasibility of dobutamine stress cardiovascular magnetic resonance imaging in children. J Magn Reson Imaging. 2009;29(2):313–9.

27. Mavrogeni S, Papadopoulos G, Douskou M, Kaklis S, Seimenis I, Baras P, et al. Magnetic resonance angiography is equivalent to X-ray coronary angiography for the evaluation of coronary arteries in Kawasaki disease. J Am Coll Cardiol. 2004;43(4):649–52.

28. Backer CL, Stout MJ, Zales VR, Muster AJ, Weigel TJ, Idriss FS, et al. Anomalous origin of the left coronary artery. A twenty-year review of surgical management. J Thorac Cardiovasc Surg. 1992;103(6):1049–57. discussion 1057–8.

29. Belli E, Roussin R, Ly M, Roubertie F, Le Bret E, Basaran M, et al. Anomalous origin of the left coronary artery from the pulmonary artery associated with severe left ventricular dysfunction: results in normothermia. Ann Thorac Surg. 2010;90(3):856–60.

30. Ben Ali W, Metton O, Roubertie F, Pouard P, Sidi D, Raisky O, et al. Anomalous origin of the left coronary artery from the pulmonary artery: late results with special attention to the mitral valve. Eur J Cardiothorac Surg. 2009;36(2):244–8. discussion 248–9.

31. Karunadasa R, Buxton BF, Dick R, Calafiore P. Anomalous origin of left coronary artery from the pulmonary artery does the management in the adult differ from that of the infant? Four cases of the bland-white-garland syndrome. Heart Lung Circ. 2007;16 Suppl 3:S29–33.

32. Mavroudis C, Dodge-Khatami A, Stewart RD, Jacobs ML, Backer CL, Lorber RE. An overview of surgery options for congenital coronary artery anomalies. Future Cardiol. 2010;6(5):627–45.

33. Wintersperger BJ, von Smekal A, Engelmann MG, Knez A, Penzkofer HV, Laub G, et al. Contrast media enhanced magnetic resonance angiography for determining patency of a coronary bypass. A comparison with coronary angiography. Rofo. 1997;167(6):572–8.

34. Brenner P, Wintersperger B, von Smekal A, Agirov V, Bohm D, Kreuzer E, et al. Detection of coronary artery bypass graft patency by contrast enhanced magnetic resonance angiography. Eur J Cardiothorac Surg. 1999;15(4):389–93.

35. Bunce NH, Lorenz CH, John AS, Lesser JR, Mohiaddin RH, Pennell DJ. Coronary artery bypass graft patency: assessment with true ast imaging with steady-state precession versus gadolinium-enhanced MR angiography. Radiology. 2003;227(2):440–6.

36. Schmitt R, Froehner S, Brunn J, Wagner M, Brunner H, Cherevatyy O, et al. Congenital anomalies of the coronary arteries: imaging with contrast-enhanced, multidetector computed tomography. Eur Radiol. 2005;15(6):1110–21.

37. Ishida M, Schuster A, Takase S, Morton G, Chiribiri A, Bigalke B, et al. Impact of an abdominal belt on breathing patterns and scan efficiency in whole-heart coronary magnetic resonance angiography: comparison between the UK and Japan. J Cardiovasc Magn Reson. 2011;13:71.

38. McConnell MV, Ganz P, Selwyn AP, Li W, Edelman RR, Manning WJ. Identification of anomalous coronary arteries and their anatomic course by magnetic resonance coronary angiography. Circulation. 1995;92(11):3158–62.

39. Post JC, van Rossum AC, Hofman MB, Valk J, Visser CA. Protocol for two-dimensional magnetic resonance coronary angiography studied in three-dimensional magnetic resonance data sets. Am Heart J. 1995;130(1):167–73.

40. Vliegen HW, Doornbos J, de Roos A, Jukema JW, Bekedam MA, van der Wall EE. Value of fast gradient echo magnetic resonance angiography as an adjunct to coronary arteriography in detecting and confirming the course of clinically significant coronary artery anomalies. Am J Cardiol. 1997;79(6):773–6.

41. Bekedam MA, Vliegen HW, Doornbos J, Jukema JW, de Roos A, van der Wall EE. Diagnosis and management of anomalous origin of the right coronary artery from the left coronary sinus. Int J Card Imaging. 1999;15(3):253–8.

42. White CS, Laskey WK, Stafford JL, NessAiver M. Coronary MRA: use in assessing anomalies of coronary artery origin. J Comput Assist Tomogr. 1999;23(2):203–7.

43. Taylor AM, Thorne SA, Rubens MB, Jhooti P, Keegan J, Gatehouse PD, et al. Coronary artery imaging in grown up congenital heart disease: complementary role of magnetic resonance and x-ray coronary angiography. Circulation. 2000;101(14):1670–8.

44. Greil GF, Stuber M, Botnar RM, Kissinger KV, Geva T, Newburger JW, et al. Coronary magnetic resonance angiography in adolescents and young adults with Kawasaki disease. Circulation. 2002;105(8):908–11.

45. Bunce NH, Lorenz CH, Keegan J, Lesser J, Reyes EM, Firmin DN, et al. Coronary artery anomalies: assessment with free-breathing three-dimensional coronary MR angiography. Radiology. 2003;227(1):201–8.

46. Su JT, Chung T, Muthupillai R, Pignatelli RH, Kung GC, Diaz LK, et al. Usefulness of real-time navigator magnetic resonance imaging for evaluating coronary artery origins in pediatric patients. Am J Cardiol. 2005;95(5):679–82.

47. Taylor AM, Dymarkowski S, Hamaekers P, Razavi R, Gewillig M, Mertens L, et al. MR coronary angiography and late-enhancement myocardial MR in children who underwent arterial switch surgery for transposition of great arteries. Radiology. 2005;234(2):542–7.

48. Takemura A, Suzuki A, Inaba R, Sonobe T, Tsuchiya K, Omuro M, et al. Utility of coronary MR angiography in children with Kawasaki disease. AJR Am J Roentgenol. 2007;188(6):W534–9.

49. Gharib AM, Ho VB, Rosing DR, Herzka DA, Stuber M, Arai AE, et al. Coronary artery anomalies and variants: technical feasibility of assessment with coronary MR angiography at 3 T. Radiology. 2008;247(1):220–7.

50. Beerbaum P, Sarikouch S, Laser KT, Greil G, Burchert W, Korperich H. Coronary anomalies assessed by whole-heart isotropic 3D magnetic resonance imaging for cardiac morphology in congenital heart disease. J Magn Reson Imaging. 2009;29(2):320–7.

51. Clemente A, Del Borrello M, Greco P, Mannella P, Di Gregorio F, Romano S, et al. al. Anomalous origin of the coronary arteries in children: diagnostic role of three-dimensional coronary MR angiography. Clin Imaging. 2010;34(5):337–43.

52. Tangcharoen T, Bell A, Hegde S, Hussain T, Beerbaum P, Schaeffter T, et al. Detection of coronary artery anomalies in infants and young children with congenital heart disease by using MR imaging. Radiology. 2011;259(1):240–7.

53. Rajiah P, Setser RM, Desai MY, Flamm SD, Arruda JL. Utility of free-breathing, whole-heart, three-dimensional magnetic resonance imaging in the assessment of coronary anatomy for congenital heart disease. Pediatr Cardiol. 2011;32(4):418–25.

Pericardial Diseases

15

Edward T. Martin

15.1 Introduction

Pericardial disease can be an important cause of morbidity and mortality in a clinical cardiology practice. However, patients with pericardial disease are not always encountered on a daily basis, and because pericardial disease can mimic other diseases, such as cardiovascular, pulmonary and pleural processes a firm diagnosis may be difficult. Frequently, pericardial involvement can be the initial presentation of a systemic disease process. Disorders of the pericardium can also have a variety of etiologies, including congenital malformations along with infectious, infarction-related, metabolic, autoimmune, traumatic, neoplastic, and idiopathic processes. Additionally, accurate diagnosis of a pericardial disorder may require the use of multiple noninvasive tests or a noninvasive test coupled with an invasive study.

This chapter will focus on the ability of cardiac magnetic resonance imaging (CMR) to accurately assess pericardial diseases. It will compare and contrast CMR's ability to diagnose pericardial disorders to both echocardiography and computed tomography (CT). The chapter will also provide rationale for the appropriate use of CMR in a patient with suspected pericardial disease.

15.2 Anatomy/Physiology

The pericardium is a relatively avascular double layered sac that surrounds the heart and extends superiorly to the origin of the great vessels and is attached to the sternum, the dorsal spine and the diaphragm. It consists of a visceral and parietal layer. In general its combined thickness is less than 2 mm. The two layers create a potential space that normally contains 15–35 ml of serous fluid which is secreted by the visceral

pericardium [1]. A variable amount of epicardial and pericardial fat is also present which can aid MRI and CT by providing enhanced tissue contrast. The pericardium is well innervated and can cause severe pain during inflammation and trigger vagally-mediated reflexes. From a physiologic perspective, the pericardium interacts with the pleural space and the ventricles. The pericardium is also involved in the interaction between the right and left ventricles. This interaction can be utilized in the diagnosis of pericardial constriction in the form of ventricular interdependence.

While the pericardium does not appear to be essential for the cardiovascular system to perform its normal physiologic function it does seem to have utility. It maintains the normal position of the heart, anchoring it to the central thorax and may also provide a barrier to infection. It also secretes prostaglandins that regulate cardiac tone. Finally, the pericardium restrains cardiac volume and enhances mechanical interactions of the cardiac chambers. Despite these important functions, absence of the pericardium does not usually result in significant problems.

15.3 MRI Examination for Pericardial Diseases

The pericardium is usually bordered by epicardial and pericardial fat, which has high signal on black blood T1-weighted images. Black blood imaging demonstrates the pericardium as a thin band of low signal due to its mainly fibrous structure and lack of water content. The normal pericardial thickness by MRI is between 1 and 3 mm and is best evaluated anatomically on axial imaging (Fig. 15.1). However scanning in two perpendicularly oriented planes through the heart optimizes the depiction of the entire pericardium. The normal

E.T. Martin, MS, M.D., FACC, FACP, FAHA
Department of Cardiovascular MRI, Oklahoma Heart Institute,
9228 South Mingo Road, Tulsa, OK 74113, USA
e-mail: martin@oklahomaheart.com

Electronic supplementary material The online version of this chapter (doi:10.1007/978-1-4471-4267-6_15) contains supplementary material, which is available to authorized users.

M.A. Syed, R.H. Mohiaddin (eds.), *Magnetic Resonance Imaging of Congenital Heart Disease*,
DOI 10.1007/978-1-4471-4267-6_15, © Springer-Verlag London 2012

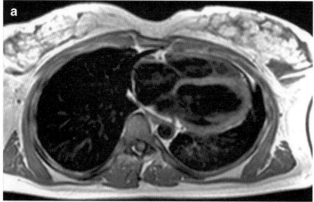

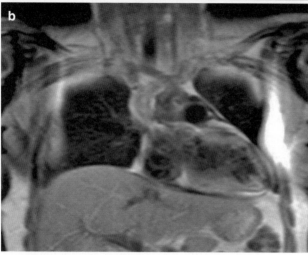

Table 15.1 Cardiac MRI strategies to evaluate the pericardium

Pericardial width/localization/extent (T1w/T2w spin-echo CMR/cine CMR)
Pericardial delineation (T1w/T2w spin-echo CMR/cine CMR, CMR/gadolinium-enhanced CMR)
Pericardial layer/fluid characterization (T1w/T2w spin-echo CMR/cine CMR/gadolinium-enhanced CMR)
Pericardial function
Motion pattern (cine CMR)
Fusion of pericardial layers and myocardial adherence (CMR tagging)
Pericardial masses (T1w/T2w spin-echo CMR/double IR with fat saturation/triple IR/cine CMR/gadolinium-enhanced CMR)
Cardiac morphology (spin-echo CMR, cine CMR)
Size and shape of ventricles and ventricles
Myocardial morphology (restrictive cardiomyopathy)
Cardiac systolic function (cine CMR)
Regional and global systolic ventricular function
Cardiac filling (velocity-encoded CMR)
Ventricular coupling (real-time cine CMR)
Ventricular septal shape and septal motion patterns
Respiratory-related septal shift
Other findings (spin-echo CMR/cine CMR/gadolinium-enhanced CMR)
Myocardial enhancement (associated myocarditis or myocardial infiltrative or storage disease)
Caval vein size
Pleural effusion/ascites
Lung processes

Fig. 15.1 Normal pericardial appearance. (**a**) Black blood axial view of the heart. The pericardium is the thin black line surrounding the heart. (**b**) Black blood coronal view of the normal pericardium. Again, the pericardium is the thin black line seen at the outer edge of the heart extending superiorly to level of the main pulmonary artery

MRI pericardial thickness is somewhat larger than the normal anatomical thickness which is 1 mm or less [2–4]. Cardiac motion and limited spatial resolution in this area contribute to this phenomenon [5].

A cardiac examination designed for evaluation of pericardial disease will include the standard sequences used in essentially all cardiac MRI. These sequences can then be supplemented by real-time, delayed-enhancement and perfusion imaging depending on the clinical condition (Table 15.1).

The CMR exam will start with a morphological assessment of the heart, pericardium and mediastinum using a black-blood, T1-weighted technique, using a fast segmented sequence. The T2-weighted half-Fourier acquisition single-shot turbo spin echo (HASTE) sequence can also be used as it allows dark blood imaging with a reduced acquisition time. There is slightly increased blurring with this technique relative to standard gated spin-echo techniques. However the resistance of the single-shot sequence to respiratory motion

artifact and cardiac arrhythmias, which frequently degrades spin-echo image quality, usually offsets this minimal disadvantage. The T2-weighted spin echo CMR sequences are useful for depicting myocardial edema, pericardial edema and fluid, as well as allowing one to differentiate pericardial cysts from other types of masses. Triple inversion recovery or double inversion recovery with fat saturation can also help in this instance as well.

Cine imaging through the entire myocardium in the short and long axis planes as routinely performed for cardiac evaluation is appropriate for the imaging of suspected pericardial diseases. Balanced steady state free precession (SSFP) gradient-echo sequences are now the standard technique used for cine imaging. They demonstrate improved image quality in comparison with segmented gradient echo imaging techniques. The signal intensity in the SSFP technique depends upon the T2/T1 ratio. Therefore, structures with a high T2/T1 ratio such as fat, fluid, and intracavitary blood demonstrate similar high signal despite their significantly different T1 and T2 properties. Cine imaging allows one to view myocardial movement in relation to pericardial movement and differentiate normal pericardial movement from a stiff immobile pericardium seen in patients with constrictive pericarditis. The cine sequences are also used to qualitatively assess myocardial and valvular function.

MRI tagging sequences can be performed to aid in identifying adhesion of the visceral to parietal pericardium in constrictive pericarditis. In this sequence, a grid of saturation bands is placed over the heart in diastole, and their deformation in systole can provide information about regional cardiac motion. The grid lines remain unbroken, as opposed to demonstrating normal disruption caused by cardiac motion, in areas of pericardial adherence.

Velocity-encoded, phase contrast CMR is also used to evaluate diastolic cardiac function by looking at the inflow patterns of the mitral and tricuspid valves as well as the pulmonary and systemic veins to help rule out myocardial restriction from pericardial constriction.

Perfusion sequences using gadolinium contrast are used to evaluate the vascularity of cardiac and pericardial masses and can be obtained in multiple imaging planes with one injection. These are heavily T1-weighted imaging sequences that can provide information on perfusion and diffusion in the myocardium or in a mass.

The contrast-enhanced inversion-recovery technique with delayed enhancement (DE-CMR), also called late gadolinium enhancement (LGE) can be employed to identify pericardial enhancement in a similar manner to identifying infarcts in the myocardium. This enhancement represents inflammation and can diagnose pericarditis. This technique can better differentiate between inflammatory and constrictive forms of pericarditis. Because the myocardium is also being assessed, myopericarditis can also be diagnosed.

Newer MRI scanners are now able to perform real-time cine image acquisitions, which obtains images without breath-holding and without segmentation. These non-gated SSFP images are acquired in real-time and can be used to assess ventricular coupling to aid in the diagnosis of pericardial constriction.

15.4   Congenital Abnormalities of the Pericardium

Congenital abnormalities of the pericardium are rare. Pericardial disorders are more commonly seen as postoperative sequelae in patients with congenital heart disease. The following section covers the pericardial disorders encountered in patients with congenital heart disease.

15.4.1 Congenital Absence of the Pericardium

Congenital absence of the pericardium is a rare entity. Complete or partial absence can occur with partial defects being more common. Other congenital abnormalities can also be seen and include anomalies of the chest wall, lungs, and diaphragm. Cardiac anomalies such as tetralogy of Fallot, atrial septal defect, mitral valve stenosis and patent ductus arteriosus can also occur in concert with congenital absence of the pericardium [5, 6].

Patients with absence of the pericardium are usually asymptomatic, and the condition may be detected on routine chest radiograph as an abnormal left cardiac contour. Symptoms occur when cardiac structures become entrapped in the defect. Herniation of the left atrial appendage through a small defect may lead to infarction of the appendage, compression of the left coronary artery during exercise and/or prolapse of the pulmonary trunk (Movie 15.1).

The diagnosis of congenital absence of the pericardium by CMR may be difficult because the partial defects of the pericardium predominantly occur on the left side of the heart where the pericardium is difficult to visualize because there is a minimal amount of fat in this location [7]. Therefore the diagnosis may rely on other signs such as an abnormal location of cardiac structures with excessive levorotation or cardiac indentation at the location of the defect [5, 8]. Functional MRI assessment may also be of use in diagnosing pericardial defects by detecting excessive mobility of the cardiac apex which is normally stationary [9].

15.4.2 Pericardial Diverticulum

This is a rare condition where there is herniation through a defect in the parietal pericardium allowing communication into the pericardial space. The most typical location of these defects is at the cardiophrenic angles. These defects resemble cysts but differ because a complete wall cannot be identified in all parts of the abnormality [10].

15.4.3 Pericardial Cysts

Pericardial cysts are thin-walled, saccular, fluid-filled and self-contained. They are usually classified as congenital, postinflammatory or ecchinococcal. They do not communicate with other structures or the pericardium. They are most often found in the cardiophrenic space. Pericardial cysts occur on the right side 70 % of the time and may calcify. When they do occur on the left they may mimic left ventricular aneurysms or a prominent left atrial appendage.

During CMR, cysts typically have low or intermediate signal intensity on T1-weighted images and homogeneous high intensity on T2-weighted images (Fig. 15.2). Triple inversion recovery sequences or double inversion recovery with fat saturation sequences may help display the cyst as bright while eliminating interfering fat signal. A line of low signal intensity may be seen surrounding the cyst representing parietal pericardium [2]. Cysts do not enhance with the administration of gadolinium chelates. Occasionally, a cyst

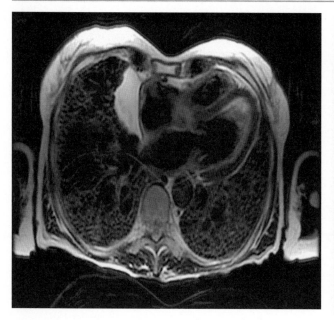

Fig. 15.2 Pericardial cyst. T2-weighted axial image showing bright signal representing a pericardial cyst lateral to the right atrium

Table 15.2 Causes of pericarditis

Infectious: viral, bacterial, fungal, tuberculosis, parasite
Myocardial Infarction (Dressler's syndrome)
Postpericardiotomy syndrome
Immunologic conditions including systemic lupus erythematosus or rheumatoid arthritis
Uremia
Malignancy – Breast, lung, lymphoma, mesothelioma, sarcoma, leukemia
Side effect of some medications (e.g. isoniazid, cyclosporine, hydralazine, warfarin, and heparin, tertracyclines)
Radiation induced
Aortic dissection
Trauma to the heart

may contain highly proteinaceous fluid, which may demonstrate high signal intensity on T1-weighted images. Pericardial cysts need to be distinguished from bronchogenic and thymic cysts as well as from coronary artery aneurysms. Pericardial cysts are distinguished from the latter in that they will exhibit no mass effect on the myocardium (Movie 15.2).

15.5 Pericarditis

Pericarditis is an inflammatory process of the pericardium that has multiple etiologies (Table 15.2). The initial presenting symptom is chest pain that worsens with inspiration or in the supine body position. Acutely, an inflamed pericardium contains highly vascular granulation tissue with fibrin deposits [11]. Chronically,

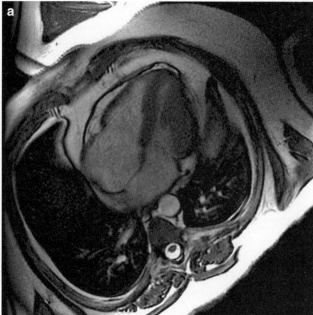

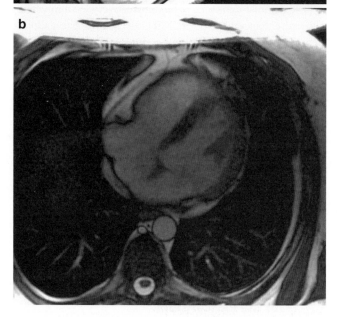

Fig. 15.3 Pericardial assessment before and after treatment for pericarditis. (**a**) Axial white blood image of a thickened pericardium in a patient with pericarditis. (**b**) White blood axial image of the same patient after treatment with steroids and plaquenil. Note the reduction in pericardial thickness

the pericardium can become fibrosed and stiffened by fibroblasts and collagen. In this acute phase there may also be a pericardial effusion and slight pericardial thickening. This process can be detected and evaluated by CMR. Response to treatment can be monitored by MRI as well (Fig. 15.3).

The pericardium can initially be assessed for thickening and fluid by both dark-blood fast spin echo techniques and by white-blood cine techniques (Fig. 15.4). The DE-CMR technique has been described as being useful for detecting

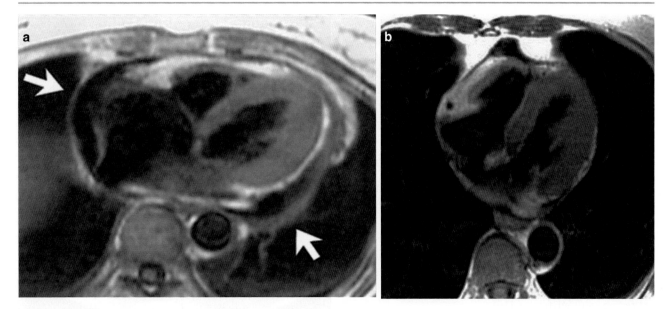

Fig. 15.4 (**a**) Pericardial Effusion – Axial Black Blood MR image. White arrows point to black space surrounding the heart, which represents a pericardial effusion. (**b**) Pericardial Effusion – Four Chamber Black Blood MR image. The white areas anterior to the right ventricular free wall and to the black space represent fat

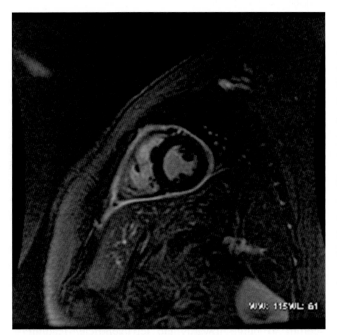

Fig. 15.5 Acute pericarditis. Pericardial enhancement is seen in a patient with acute pericarditis using the delayed enhancement sequence following the administration of gadolinium

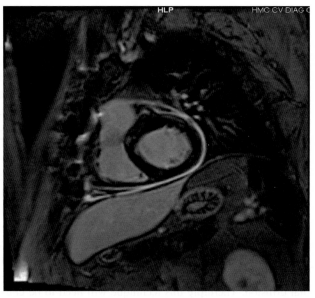

Fig. 15.6 Myopericarditis. In addition to the ring enhancement of the pericardium small islands of gadolinium are seen in the myocardium especially in the anteroseptal and inferoseptal walls. This represents concomitant myocarditis along with pericarditis

pericardial inflammation [11, 12]. The normal pericardium, being relatively avascular does not enhance. However when the pericardium is inflamed acutely with vascularized granulation tissue the pericardium will enhance (Fig. 15.5).

Sometimes there is concomitant myocarditis with pericarditis and vice versa. In one CMR study for the detection of myocarditis, 9 of 20 patients with myocarditis also had peri-

cardial enhancement [13]. With DE-CMR this phenomenon is easily diagnosed and characterized [12, 13] (Fig. 15.6).

The initial acute inflammatory reaction within the pericardium also contains an increase in free water content due to lymphocyte infiltration. This can cause T2 relaxation time prolongation. Therefore one can also use a short τ-inversion recovery T2-weighted sequence looking for a hyperintense signal from the pericardium representing edema [14].

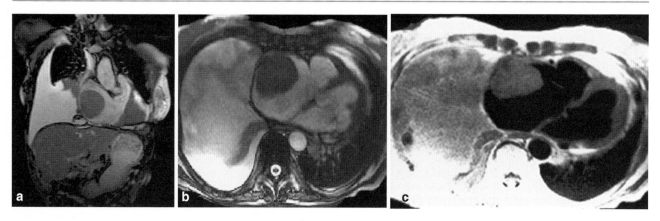

Fig. 16.1 Large mass in the right atrium. Mass has well defined borders and is isointense with myocardium on black blood T2 image. Right atrium is severely dilated. This is an example of a large thrombus in the right atrium in a patient with Ebstein's anomaly (**a**, **b** are SSFP images and **c** is black blood T2w spine-echo image)

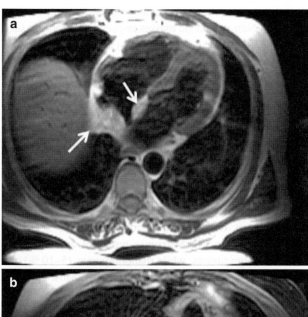

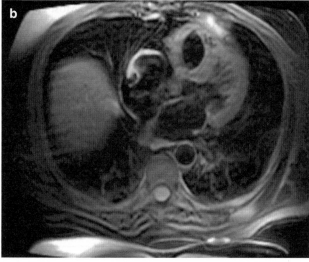

Fig. 16.2 Lipomatous hypertrophy of interatrial septum. The fatty mass is "dumb-bell" shaped and spares the fossa ovalis (**a**, *arrows*). On T1 weighted fat saturation image the fat is saturated and mass appears dark confirming fatty tissue (**b**)

extension from adjacent tumors, hematogenous and/or lymphatic spread, and transvenous invasion. Common tumors metastasizing to the heart are shown in Table 16.2. Direct extension occurs from lung, breast, esophageal or other mediastinal tumors. Venous extension occurs through the inferior vena cava, superior vena cava or pulmonary veins.

Primary malignant tumors account for approximately 15 % of primary cardiac tumors and can broadly be divided into sarcomas, lymphomas and pericardial malignancy [6]. Sarcoma is the most common primary cardiac malignant tumor and are extremely rare, usually described in isolated case reports or reviews. Virtually all types of sarcomas have been reported in the heart. Angiosarcomas are the most common form of cardiac sarcoma arising predominantly in the right atrium. Other most frequently described sarcomas include rhabdomyosarcomas (most common primary cardiac malignancy in children), fibrosarcomas and leiomyosarcomas.

According to one recent report, primary cardiac lymphoma histology has become the most common histology type after 1992, representing 39 % of primary cardiac malignant tumors by 2003 [7]. Primary cardiac lymphomas are aggressive B-cell lymphomas with higher incidence in immunocompromised patients. The right atrium is the commonest site of origin with frequent involvement of more than one cardiac chamber and pericardial invasion.

16.3 Cardiac Tumors in Children

Cardiac tumors are also rare in children, with reported incidence of 0.03–0.08 % [8, 9]. In a recently published multicenter international CMR study of 78 cases in children, tumors were found in all cardiac chambers and extracardiac locations with most common location being the ventricular myocardium [10]. Most common tumor was fibroma (38 %)

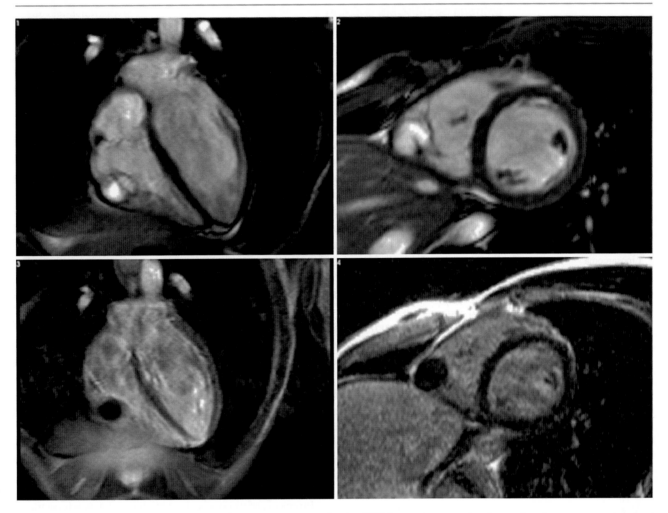

Fig. 16.3 Hydatid cyst in the right ventricle. A cystic mass is seen on the cine SSFP images (*upper row*) and non-enhancing mass on post-contrast images (*bottom row*)

followed by rhabdomyoma (18 %), malignant (16 %), hemangioma (12 %), myxoma (4 %) and teratoma (3 %). Malignant tumors included osteosarcoma (n = 3), rhabdomyosarcoma (n = 2), and 1 case each of angiosarcoma, B-cell lymphoma, desmoplastic round cell tumor, melanoma and medulloblastoma. Other series have reported rhabdomyomas as the most common cardiac tumor in children which likely represents a referral bias to MR imaging as these tumors are usually diagnosed by echocardiography due to their typical appearance and not referred for MR imaging [11].

16.4 Clinical Presentation

Many tumors are found on cardiac imaging studies investigating other pathology and may remain clinically silent while others present with early symptoms. Symptoms of cardiac tumors are highly variable and are typically secondary to their effect on normal cardiac geometry and function. Symptoms also depend upon mass size

and location. Arrhythmias, particularly sudden death and abnormal atrioventricular conduction, are common because of tumor disruption of the conduction system. Cardiac tumor should be considered in the differential diagnosis of any patient with an embolic phenomenon or signs or symptoms of inflow or outflow obstruction with left or right-sided heart failure.

16.4.1 Symptoms and Signs

- Heart failure: left and/or right ventricular failure can be caused by cardiac chamber obliteration by tumor or abnormal myocardial function secondary to intramyocardial tumor growth. Tumor growth can also cause left or right ventricular outflow tract obstruction (Fig. 16.4). Valve function can also be impaired due to tumor compression or growth causing stenosis or regurgitation.
- Palpitations: tumor involvement of the conduction system might cause palpitations or syncope.

16.6.2 Malignant Tumors

16.6.2.1 Angiosarcoma

Angiosarcoma is the most common malignant tumor of the heart and accounts for less than 10 % of all primary cardiac tumors [27]. Angiosarcoma is characterized by rapid growth, local invasion and distant metastasis and has a predilection for the right atrium (>90 %) but other cardiac chamber involvement has been reported (Fig. 16.8). Angiosarcoma grows rapidly and metastasis is usually present at the time of presentation with lung being the commonest site [28]. Pericardial effusion and tamponade is often present. CMR findings include broad base of attachment, lack of pedicle, presence of hemorrhage or necrosis, vascularity and invasion of surrounding structures [13]. Heterogeneous signal intensity of the mass on T1 and T2-weighted fast spin echo is consistent with areas of tumor tissue, necrosis and hemorrhage in the tumor which is a feature of cardiac angiosarcoma [29]. Right atrial location is a distinguishing feature from other forms of sarcomas that tend to arise from the left atrium [30].

16.6.2.2 Lymphoma

Primary cardiac lymphoma is extranodal non-Hodgkin's lymphoma located in the heart and/or pericardium. This neoplasm has increased prevalence in immunocompromised patients and is rarely seen in immunocompetent patients. This is an aggressive neoplasm presenting with heart failure, pericardial effusion/tamponade, syncope or arrhythmia. There are no pathognomonic imaging features (Fig. 16.9). Primary cardiac lymphoma typically involves the right heart chambers and/or pericardium. Pericardial effusion, outflow obstruction, and infiltration of adjacent tissues are usually seen. Histological and immunohistochemical examination of the involved tissue is always required to confirm diagnosis as chemotherapy ± radiation is the main therapeutic approach [31].

16.6.2.3 Other Sarcomas

Virtually all types of sarcomas have been reported in the heart (Fig. 16.10). In one review, undifferentiated sarcomas accounted for 25 % of all primary cardiac tumors, however, with improved immunohistochemistry techniques this frequency is decreasing as they may now be assigned a specific subtype [32]. Leiomyosarcoma arise mostly in the left atrium infiltrating the pulmonary veins. Fibrosarcomas arise in the left atrium in 50 %, either ventricle in 30 % and pericardium in 20 %. Liposarcomas do not have a predilection for any cardiac chamber while osteosarcomas always originate from the left atrium invading into the pulmonary vein ostia and mitral valve [32]. The CMR tissue features of these sarcomas are non-specific with heterogeneous signal intensity on post-contrast imaging. Cardiac CT can better delineate the calcific components of osteosarcoma providing a complimentary role to CMR imaging.

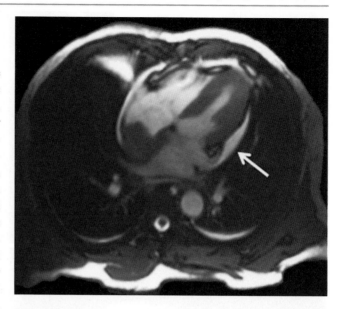

Fig. 16.8 Angiosarcoma of the right atrium. Cine SSFP image shows infiltration of right atrial wall and pericardial effusion (*arrow*), which are signs of a malignant tumor

16.7 Comparison with Other Imaging Modalities

16.7.1 Echocardiography

Transthoracic echocardiography (TTE) is usually the first line imaging modality used in the evaluation of cardiac masses. However, TTE has significant limitations from dependence upon availability of good acoustic windows particularly in patients with obesity, emphysema and chest deformities. TTE also has limited field of view and ability to characterize tissue structure. TTE is therefore not a reliable method for characterizing the cardiac mass. The tissue characterization can be improved by utilizing contrast echocardiography to distinguish thrombus from tumor. Most malignant tumors have abnormal neovascularization with increased blood supply, while thrombi are avascular. Mansencal et al. have shown that with microbubble contrast administration, a complete lack of enhancement is suggestive of thrombus; partial or incomplete enhancement suggests myxoma and complete enhancement suggests tumor [33].

Transesophageal echocardiography (TEE) is also routinely performed for cardiac mass evaluation. Compared to TTE, TEE can provide more detailed assessment of small masses, masses in atria particularly left atrial appendage and masses associated with valves. However, TTE is better than TEE in evaluating mass in left ventricular apex. Despite using microbubble contrast agents, both TTE and TEE remain limited in their tissue characterization of cardiac masses and confident differentiation between thrombi and benign and malignant tumors may not be possible.

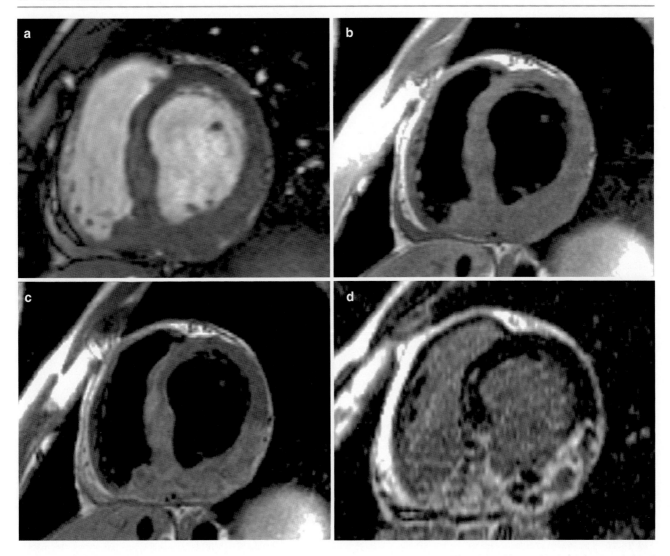

Fig. 16.9 Lymphoma involving the left ventricle. Cine imaging (**a**) shows irregularly thickened myocardium in the septum, inferior and inferolateral segments and a mass in the right ventricle adjacent to the inferior RV insertion site. T1 black blood (**b**) does not show any significant signal intensity difference between the abnormal and normal myocardium, however, T2-weighted image (**c**) shows increased signal intensity in the abnormal myocardial segments suggesting increased water content. Late gadolinium enhancement shows diffuse, patchy enhancement suggesting necrosis (**d**)

16.7.2 Computed Tomography

Electrocardiographic (ECG) gated multidetector computed tomography (MDCT) has evolved into an important cardiac imaging technique particularly for the assessment of coronary arteries. MDCT provides high spatial resolution and can be a valuable tool for assessing a cardiac mass, particularly when a patient can't undergo CMR due to contraindications. CT scanning is often performed during an evaluation for a possible thoracic malignancy where an incidental cardiac tumor may also be found. MDCT can be complimentary to CMR imaging particularly in the evaluation of calcified masses [34]. The wide field of view and multiplanar reconstruction capabilities are useful in providing a detailed evaluation of cardiac and pericardial masses and adjacent structures [35]. Non-contrast images are diagnostic for detecting calcification, e.g. central calcification suggestive of a cardiac fibroma or identifying caseous variety of mitral annular calcification. Contrast enhanced images may help identify the nature of the mass similar to contrast echocardiography and perfusion CMR, however, this requires specialized acquisition protocols for perfusion CT.

MDCT require the use of iodinated contrast agents and exposure to radiation. The temporal resolution is also limited requiring the use of beta-blockers to slow the heart rate for better image quality. Imaging of the heart necessitates the use of MDCT scanners with ECG gating capabilities. The

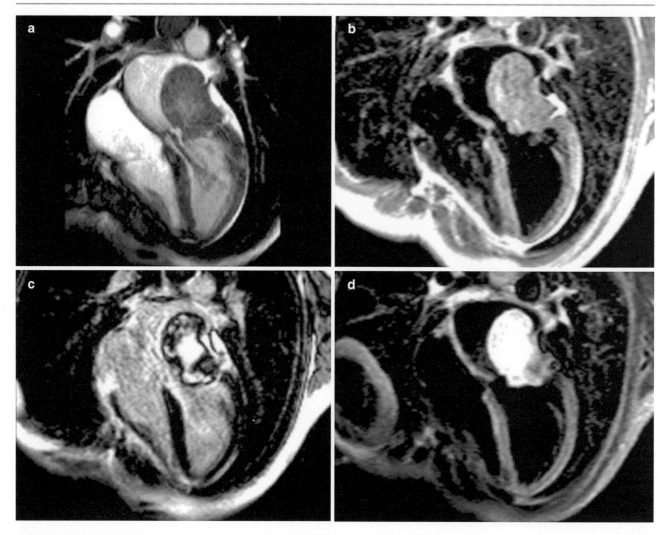

Fig. 16.10 Sarcoma (undifferentiated) of the left atrium obstructing the mitral inflow (**a**). Black blood spin-echo imaging shows the mass is isointense on T1 (**b**) and hyperintense on T2W spin-echo image (**d**). Patchy enhancement is seen on late gadolinium enhancement (**c**)

tissue characterization properties of CT are inferior to CMR, however, CT has an important role when MR imaging is contraindicated or not available.

16.7.3 Positron Emission Tomography

Positron emission tomography combined with computed tomography (PET-CT) is increasingly available and has become an important tool for assessment of myocardial ischemia, viability and malignant disease. With the use of 2-[18F] Flouro-2-deoxy-D-glucose (18-FDG) PET can distinguish benign from malignant lesions, accurately stage malignancies and assess response to therapy [36]. An increased 18-FDG uptake by a mass is suggestive of a neoplasm, however, increased uptake can also be seen in the presence of brown fat, e.g. lipomatous hypertrophy of atrial septum [37]. PET-CT is not routinely utilized for cardiac mass evaluation,

perhaps due to easy availability and use of echocardiography, MRI and CT imaging.

16.7.4 Angiography with Cardiac Catheterization

In the current era of high resolution, 3 dimensional non-invasive imaging, cardiac catheterization has limited role in the evaluation of patients with known intracardiac mass. Ventriculography is relatively contraindicated in patients with known intracardiac mass because of the risk of catheter-induced tumor embolization. In other patients, ventriculography might demonstrate filling defects suggestive of an intracavitary mass. If a mass is found as an incidental finding during angiography, strict care is required to minimize disruption of the mass to avoid causing a systemic embolic complication. In patients who are at high risk for concomitant coronary disease and are undergoing surgical treatment, coronary angiography is usually necessary. Coronary angiography may also demonstrate neovascularization of the cardiac mass [38].

16.8 CMR Role in Treatment Decision Making

Treatment of cardiac mass is dependent upon accurate localization and diagnosis. CMR can provide localization and tissue characterization non-invasively. Black-blood imaging, first pass perfusion and LGE with long inversion can accurately differentiate tumor from thrombus and obviate the need for additional invasive procedures. Fatty masses are well characterized by black-blood sequence with fat saturation prepulse. Vascularity of cardiac mass is suggestive of tumor and is evaluated by first pass perfusion and LGE.

Malignant tumors (Fig. 16.11) can be differentiated from benign tumors by some specific features that include invasion of extra-cardiac tissues, involvement of more than one cardiac chamber, right sided location, poor border definition and the presence of pericardial effusion [39].

It's important to know that there may be significant overlap between biologic properties of different neoplasms, and therefore, decisions regarding chemotherapy or radiation treatment generally cannot be made solely on the basis of CMR imaging but rather require a tissue diagnosis. CMR imaging provides an excellent anatomical assessment of cardiac tumors and its relationship to extracardiac structures that is useful for surgical excision planning.

Conclusion

CMR imaging is currently considered the modality of choice for evaluating suspected cardiac tumors. A comprehensive CMR evaluation of cardiac tumors includes accurate localization, delineation of anatomical extent, assessment of associated functional consequences and complications and characterization of cardiac mass tissue into pseudo-tumor, benign and malignant neoplasm.

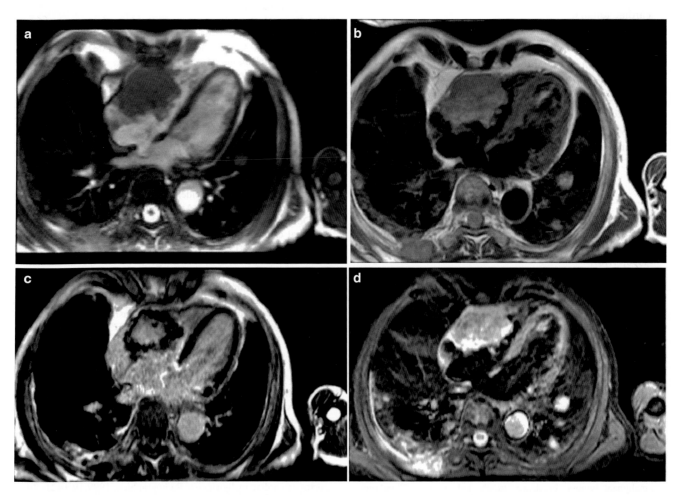

Fig. 16.11 Cardiac metastasis from gastric carcinoma. Tumor involves the right atrium and right ventricle and is infiltrating the myocardium. Tumor is isointense on precontrast SSFP (**a**) and T1w spin-echo image (**b**) and hyperintense on T2w STIR image (**d**). Patchy enhancement is present on late gadolinium enhancement imaging (**c**)

is suggested to outperform contrast enhanced angiography for visualisation of the cardiac chambers, proximal coronary arteries, pulmonary trunk and aortic root [24].

As noted above, imaging may be performed in either the systolic or diastolic rest period. The end diastolic pause is generally longer than that at end systole [25] (152 ± 67 vs. 98 ± 26 ms) and would therefore allow the scan to be completed more quickly. However, for subjects with an irregular heart rate, systole is more consistent and imaging in the systolic rest period may be preferred. We have also found systolic imaging helpful at faster heart rates including for studies when patients are in the index atrial tachycardia at CMR attendance awaiting ablation (Figs. 19.5 and 19.6).

When considering the timing of the acquisition, consideration should also be given to flow inducing artifacts. For pulmonary vein imaging for example, mid-diastolic imaging when pulmonary vein flow is high results in signal voids in the left atrium which may be reduced by imaging in late diastole [22]. In congenital heart disease there are likely to be other sources of turbulent flow from valvular regurgitation or flow accelerations in partially obstructed pathways and timing of the acquisition needs to account for these effects. Where several flow effects may be seen, the flow effects which summate to the least negative impact on the clear delineation of the chamber(s) of interest for the planned EP procedure should be chosen.

Diaphragmatic navigators allow the acquisition to be respiratory gated so that only data acquired when the diaphragm position is within a narrow window centered on the end-expiratory pause position are accepted [26]. These techniques are inherently inefficient, with the data acceptance rate (or respiratory efficiency) typically being around 40 % for a 5 mm acceptance window. Furthermore, in cases where the respiratory pattern is irregular or unstable, the respiratory efficiency may drop so low that the acquisition must be abandoned. Improved respiratory gating techniques, such as those implementing real-time motion correction with subject-specific motion models [27], potentially improve the respiratory efficiency and reduce acquisition duration. These models are derived from a short pre-scan and have also been used to generate dynamic roadmaps that vary with respiration [28]. Another option for increasing the respiratory efficiency of an acquisition is to use a real-time and fully automatic algorithm to determine the optimal placement of the navigator acceptance window so as to maximise efficiency (CLAWS [29]).

19.5 Role for Ventricular and Atrial Scar Imaging in ACHD EP

Intravenous gadolinium contrast lingers in scarred regions of the heart. CMR imaging can then be used to visualize scarred myocardial regions enhanced with gadolinium that appear different from neighbouring normal myocardiaum.

Late gadolinium enhancement (LGE) CMR is the gold standard imaging method for non-invasive measurement of myocardial infarction and fibrosis [30]. LGE CMR evidence of fibrosis has been documented in varying extents and patterns in a number of heart diseases [31]. It predicts outcomes in ischaemic heart disease [32], dilated cardiomyopathy [33] and hypertrophic cardomyopathy [34]. Whether these findings can be extrapolated to patients with congenital heart disease remains the subject of current study.

19.5.1 2D Late Gadolinium Enhancement Imaging Methods

LGE imaging is usually performed as a 2D stack of breath-hold inversion-prepared segmented gradient-echo acquisitions [35] with inversion time (TI) adjustment to compensate for gadolinium wash-out throughout the study. Imaging is generally performed with alternate R-wave gating which allows for almost complete recovery of the longitudinal magnetization between sequence repeats and improves contrast between normal and abnormal tissue and reduces the effects of cardiac arrhythmia [36]. In patients with faster or irregular heart rates, gating on every third or even fourth R wave may improve image quality. In-plane resolution is typically $1.2–1.8 \times 1.2–1.8$ mm, with a slice thickness of 6–8 mm in a breath-hold of ~12 s. The inversion time varies from patient to patient and depends on the dose of gadolinium and the time after administration [37]. For experienced operators this individualized approach with meticulous inversion time adjustment remain the best [35]. The inversion time can be estimated by visual inspection of an inversion recovery cine scout acquisition [38] and then shifted upwards as the study progresses to account for gadolinium wash-out. Alternatively, phase-sensitive reconstruction of data acquired with a nominal TI eliminates the need for precise setting [39] and has demonstrated better contrast between viable and non-viable myocardium at sub-optimal TI [40, 41]. It also eliminates the 'dark rim' artifact apparent in magnitude reconstructed images [42] when the TI is too short, which may aid the depiction of thin-walled structures such as the right ventricle [43] or the atria. Imaging is performed in diastole, when the heart is relatively still, and the number of lines of data acquired per cardiac cycle is reduced in tachycardic patients as the length of this quiescent period is shortened. Recent studies have shown that imaging at higher field strength improves both the signal-to-noise ratio (SNR) and, because of the field dependency of longitudinal relaxation times, the contrast-to-noise ratio (CNR) [44–46]. BSSFP is an alternative to segmented gradient-echo and has a shorter TE and TR, enabling more lines to be acquired in the cardiac rest period and consequently, a reduced imaging time. However, the contrast achieved between viable and

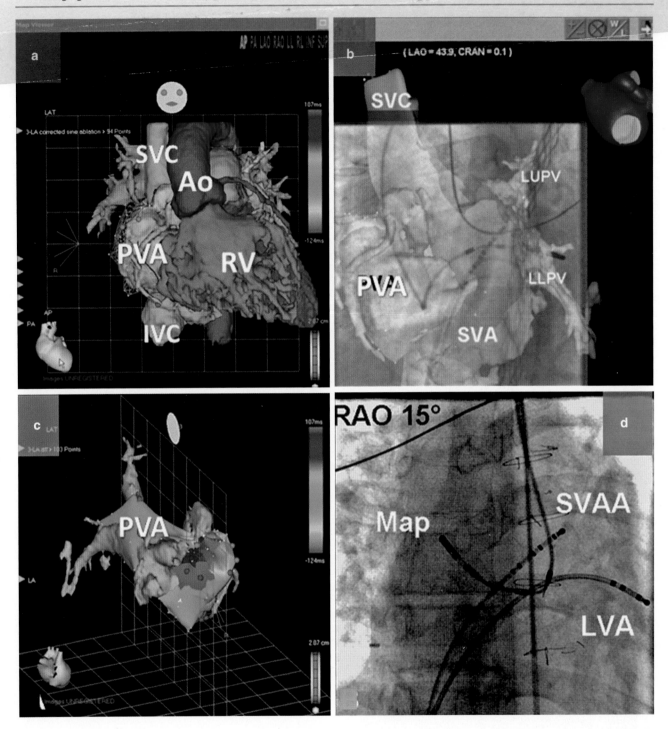

Fig. 19.5 3D bSSFP for 3D volume reconstruction and image integration with 3D EP mapping systems to facilitate a retrograde approach and avoid puncture of baffled atrial pathways after Mustard operation for transposition of the great arteries. This patient followed up after Mustard operation for transposition of the great arteries presented with atrial tachycardia requiring cardioversion. His CMR study was performed in sinus rhythm and 3D bSSFP was timed in systole. (**a**) 3D bSSFP imaging was performed and subsequently segmented with CARTO. The subaortic (*red*) heavily trabeculated RV (*purple*) is shown. The pulmonary arteries are colored *orange* and the subpulmonary LV brighter *purple*. The systemic venous baffled atrial compartment (*turquoise*) and pulmonary venous atrial compartment (*yellow*) were separately segmented. A rotating movie can be seen (Movie 19.1). (**b**) 3D CMR reconstructions of the systemic venous compartment (*SVA*) and pulmonary venous atrial compartment (*PVA*) were displayed and merged to the local activation time map. The CMR roadmap of all the heart chambers was merged with the EP maps and displayed superimposed on fluoroscopy. (**c**) Low voltage (*grey*) scar was found in the pulmonary venous (PVA) compartment. The *dark red* tags depict the ablation sites. (**d**) This site in the left inferior pulmonary vein was reached using retrograde access from the femoral artery and avoiding puncture of the surgical baffle. Retrograde manipulation was made possible by the combination of CMR image integration and remote navigation EP using magnetic navigation allowing several S bends of the catheter. The "MAP" catheter is shown and the retrograde path to reach the site of ablation can be appreciated on the fluoroscopy image. The other two catheters are in the LV apex (*LVA*) and systemic venous atrial appendage (*SVAA*) respectively. *SVC* superior vena cava, *AO* aorta, *PVA* pulmonary venous atrium; *RV* right ventricle; *IVC* inferior vena cava; *SVA* systemic venous atrium; *LUPV* left upper pulmonary vein; *LLPV* left lower pulmonary vein; *SVAA* systemic venous atrial appendage; *LVA* LV apex

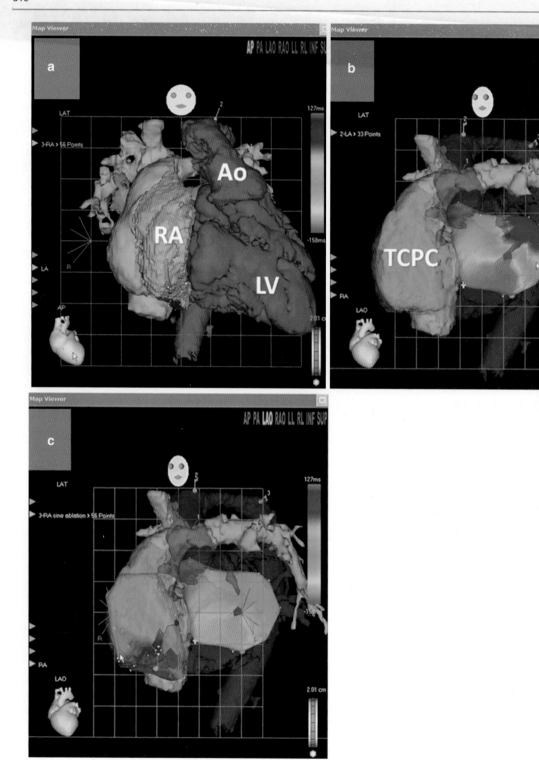

Fig. 19.6 3D bSSFP for 3D volume reconstruction and image integration with 3D EP mapping systems to facilitate a retrograde approach and avoid puncture of lateral tunnel total cavopulmonary connection and integrated EP activation map. A patient with single ventricle physiology presented clinically with recurrent atrial tachycardia status post lateral tunnel total cavopulmonary connection (*TCPC, blue*). The TCPC was performed for situs solitus, discordant atrioventricular connections, double inlet left ventricle, transposed great arteries and pulmonary stenosis. The CMR was performed in established atrial arrhythmia and 3D bSSFP was timed in systole. (**a**) 3D reconstruction of 3D bSSFP CMR imaging showing the lateral tunnel total cavopulmonary connection (*TCPC, turquoise*) and the remaining native RA (*yellow*). The underlying anatomy was double inlet LV (*purple*). A rotating whole heart structure can be seen in the attached movie (Movie 19.2) whereby the aorta is red, and left atrium dark blue. (**b**) In this image the ventricular mass has been masked. Re-entrant tachycardia was mapped in the residual RA with counterclockwise activation around the tricuspid annulus. (**c**) There is bystander activation of the left atrium. *AO* aorta; *RA* right atrium; *LV* left ventricle; *TCPC* total cavopulmonary connection

non-viable myocardium may be different, as may the artifacts generated. Its use for LGE imaging has generally been limited to single-shot acquisitions in patients with frequent arrhythmias or in those who cannot hold their breath [47], but generally, these studies have compromised spatial resolution and much increased acquisition windows [48–51]. More recently, parallel imaging has been used to reduce the long acquisition windows with rigid [52] and non-rigid [53] image registration of multiple free-breathing images being performed to improve SNR.

19.5.2 3D Late Gadolinium Enhancement Methods

With conventional 2D LGE imaging, the spatial resolution is limited by the need to acquire the complete data set within the duration of a comfortable breath-hold period. For high spatial resolution, respiratory gated 3D acquisitions may be performed during free-breathing [54, 55]. Registering the LGE images with 3D electrical maps and fluoroscopic images within a catheter navigation environment may guide ablation studies [56–58] potentially increasing procedural success and reducing radiation exposure to patients. High resolution imaging may also facilitate atrial fibrillation ablation procedures by improving planning and assessing the adequacy of ablation. Scarring resulting from radiofrequency ablation has recently been demonstrated in the atria [59–64], and its spatial distribution and extent appears related to the likelihood of arrhythmia recurrence [65–68]. Radiofrequency ablation -induced scarring has formed by 3-months post ablation [67]. Such imaging could help predict recurrent arrhythmia in future and help guide ablation procedures in patients with recurrent atrial or ventricular arrhythmia (Fig. 19.7).

For 3D imaging, typical parameters include spatial resolution of 1.25–1.5 × 1.25–1.5 × 4 mm (before zero-filling) with 32 slices covering the atrial chambers, more being required if whole heart imaging is required. Acquisition duration is reduced by using parallel imaging with a ×2 acceleration factor, the resulting SNR decrease being mitigated by the thick slab excitation. For segmented gradient echo imaging at 1.5 T, selecting a TE of 2.4 ms ensures that fat and water are out of phase at the time of echo formation which reduces partial volume effects around the thin walled atria and right ventricle. In addition, fat saturation is used to suppress the fat signal. Acquisitions are typically performed within a window of approximately 120 ms in diastole, the exact timing being determined from atrial cine acquisitions. Using alternate R-wave gating, as for 2D imaging, would result in the acquisition duration being prolonged unacceptably. As well as being difficult for the patient, the gadolinium wash-out during this period would result in poor nulling of

the normal myocardium and any scarring would be seen with reduced contrast. Consequently, 3D acquisitions are performed with single R-wave gating with the TI used being reduced to compensate. However, although this is necessary to reduce the acquisition duration, incomplete magnetization recovery between sequence repeats on every heart beat results in the sequence being very susceptible to changes in the RR interval, resulting in ghosting and poor nulling of the normal myocardium. In the atrial fibrillation population for example, image quality can be poor [61], with up to 40 % of studies being unsuitable for further analysis [64]. The most common cause of a failed acquisition is poor rate control in patients presenting with atrial fibrillation during the scan [68]. Typical acquisition durations are 4–8 min, depending on volume coverage, spatial resolution and respiration and heart rate. Endo and epicardial atrial borders may be segmented and the extent of atrial scar determined using a threshold-based algorithm [64]. The amount of left atrial scar calculated in this way has recently been used to stage atrial fibrillation and to allow a more tailored approach to management [69].

As for the roadmap studies discussed above, respiratory gating is generally performed using navigators. These navigators consist of 'pencil-beam' or 'crossed-pair' excitations which create an inflow artifact in the right pulmonary veins and atrial wall which may obscure detail. This has recently been reduced by using a large slab right hemi-diaphragm navigator [70]. In congenital heart disease patients, effort must be taken to place the navigators carefully. The navigators and their localized artifact should not be placed such that they impair imaging of enlarged heart chambers. In some cases such as dextrocardia the left hemidiaphragm needs to be chosen.

19.5.3 Clinical Application of LGE CMR in Congenital Heart Disease Risk Stratification

LGE CMR has been applied to the RV and LV in congenital heart disease. RV LGE evidenced RV fibrosis related to markers of adverse clinical risk and clinically documented atrial or ventricular arrhythmia [71, 72] (Figs. 19.8 and 19.9).

In the systemic RV after Mustard operation for transposition of the great arteries, the presence of LGE was associated with older patients with longer follow-up and adverse clinical risk markers such as right ventricular dysfunction, incidence of atrial arrhythmia and prolonged QRS duration and QT dispersion which are markers for sudden cardiac death in this population [71]. Whilst there is suggestion that RV LGE may have a prognostic role, the study design was cross-sectional [31, 71, 72]. Subsequent studies have also documented the

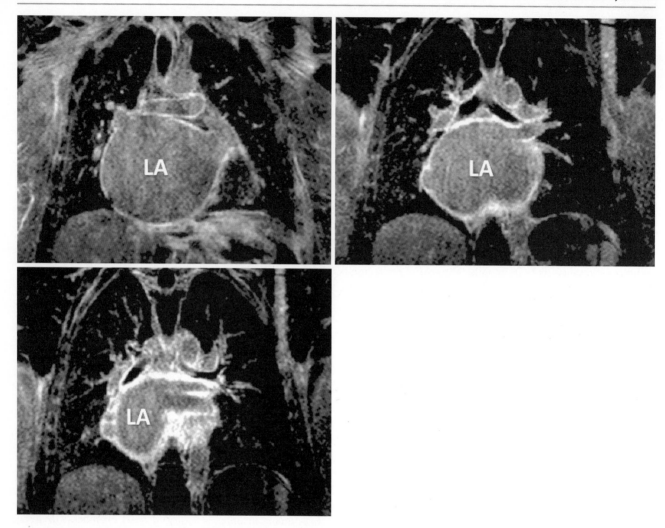

Fig. 19.7 3D LGE images in atrial fibrillation and dilated left atrium due to congenital mitral valve disease. This young woman had mitral valve replacement for congenital mitral regurgitation. The left atrium is markedly dilated and measures 92 × 88 mm in the *left hand image*. The giant nature of the left atrium in relation to the chest cavity can also be noted. Of note, the pulmonary veins are not severely dilated. In this case there is striking diffuse late gadolinum enhancement and thickening of the atrium in a global distribution. Even if the patient underwent pulmonary vein isolation there may be multiple triggers outside the pulmonary veins and sufficient left atrial body fibrosis for atrial fibrillation maintenance. *LA* left atrium

presence of RV LGE [73, 74] including in unoperated patients with systemic RV in the context of congenitally corrected transposition of the great arteries as well as those after atrial redirection surgery suggesting that the etiology of RV LGE is not confined to perioperative myocardial protection [73]. This study also showed that systemic RV LGE correlated with objectively assessed impairment in cardiopulmonary exercise capacity [73].

RV dysfunction, arrhythmia and sudden cardiac death remain problematic long-term for the growing population of repaired tetralogy of Fallot (rToF) patients under follow-up LGE CMR may be a future tool to help refine existing risk stratification in these patients.

RV LGE is a ubiquitous occurrence in older, operated rTOF patients but the exact locations and extent of RV myocardial fibrosis varies (Fig. 19.9). Sites of RV LGE may relate to incisions and interventions at the time of intracardiac surgery such as ventriculotomy or areas of VSD and outflow tract patching. More modern surgical techniques with more limited extent and depth of RV outflow tract myocardial resection may result in younger patients having less marked outflow tract fibrosis. RV LGE has additionally, however, been demonstrated in areas remote from surgical incision which relates to a higher incidence of clinical arrhythmia [72]. Extent of LGE may be important in predicting arrhythmia. Expected site LGE may have differing significance to non operative incisional LGE. The degree of heterogeneity will also likely have an impact on arrhythmogenic propensity.

In rToF patients, expected LV LGE was demonstrated [72]. Commonly, evidence of peri-operative apical vent insertion was seen underlining the technique's sensitivity but other unexpected non-apical vent LV LGE was also seen in a smaller number of patients. The latter, when more

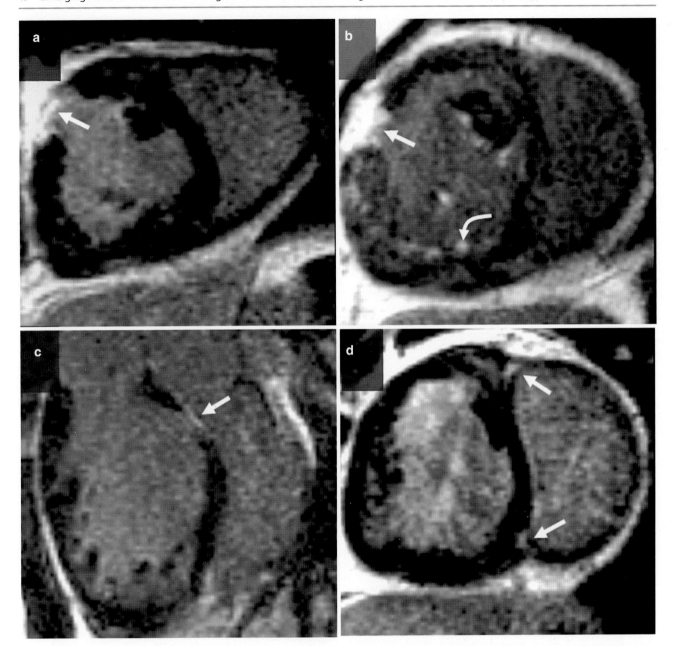

Fig. 19.8 RV LGE in the systemic RV after Mustard operation for transposition of the great arteries. (**a**) Full thickness late gadolinium enhancement of the anterior wall of the RV (*arrow*). (**b**) RV anterior wall enhancement (*arrow*) and multiple foci of late gadolinium enhancement suggesting fibrosis of the RV trabeculae (*curved arrow*). (**c**) Late gadolinium enhancement of a spontaneously closed perimembranous VSD (*arrow*). (**d**) Superior and inferior LV and RV insertion point enhancement (*arrows*) (With kind permission from Babu-Narayan et al. [71])

extensive seemed to be anteroapical (Fig. 19.10), but LV LGE confined to very small mid LV wall areas and papillary muscle, was also seen [72]. The extent of RV LGE related to adverse clinical markers including ventricular dysfunction, objective exercise intolerance and neurohormonal activation and also to the incidence of clinical arrhythmias which may therefore shed light on the pathophysiological substrate of arrhythmia and ventricular dysfunction in rTOF patients [72]. Whether RV LGE reflects

a single early insult or progressive change with time, in rTOF patients is uncertain. In future LGE CMR may contribute to risk stratification and decision making on the timing of arrhythmia intervention or hemodynamic surgery such as pulmonary valve replacement but as yet such a role remains to be determined. A potential role for LGE CMR in risk stratification in congenital heart disease is also suggested by other groups correlating absence of LGE with negative EP ventricular stimulation studies [75].

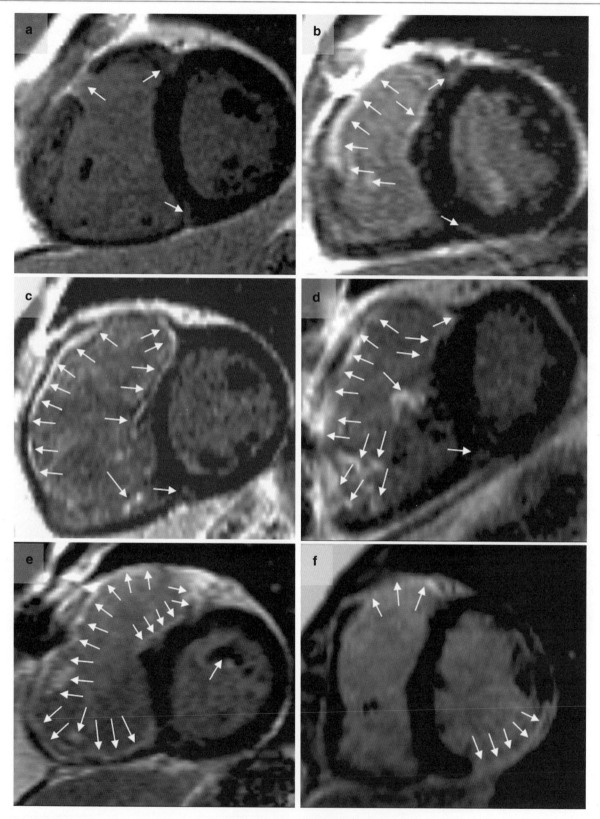

Fig. 19.9 RV LGE in the subpulmonary RV after repair of tetralogy of Fallot. Six different patients (**a–f**) are shown. *Arrows* indicate areas of LGE including the commonly seen faint RV insertion point LGE. The regions of RV LGE are more extensive progressing from patient (**a–e**) and illustrate the range in extent of RV LGE that can be documented in the adult repaired tetralogy of Fallot population. In (**f**), there is transmural LV LGE in addition to RV LGE which was a relatively more unusual finding in the patients studied [72] and related to age, early era surgery, raised neurohormones, redo surgery and in this patient anomalous unobstructed coronary arteries (With kind permission from Babu-Narayan [31]).

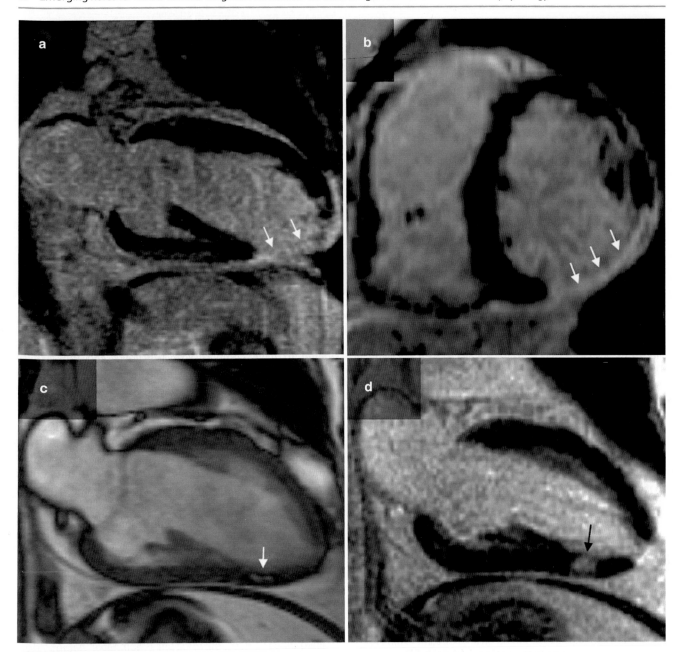

Fig. 19.10 Examples of LV LGE late after tetralogy of Fallot repair. Images illustrating unexpected LV infarction (*arrowed*) in two different patients (**a** and **b**) A further example of localized LV LGE in another patient is shown. The cine frame in (**c**), and corresponding LGE image in (**d**) suggest fibro-fatty change in this region (With kind permission from Babu-Narayan et al. [72]). The white arrow shows phase cancellation effect suggestive of fatty change in steady state free precession cine imaging. The black arrow shows late gadolinium enhancement in a slightly larger region. Together there is suggestion of both fat and fibrosis

Patients after Fontan palliation for univentricular physiology have also been studied with late gadolinium CMR [76] and important cross-sectional correlations with adverse ventricular mechanics and a higher presence of non-sustained ventricular tachycardia.

As previously mentioned, there is also overlap in clinical presentations, such that patients presenting with atrial arrhythmia are at higher risk of ventricular arrhythmia [1]. It is not known whether a similar fibrotic pathogenesis occurs in both atria and ventricles in these conditions, or whether

this can be used clinically to predict outcomes and guide treatment. Left atrial LGE CMR has been proposed to help identify patients who will benefit from atrial fibrillation ablation [64, 67]and those at risk of recurrence [77]. Congenital heart disease patients often present with right ventricular or right atrial arrhythmia and imaging both chambers for LGE evidence of fibrosis is therefore of interest. Post processing may help to improve demonstration of fibrosis (Fig. 19.11). Subtraction of pre and post ablation images may also help define the effects of ablation. With future, high resolution

Printed by Printforce, the Netherlands

GREYSCALE

BIN TRAVELER FORM

Cut By _A.Lelef_   Qty 30   Date 11/06/24

Scanned By _____   Qty _____   Date _____

Scanned Batch IDs _____

Notes / Exception

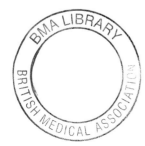